Biomedical Research: An Insider's Guide

Seward B. Rutkove

Biomedical Research:
An Insider's Guide

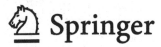 Springer

Seward B. Rutkove, MD
Professor of Neurology
Harvard Medical School
Beth Israel Deaconess Medical Center
Boston, MA, USA

ISBN 978-1-4939-3653-3   ISBN 978-1-4939-3655-7   (eBook)
DOI 10.1007/978-1-4939-3655-7

Library of Congress Control Number: 2016935412

Printed on acid-free paper

This Springer imprint is published by Springer Nature
The registered company is Springer Science+Business Media LLC New York

For Elena and Sophie

Foreword

Research. The term often seems to be bandied about with a certain reckless glamour. This thought struck me while I was recently touring colleges with my high school daughter. As we sat in one information session after another, in dimly lit halls filled with hundreds of anxious students and their equally distressed parents, the presenters, usually university admissions officers, each suggested that their school made a special effort to ensure anyone who wanted to do research could do it. What was meant by research and what the students would be doing, of course, was left intentionally vague, in part, because there are so many types of research possible, especially to an undergraduate who is still uncertain as to whether she wants to study biology, women's studies, or engineering. I suppose the idea is meant to conjure up the image of sitting in a laboratory teasing apart data, hoping to find a new subatomic particle, or perhaps it is meant to invoke being lost deep in the stacks of some mammoth library finding a long-forgotten volume that suddenly reveals a new insight into a great author's writings. Whatever the case, it is the general concept that you will be opening a door into some new frontier or happening upon that "undiscovered country" that had been there all along but invisible to nearly all that makes the general concept of research so enticing.

In many respects, my own personal experience of research in college fell exactly along those lines. It all started when I applied for a position at Memorial Sloan Kettering Cancer Center as a summer intern after my freshman year at Cornell. That summer of 1982 started out fairly mundanely for me. There was no response from the center, and so I found myself working as a short order cook in an amusement park in Rye, New York. I worked the deep fryer and actually discovered that I was pretty adept at cooking those frozen fries to near-perfect gold-brown crispiness. Although the work was not what I was after, there was something simple about it and customers seemed happy enough with my efforts. That was until one day in mid-July when I received a phone call saying that a researcher at Sloan-Kettering needed someone to help out in the lab for a couple of months. And just a few days later, I found myself cleaning glassware over a large granite sink in a coolly lit organic chemistry lab at the Memorial Sloan Kettering Cancer Center Annex in

Rye, New York. While strictly speaking cleaning glassware was not exactly a huge leap up from cooking fries (one even might argue the latter required greater skill), I found the environment seductive: chemical powders in brown glass bottles and white plastic jugs, long shelves containing liquids with complex names, and people walking down dimly lit halls in coats speaking in hushed tones. And then, there was the overall sense that I was now, albeit peripherally, involved in a larger effort toward discovery and world betterment. Those fries quickly seemed like a distant past. Indeed, my reflection in those shiny pieces of glassware revealed a young man with unkempt hair, aviator spectacles, and a persistent grin.

And when the following summer arrived, the laboratory wanted me back to help out for the summer. But this time, having finished organic chemistry and organic chemistry laboratory, I could actually help out in a more substantive way. So I was put to work in the chemotherapy development lab of Dr. Joseph Roberts, helping to design a new chemotherapy agent based on a couple of older ones that worked but were broken down (hydrolyzed) in the blood. The actual scientific concepts entailed were even straightforward to a rising junior in college. Basically, the antimetabolites are a group of anticancer drugs that work by inserting themselves into the normal biochemical pathways of the cell but not interrupting the normal metabolic pathways. They are agents that looked like normal molecules but that were modified in some way so as to make them injurious to a growing cell. Since cancer cells grow more rapidly than normal cells, such drugs impact the cancerous cells and kill them more readily than healthy cells (though a few healthy cells are certainly taken along the way as well). My job would be to synthesize a drug that mimicked L-tryptophan, one of the amino acids. Others had initiated this work a number of years earlier, by attaching a large alcohol chain to the acid moiety and thus turning the molecule into an ester. Such a molecule would look like L-tryptophan but could not be incorporated into proteins. In fact, in the earlier work, in cell cultures, these molecules were found to be highly toxic and destructive to a variety of tumor cells. The only problem was that body had natural defenses to such esters. The blood was filled with enzymes called esterases whose job was to break down esters into their composite acids and alcohols, rendering them harmless.

Thus, my job was to create a tryptophan ester that could not be destroyed by these enzymes. The way to do this was to build an ester that was "sterically hindered." In other words, the molecule would have some additional components to it that would shield the ester bond from destruction by these esterases. It was akin to creating a molecule with a defensive shield around it. Although Dr. Roberts was not an organic chemist, he understood these basic concepts and suggested that I figure out how to build such a molecule. Although I probably wouldn't be able to get it completed in 10 weeks over the summer, his hope was that I could bring this project back to Cornell's chemistry department where I could get a serious organic chemist to help me with it. And with the support of a couple of other people in the lab, by the end of August, we had made some tentative progress toward identifying the appropriate synthetic pathway, but we were nowhere close to the creation of this new compound.

So in the fall of that year, I talked to one of the organic chemistry professors, Dr. Charles Wilcox. He was happy to have me work on this project. He conferred a bit with Dr. Roberts by phone, and then he pretty much let me have free reign in his lab, though under the direct guidance and supervision of several of the graduate students. One of the lessons I learned early on was from Erik Farley who told me that "a day in the library is worth a month in the lab." And so I spent weeks looking through the literature to help guide me to the best pathways for making the drug. Then I was back in the lab, often late at night and on weekends, when other academic demands were not overwhelming, trying to work on designing this sterically hindered tryptophan ester. Weeks turned into months, but late in my junior year, somewhere well past midnight, Erik and I sat by the NMR machine watching as the pen drew squiggles on a sheet of paper. And there it was. The telltale sign: two neighboring spikes indicating that the two methyl alcohol groups were each unique, conferred on them by the asymmetry of the L-tryptophan molecule. The next day Erik and I showed the tracings to Dr. Wilcox who confirmed that we had indeed created the new drug. I had a feeling of satisfaction and achievement that I do not believe I have had again to this day. I had achieved something seemingly miraculous: I had virtually single-handedly created a molecule that had likely never existed in the history of the universe.

But then it was pretty much all downhill from there. While I had managed to synthesize it, we quickly discovered that it was highly unstable in air and needed to be stored under nitrogen. If that storage process was not carefully performed, the white power would turn into a brown goo over several days. Moreover, the synthetic process was extremely difficult and costly and the yield was very poor. I tried a few different approaches for improving the synthesis, but they were all equally challenging and by and large unsuccessful. I did have two more minor successes: we were able to show that the drug was resistant to blood esterases as we had predicted. And then when we injected a small amount into a handful of mice with colon tumors, the tumors shrank dramatically. But in the end, the challenges of its synthesis and its poor stability made it a loser. While the project did serve as the subject of my honors thesis at Cornell and ensured me a "magna cum laude" title, the effort had proven a fruitless dead end. Perhaps my cooking more fries to serve to all those hungry fairgoers would have been a more worthwhile effort.

And yet here I am decades later, more deeply ensconced in research than ever. Not synthesizing chemotherapy agents—no, I chose neurology over oncology in the end. Rather, I have moved more into the realm of engineering and technology and physics over that of the crystals and colorless solvents of organic chemistry. But like that college student that I was three decades ago, I still find myself constantly drawn to the mystery of discovery, hoping to create something novel and new from the ether. But along with it, I have also acknowledged that like most worthwhile efforts, much of the time and work ends up being a footnote to a footnote or, worse yet, entirely unsuccessful. The successes and inevitable failures are only a small part of the story of most research. There is the money side and the policy side. Those aspects of the work, so invisible to a college student, become front and center to a principal investigator running a lab, buying equipment, treating patients, caring for animals, and employing a dozen people. Money, in many respects, ends up becoming a constant preoccupation as one tries to move one's research forward. Indeed, in research you really need only need two things: a mission and money.

The goal of this book is not to provide a definitive treatise on how to become a successful researcher. I don't think anyone has sufficient experience and skills to offer such advice to a broad audience. Rather, this book is meant to serve as a guide to help introduce people at all levels of training—undergraduate students, graduate students, medical students, residents, and fellows—as well as junior faculty to the basic joys and pains of research in order to help people determine for themselves whether or not research is really for them. By understanding the process, I would like to think that it may become possible to make better informed decisions about their future careers, as well as providing a basic set of instructions to help initiate their careers in research. Importantly, this book is also not a treatise on how to most effectively institute the scientific method—you'll have to figure that out for yourself, hopefully with the help of your own mentors.

This book is intended for a fairly wide audience, and I hope that people at any stage of their training or career will glean something useful from it. Accordingly, I don't think you need to read it end to end and I've divided book into several sections that may be helpful to the reader. The first focuses on decision points regarding whether one wants to enter into research and which type for which type of person— basic, clinical, or translational. The second section focuses on some basic practicalities of pursuing medical research with which you are sure to become familiar, including institutional review boards and animal care committees, as well as general suggestions regarding idea generation and collaboration. The third section focuses on something you will be doing a lot of if you go into research: writing. This section focuses on both writing grants and papers. Although very different, they share some commonalities, and it useful to think of them as connected in a fashion. The fourth section runs through a hodgepodge of issues, including everything from conferencing to patents to industry to philanthropy. The final section deals with broader life issues from job choices to thoughts on trying to keep the big picture front and center as you move through your career.

This book represents only one person's view of the world of biomedical research and paths to success. My hope is that I will learn valuable things from readers' responses to this effort and that, like my own research efforts, the second edition will be better than this first effort. But I hope one message comes across loud and clear: biomedical research, despite of or perhaps because of its multitude of challenges, is truly and inexplicably fun. I cannot imagine having made a better career choice.

Boston, MA   Seward B. Rutkove
November 2015

Acknowledgments

Without the National Institutes of Health and their generosity, this work would never have come to be. In fact, I proposed the creation of this book as part of my K24NS060951 grant application in 2013, and it is that grant that has provided the time for me to complete this. So thank you once again NIH for making another dream become reality. Hopefully, those taxpayer dollars will be considered well spent.

I must also acknowledge the wonderful and warm work environment that I have had the privilege to be part of at Beth Israel Deaconess Medical Center in Boston. The hospital has been welcoming and generous since I first stepped through the door as a newly minted neurology resident in 1991. And much of that warmth has been a product of my colleagues with whom I have worked all these years and who have put up with me, including Elizabeth Raynor, Rachel Nardin, Pushpa Narayanaswami, Andrew Tarulli, Courtney McIlduff, and Aimee Boegle. And there is, of course, my chairman, Clifford Saper, to whom I am especially indebted for his providing a uniquely supportive atmosphere and for giving me ample opportunity to find my own way.

There are many other collaborators and mentors who have taught and continue to teach me not only about doing good research but also about life. Foremost among them is Jeremy Shefner who has served as a constant friend and supporter and who served as an early role model of someone engaged in neuromuscular research. Eric Logigian, David Preston, and Martin Samueuls also served as valuable mentors.

I also want to offer special thanks to my readers: Bernard Chang, Tom Geisbush, and Courtney McIlduff for giving me invaluable feedback and helping the final product become a bit more focused and "appropriate."

Although they may never read this, I also owe a great deal of debt to my first research experiences in the Department of Chemistry at Cornell University that I described in the foreword: Dr. Charles F. Wilcox and his team of graduate students, Erik Farley, Kevin Lassila, and David Blain who all helped nurture my original love of research. I look back upon those days very fondly.

No acknowledgment section would be complete without including my parents, Edith and Lowell. They have encouraged me to pursue my dreams from as early as I can remember.

Finally, I owe the deepest thanks to my daughter, Sophie, and my wife, Elena. Both have boundless love, creativity, and vision, and there can be nothing more wonderful than living in such an artistic, imaginative, and warm household. Thank you both, so, so much.

Contents

About the Author

Dr. Rutkove is Professor of Neurology, Harvard Medical School and serves as Chief of the Division of Neuromuscular Disease in the Department of Neurology at Beth Israel Deaconess Medical Center. He received his medical degree from Columbia University's College of Physicians and Surgeons, and his bachelor *magna cum laude* from Cornell University, College of Arts and Sciences. Dr. Rutkove's research focuses on the application of innovative techniques for the assessment of neuromuscular disease with an emphasis on electrical impedance and ultrasound methodologies. This work has been supported by numerous grants from the National Institutes of Health and multiple foundations and has resulted in nearly 150 peer-reviewed publications. He is currently serving as an associate editor for *Annals of Neurology*. Dr. Rutkove is also a co-founder of Skulpt, Inc, a company commercializing muscle impedance tools for clinical care and consumer use. In 2011, he was awarded the Biomarker Challenge Prize from the non-profit foundation Prize4Life, Inc for his work demonstrating that electrical impedance measurements of muscle could speed clinical therapeutic studies in amyotrophic lateral sclerosis.

The original version of this book was revised. An erratum to this book can be found at DOI 10.1007/978-1-4939-3655-7_42

Part I
Basic Considerations

Chapter 1
So Do You Really Want to Pursue Research?

I am not a psychiatrist, psychologist, or social worker. But if you speak with any person deeply involved in research, I can guarantee you that they will tell you that he will view himself as "atypical" in his approach to his interests, career, and long-term life goals. Admittedly, none of us think of ourselves as typical or average, yet I do believe that most people who pursue biomedical research are not content with having a job where the day-to-day work is at all predetermined or in any way mundane. Accordingly, I believe that there are a number of personality traits common to many researchers. The degree to which any of these traits predominate, of course, varies considerably among people and is undoubtedly one of the factors that leads to a rich and varied group of people involved in scientific research. It is also one reason why there are so many arguments, dislikes, petty controversies, big controversies, and occasional intentionally malevolent acts.

So in the following section, I list what I consider to be some of the more common personality traits shared by researchers with a short description after each. Clearly, putting forward such a list may generate some disagreement and may be considered politically incorrect in some fashion. However, I think it is worth stating outright some of the often-thought but rarely expressed ideas that many of us in the research realm hold that might differentiate us from those who are more content with jobs in which outcomes are relatively predictable. And of course, any list like this is going to be quite incomplete. But I hope it provides a starting point and something for those considering pursuing a career in research to reflect upon.

1. **Tenacity and persistence**. This is perhaps one of the most obvious and important characteristics. One cannot go into science and hope for easy success—every idea and every experiment are full of one challenge after another. One must embrace and accept rejection and criticism again and again and again. If a grant doesn't get funded and the reviews are nasty, one has to digest that result and move forward. If an experiment doesn't work out because of technical problems, one doesn't give up, but rather gives it another go or pursues a different tack. Tenacity is a critical feature of nearly every successful researcher. It is related to both passion and obsession discussed further below.

© Springer Science+Business Media New York 2016
S.B. Rutkove, *Biomedical Research: An Insider's Guide*,
DOI 10.1007/978-1-4939-3655-7_1

2. **Compulsiveness, but not too much**. Attention to detail, almost to the point of obsession, is typical among most researchers. It is often in the details that the greatest discoveries are found and also in the details that the potential breakthroughs are ultimately dismissed as nothing more than spurious data. As any researcher will tell you, "The devil is in the details" but at the same time the other aphorism "God is in the details" often is just as valid. One must embrace the details, whether they are the finer points of a comprehensive data analysis plan or ensuring that you complete all the boxes in your grant application and the institutional review board forms. In fact, ignoring a single detail can be the death of a project. One cannot be too paranoid about such details.

But there is a flip side to this. The details are critical *up to a point*. What one does not want to do is to become paralyzed by the details. Large data sets can be mind-numbing and absolutely confounding. Finding ways to simplify and reduce data sets to manageable size can be critical. No matter how brilliant any of us may be, huge data sets are almost always daunting, and simplification is often key if you hope to make heads or tails out of the data.

And the extreme of compulsivity is perfectionism. Simply put: research is not perfect. One expression that I often remind my staff is that we "cannot let perfection be the enemy of the good." Is it worth repeating a lengthy, costly experiment because of a minor flaw in the design? It may be, but it may also not be. The point of science is not necessarily to solve riddles, but rather to improve our understanding of nature and the world around us. We don't necessarily have to get it all exactly right the first time out of the gate—in fact we should never expect that. But it may still be better than never getting out of the gate at all. You can always let the next experiment improve upon the past one or hope that some other soul will pursue a line of research that you have initiated.

3. **Passion and obsession**. One cannot be a part-time researcher. It is a full-time effort and it is an effort that must be allowed to seep into all parts of your life. That is not to say it has to be at the exclusion of anything else. It is just that it is very hard to do research according to some strict schedule (e.g., 9–5), especially in today's world. One develops research relationships that are not confined to localities or time zones. Collaborations easily stretch across the country and more often than ever, across the globe as well. Conferences are becoming more and more international. Accordingly deadlines may not fit with school vacations and critical experiments may run longer than you anticipate.

This does not mean that you need to be a workaholic. It doesn't mean that you can't go on vacation or spend two uninterrupted hours per day practicing piano. But it does mean you will need to allow it to become part of the fabric of your life. But I can guarantee you this: that will not be a problem, if you have chosen your research career well, you will always find yourself happily occupied, whether it is reviewing someone's grant applications or tweaking a figure for improved clarity prior to a presentation.

4. **Risk-taking**. Risk is a natural aspect of research. You have to take risks from the very first paper you try to write. But research is also not gambling nor is it Olympic skiing. It is its own unique form of risk-embracing behavior. Every

hypothesis to be tested, every idea you generate, every piece of data you gather may amount to absolutely nothing or may be just plain wrong. Unlike seeing patients in the office or manufacturing a product or accounting, each of which has its own risks, of course, there are no guarantees that anything you are doing is even going to be remotely worthwhile. But on the other hand, risk-taking can also have big payoffs. Those big payoffs are things we hope for but seldom achieve.

5. **Outgoing**. I don't think you can be a successful researcher if you are naturally shy and very introverted. If you can control your diffidence and displace it to the background during your day, that is all you need. You certainly do not need to be an absolute extrovert. Yet at the same time the ability to work with many people, to not be afraid to speak in front of crowds, to reach out to people you don't know on a regular basis, and to be comfortable and collegial in large groups is really critical to becoming a member of the greater research community and seeing your work succeed. Research is definitely not a single person struggling alone in a lab. It is a group effort and you need to be sufficiently outgoing so as to be a member of that greater community constantly contributing and actively participating in it.

6. **Love of writing**. If you want to pursue research in a serious way, you will need to enjoy writing and not simply tolerate it. I think most researchers generally have a sense of a need to express themselves and their ideas through writing. Of course writing can sometimes be a chore for even the most extreme word lovers (and this very much includes me, despite the creation of this book). But if you really dislike writing, then every grant and every paper and every review article will be a nuisance to produce. If there were any one measure that I think is a simple do or don't, this one is it. *If you hate to write, please, please, don't pursue a career in research.*

7. **Don't do it for fame and fortune**. It may be obvious, but the vast majority of researchers never reach the heights of a Salk or a Kandel. In fact, even if you were to win the Nobel Prize, most people will still not know who you are when you attend dinner parties or go to your grandchildren's birthday parties. Such extreme prizes are the exception and not the rule. You have to enjoy the journey and not the achievement of any specific goal itself. And as far as wealth goes, the granting agencies are not looking to make millionaires out of their grantees, so don't expect that. If you are lucky, you might win a prize of some sort, start a successful company in which you will have equity, or perhaps obtain an endowed chair at your institution, helping to offset the plentiful financial stressors.

8. **Confidence/ability to shrug of criticism and move forward**. Criticism always hurts, and few things can be more painful than receiving the critiques on a rejected grant or paper. Fortunately, most reviewers are reasonably kind and are sufficiently self-aware so that they thoughtfully word their critiques. But sometimes a specific criticism on a grant or a paper may hit a raw nerve, and it will feel the like the reviewer has a personal vendetta against you. Still, one needs to know how to accept those criticisms, as some may certainly be justified, and move forward. And others really may not. One must keep trying again and again and realize that there is almost never a true knockout punch to any line of research. Clearly, the ability to accept such criticism and not give up requires a strong sense of self-confidence—

both in one's ability to see beyond the criticisms of one small grant or paper or presentation to the bigger picture of what you are trying to achieve. As an important corollary to this idea, there is also very much a need to be able to learn from past experiences. One of the main reasons that Lincoln placed Ulysses S. Grant in charge of the Union forces in 1864 was not because Grant was such a skilled military strategist or brilliant thinker; in fact, people were very critical of his background and reputation for imbibing. Rather, it was Grant's ability to learn from his past mistakes and to develop new, more enlightened plans based on past errors that ultimately won Lincoln's favor.

9. **Self-criticism/self-skepticism**. These two ideas can be thought of reflecting two sides of the same coin. One needs to be comfortable being self-critical and not always interpreting one's data in the most positive light. A researcher needs to constantly understand the limitations of what is found and question all the results, *especially* those that are simply too good to be true. At the same time, one should probably have that same attitude when reviewing others' work. One should not take what one reads or hears for granted. One needs to question everything, whether it is a criticism of one's own work or, perhaps more importantly, an endorsement of it. You can be both respectful and skeptical at the same time.

10. **Generosity and open-mindedness**. In many respects, biomedical research is a selfless act. Always thinking you are correct and everyone else is wrong is no way to go about research. We, frankly, should respect all our colleagues for jumping into the fray with us and helping to decipher some the greatest intellectual challenges that the modern world and science have to offer. But it is often hard for us to keep that generosity of spirit alive, especially after your grant has been soundly rejected or you feel that a researcher is unfairly judging you or your ideas. An ability to always take the high ground and not sink to the lowest depths of behavior is always valuable.

11. **Capability of being a manager and being able to delegate**. One of the greatest stumbling blocks I have witnessed among my colleagues who exclaim their interest in pursuing research and yet they're being stymied, is the inability to delegate and trust implicitly those who work for them. If success comes your way, it will be through the efforts of a team. All recent great inventors and researchers have had teams of associates, and the ability to manage them and to effectively guide them to success in their work is a critical part of that. Importantly, it is necessary to ensure that each person in one's team has enough freedom to pursue his or her own ideas while still having enough practical information and enough oversight to make sure they aren't going in a wrong direction. I'll discuss more on management of a laboratory in Chap. 12.

12. **Integrity**. I have left what I consider the single most important attribute for last. Integrity and honesty are critical features for any successful researcher. Pursuing work for glamor, fame, or money is meaningless. If what you do is false or a gross exaggeration, you will be eventually discovered. Being honest in all of your dealings is critical. If a mistake is made, take responsibility immediately. It is better to admit a wrong than to deny it when you know it is true. If you are unsure and need sympathetic advice, talk to a trusted friend or colleague. Simply by

verbalizing your concerns, you may reach a resolution to a problem with which you had been struggling. There are times when anyone can get a little mixed-up as to what qualifies as honest and what as dishonest—and there are definitely some areas of a distinct shade of gray. I will deal with this more completely in Chap. 29. But the bottom line I want to underscore here is to always be true to yourself and remember that what you are doing is for the greater good and not just for your own personal benefit. That greater good should always be the driving motivation. And do not take credit when credit is clearly due to another person or group of people, even if others are prepared to shower you with praise. There is no better feeling than sharing the achievement with others and even, occasionally, giving them all the credit.

Chapter 2
What's in Store: The Brighter Side of Medical Research

Research in the biomedical field is full of a variety of pros and cons. In this section, I will provide an outline of what I view as the true joys of being in the world of biomedical research. In the following chapter, I will discuss some of its darker aspects.

It is useful to recall, however, that we are not static once we have reached adulthood. Our minds continue to change and our interests and needs also gradually evolve over time. In fact, studies have shown that an individual's perception of himself or herself in earlier years is often quite wrong—there is a simplistic general tendency to extrapolate backward from your current cognitive state to your past with the road to your current situation somehow seeming inevitable. In reality, the changes that happen to us, both from within and from without, alter us as we age. A woman beginning a research career at the age of 25 is likely to see and understand the world and her relationship to it in a very different way when she is 55. And one of the beautiful things about a career in research is the possibility of allowing for that change. You can slowly change your focus, interests, and ideas in sync with your own personal transformations.

Here is a short list that attempts to capture some of bright the lights that make biomedical research such a wonderful career choice:

1. **You can follow your passion and creativity**. Perhaps what drives most people into research is the possibility of being creative. One is not forced to follow a rulebook, but rather is placed in the position of actually creating the rules themselves. You have the opportunity to explore new concepts and build them from their very foundations. There are literally daily discoveries, and you can think again and again to yourself that you are the first person in the history of the world to do this or do that. There is always the possibility that you will discover some great new pathway or technology that will make everyone think in a new way. You have the opportunity to work on creating beautiful graphics or figures or developing novel and exciting ways to get your point across in print, the Internet, or during presentations at conferences. The opportunities for creativity are virtually endless, and they can

© Springer Science+Business Media New York 2016
S.B. Rutkove, *Biomedical Research: An Insider's Guide*,
DOI 10.1007/978-1-4939-3655-7_2

happen at any moment, whether it be a better way to collect data, a novel approach to analysis, or a startling new hypothesis.

2. **Making a big difference in a big way—not just on a single-person basis**. I think closely tied to the creativity piece is the idea that your ideas may end up changing the world in some big way. While it is true that most research does not create a dramatic paradigm shift in our understanding of the universe or basic physiology, it does contribute in some small way to the building of a greater structure. As Newton said (admittedly rather disingenuously), regarding his invention of the calculus, he was only able to do so by standing on the shoulders of giants. Or another way of thinking about it is that every little bit we uncover adds to the greater societal good. Perhaps your own discoveries will not change the world, but they may lead to other discoveries that eventually lead to others that do. I don't view research as being a footnote to a footnote. That idea is depressing. It should be envisioned, rather, as each of us contributing critical building blocks to a great structure.

3. **Always new challenges and ideas**. Nothing is ever the same in research. If it is, you are not doing research anymore. You will constantly be introduced to new ideas. You will find yourself needing to learn about new areas of science, new statistical methodologies, new technologies, or new models that will change the way you do things every day. You are forever a student when doing research and this is perhaps one of the greatest joys. It makes one feel eternally young to be learning about fresh ideas or, sometimes, rediscovering old ideas with a new potential application. To always feel like you are on the forefront of discovery and knowledge is an exciting place to be—the event horizon of modern-day medical science.

4. **An opportunity to become a public figure and obtain broader recognition for one's work**. In high school and college, the thought of getting up on a stage and speaking filled me with great trepidation. That was also true during the early years of my academic career. But slowly, with repeated opportunities to give talks and with increasing confidence in what I was actually speaking about, all that fear began to fade, and I now truly enjoy all opportunities to present my work publically. I like trying to tell a good story and seek to maintain the talk on a high level of complexity while not forcing the audience into a deep sleep. The opportunity to stand up and be known for one's work is truly an honor and privilege and very rewarding in itself. Occasionally, your work may even be recognized by an award—perhaps a society will give you an honorary membership (preferably before you die) or you will win a monetary or other award of recognition for what you have accomplished. Such success usually comes after much toil and with some luck—even though your moment in the spotlight is short lived.

5. **Financial rewards sometimes including possible commercialization**. While most people don't go into academic research focused on becoming wealthy, there is no question that occasional people do strike on to some new drug or technology that has the prospect of transforming the world. This could mean filing patents and creating a start-up company with goal of commercializing your efforts. It is sometimes only through commercialization of an aspect of one's work that a new technology or idea can be fully deployed. These commercialization efforts may bring about large financial rewards. However, such work also entails the challenges of dealing

with often-complex conflicts of interest that may interfere with one's own ability to perform research on the same subject matter. Plus it also almost always means acquiring an entirely new skill set in the field of business. More on this later. But for the moment, the most important thing to remember is that one of the joys about research is that it sometimes takes you into directions that may prove unexpectedly financially profitable.

6. **Work hour/location flexibility**. When I see patients in neurology clinic, I am restricted to specific hours on specific days on a specific floor to a specific room. If I start to run late, my day will turn into a huge mess. Not only do the patients become irritated and annoyed, but the support staff will undoubtedly want to throttle me since they are the ones on the firing line and dealing with the angry patients and their families. And God forbid if my clinic room is booked by another physician immediately after I am scheduled to finish my set of patients, and I am running late. I will have their wrath upon me. My patient-care life is rigidly fixed.

Medical research is virtually the diametric opposite. I can work virtually anywhere, at any time. In truth, one of the great joys I personally find about research is the tremendous flexibility it provides in terms of the flexibility of work location and time. But that wasn't always the case. When I had first entered the field in the early 1990s, the Internet was still in its infancy. If I needed to research a paper, I'd have to go to the library and start hunting for it down deep in the stacks. If I needed to review data, I would have to sit down with my research assistant in front of *their* computer. Today, though, I can work on papers at 2 AM at home or at 3 PM in the afternoon across the world. If I am away, I can Skype with my lab to make sure everything is moving along according to plan. My research assistants and postdocs can choose to work from 10–6 or 8–3 (they usually choose the former for some odd reason). About the only limitation we have is that if we are doing clinical research, we do need to try to stick to some kind of normal schedule, perhaps obtaining data on patients during regular office hours. But that freedom to pursue your work wherever and whenever you choose is truly liberating. It also means that you can be with your family and share childcare responsibilities more readily. That flexibility can go a long way to make for a good and happy home life.

7. **Make friends across the country and around the world—with endless opportunities to travel**. One of the other major pleasures of research is making new friends. It is a true pleasure to meet and interact with interesting and intelligent people from all over with a similar set of interests as your own. Even if your meetings may be only at semiannual conferences or via conference calls, there is real joy in getting to know many different often like-minded people. After all, you have all somehow found yourselves in the same area of science, so there might be a hidden commonality that binds you all together. I look forward to conferences to chat with friends and make new ones. And with that, of course, goes an opportunity to travel. Seeing all the major US and European cities is almost a certainty today for any active researcher, and increasingly we are also drawn to Asia and South America; I'm sure Africa and the Middle East will soon follow as well.

8. **An opportunity to train and teach others/working as a team**. In some respects I think this final aspect of research is perhaps the most exciting. One of my

previous fellows, who had once been a professional gymnast, described research as a "team sport." And I think that is exactly right. We all work together and try to make something greater than the sum of our parts. No one of us is a winner—we all participate together—for the greater good of the overall project. I try to encourage my group to work together and help each other whenever possible, and I constantly strive to hire real team players. In contrast, when we see patients we are often alone in the process. And it is true there are many lonely hours as a researcher—whether it is writing grants late at night or performing a tedious multi-hour experiment. But even in those situations, there may be late-night phone conversations with research staff or postdocs or early morning telephone calls to finalize a project. The paper that gets submitted, the grant that gets funded, and the presentation to a large crowd are all the results of a group effort, and the more a principal investigator can get her team to realize it was all their doing, the better. The camaraderie, the mentoring, the group beer nights, the popcorn-filled group meetings—they are all proof that it really is a team effort. And in many respects that is the best part of the whole research adventure.

Chapter 3
What's in Store: The Darker Side of Medical Research

Now, having provided some thoughts on the positive aspects of pursuing a career in research, we will explore the flip side—all those potentially awful things you will need to digest and contend with as you slowly establish yourself and, then, hopefully succeed in a research career.

1. **There is no road map**. Tuesdays are my clinical days. These are the days that I see patients in the office pretty much from 8 to 5 PM, with a short, often nonexistent break for lunch. I have the opportunity to see a variety of follow-up patients with established neurological problems which are generally well described and for which there are established or developing therapies. The patients tell me about their problems and symptoms, I examine them briefly, I modify or renew their prescriptions, and I set a follow-up appointment a few months hence. I see a few new patients as well, usually ordering tests to help elucidate what may be causing their numbness, tingling, or weakness.

The day is fairly regimented. The people at the front desk know what to do when the patient shows up for the appointment, I understand the process of evaluation, and I am practiced at the process of making a tentative diagnosis, ordering appropriate tests, and prescribing hopefully effective medications. And our nurse assistant and my administrative assistant help to ensure that everything is running smoothly. Occasionally, there are glitches—a patient shows up at the wrong time but still hopes to be seen, or because the new patient I am seeing doesn't speak English and the interpreter is late, I fall behind and find myself playing catch up all day long.

In research, however, there is no plan, no schedule, no road map. Every day (basically the other 4 work days of the week for me) presents itself as a tabula rasa, a blank slate, from which I need to create structure and ideas. Should we hold a research meeting? Which paper should I work on? Are we analyzing the right results? Is it time to call off a line of investigation and cut our losses, or do we pursue it regardless on the off chance if we proceed we will ultimately succeed? Is it time to submit a grant application? What should it focus on? Or maybe that foundation's grant opportunity would be a better way to go?

© Springer Science+Business Media New York 2016
S.B. Rutkove, *Biomedical Research: An Insider's Guide*,
DOI 10.1007/978-1-4939-3655-7_3

And there are glitches and problems all over the place. You find that a reagent you used in an experiment just didn't work when it had perfectly 3 months earlier. Or you find that your recently hired research assistant who seemed so bright and energetic at the time you interviewed him is deeply mired in a problematical relationship that has cast him into a severe depression. Or perhaps you find yourself inadvertently being noncompliant with an institutional review board regulation and finding your entire project being placed on probation.

While there is a joyous side to not having a detailed, regimented daily schedule, it can at times be disconcerting. You are constantly having to create your days from scratch, choosing the most promising directions to pursue, which grant applications to frame, and which papers to bother resubmitting to another journal for review after being rejected from two others. For each decision, you have limited data/insight, and, in the end, you must simply hope for the best.

There is a reason I enjoy my Tuesdays. They are the days I can just follow the rules. Not having a system in place that dictates your activities can create an omnipresent sense that you could be and should be spending your time more effectively—but you have no idea how.

2. **There is no schedule**. We don't schedule patients in clinic on Sunday mornings nor at 11 PM on a Tuesday night. And if you are an emergency room physician, you work 8 or 12 hours shifts and then are free to go about your life—getting home in the AM to cook breakfast for your kids or to take a trip to Target to buy some new towels. You turn "off" the past clinical shift and turn "on" another part of your life. And even if you are a surgeon and find yourself at the whim of any medical emergency, you generally still have a call schedule. There are days that you know you'll have nothing to do, except veg out and watch a football game or go for a long workout at the gym. You can turn off your work life, at least for the most part, just like that.

But research does not work that way. Just as there is no specific agenda, work has a way of flowing into every crevice of your day and night, your weekends, and even your vacations. You may find yourself obsessing over a data set that just does not make sense that flies in the face of all of your long-standing hypotheses. Or you may be reluctantly checking your email in the hotel lobby in the south of France to discover that the animal facility is freaking out over the health status of your mice, and that they're contracting an infection. Or, most commonly, you have a grant due in just a few days, and you are working 24/7 trying to put the final touches on the thing to ensure that it is as possibly good as you can get it, forcing you to cast virtually all the other parts of your life, family, friends, and perhaps even your personal hygiene, aside.

In short, it is very, very, very hard to simply flick the switch and turn it off. Sure you can take vacations, you can go out to nice dinners, you can spend lots of time with the family, but you have to be prepared for interruptions that are both internally and externally generated. This is the flip side of the flexibility I described in the last chapter—the work can be inescapable.

3. **Credibility and incredulity**. Research is not a picnic and people don't always play nice. In fact, you may learn the darker side of human nature as a researcher. I

don't mean that researchers are nefarious creatures. In fact, that is probably the farthest thing from the truth. But when you are dealing with a group of people who have their own ideas, own interests, and all want to succeed, you are sure to get head banging, disagreements, name-calling, and sometimes, rarely, outright cheating.

You have to be prepared for severe criticism when you present your work. Someone may simply not believe your data or your conclusions. Or they will question why you are bothering in the first place. They will call your work "incremental" or illogical or simply poorly considered. You will not only hear these people say such things in public (in fact, many of us have seen shouting matches erupt in conferences where someone, whose data conflicts with that of the presenter, stands his ground, while the presenter is equally determined to get her point across) but also in response to the submission of a research paper or on the critique of your grant application. In fact, the anonymity of the grant and paper review process affords the opportunity for the reviewers to be extremely critical—no holds barred.

And if that is not unpleasant enough, these are all at least legitimate and perhaps "healthy" discussions. But the fight for limited grant dollars also means that people who simply have a different line of research may try to negate your research simply because you are studying the same question, but with a different approach. While this may be frustrating to deal with when discussing your results at a meeting, it takes on a much more sinister appearance when that person is reviewing the grant application that you worked on for 4 months. This is no small issue.

But things can get even worse than that. Some people may lie and cheat and even steal. Fortunately, the few miscreants who partake in these pathologic behaviors are rare, but I have heard horror stories of people stealing each other's ideas and experimental results. People will also change data to improve their results in obvious and clearly illegal ways. I will discuss this more in the chapter on research integrity.

4. **Paperwork, administration, organization**. As one day you may discover, being a principal investigator and running a research lab, whether it is a basic science lab with five postdocs and ten research assistants or participating in a multicenter drug trial funded by a pharmaceutical company in which you are working with a single nurse assistant, you have just entered into a new world of endless paperwork, reviews, and administration.

Mind you, doing virtually any form of work has its associated paperwork. But research has its own unique set of seemingly endless forms and reports. There are budgets to track, hours of your research assistants to manage, case report forms to complete, laboratory safety surveys, intermittent inspections of your clinical animal work, appropriate disposal of toxic or addictive medications, intermittent chart reviews by the companies paying for the study drug, annual or semiannual progress reports due to the funding agencies, and online training examinations that need to be "refreshed" on a regular basis. And that is not even discussing the actual process of institutional review board or animal care and use committee applications.

Fortunately, you will have some help with these things. Usually institutions will assign you a research administrator who will help with some of the paper work, including budgeting on grants and the hiring process of new employees. But do not underestimate the immense burden that you will need to deal with regularly. And putting this stuff off only leads to trouble and added work and headaches. So until you retire, it becomes an ongoing and regular effort that cannot be easily curtailed. One has to learn to embrace it, as difficult as that may seem.

5. **Funding, money, and stress**. When you enter into the world of research, you also will find yourself suddenly facing the need to pay for it to keep it moving along. Very little can be completed without dedicated funding, short of writing simple case reports or review articles. If you really want to pursue serious research, whether it is clinical, basic, or translational, you will have to pay for it, and finding that money to fund it can be a full-time occupation in itself. You will need to apply repeatedly for grants, get used to rejection, and recognize that you may need to seek other sources of funding such as grateful patients who will provide modest amounts of philanthropy or industry dollars to help participate in a clinical therapeutic trial or to perform some basic research that will benefit them. Regardless of the funding source, ensuring a steady stream of money is a critical feature to any successful research endeavor and that means not only planning for this year or next, but really trying to foresee where you'll be in 5 years or so and plan grant applications accordingly.

Once you actually obtain funding, you cannot rest on your laurels. In fact, you must quickly turn around and keep applying to help ensure continuous funding for years to come. Ideally one is able to stagger grants so that you can be in the process of renewing one, while the other is midway through. But achieving that is not easy.

It is also important to realize that as you start receiving grants, you will start to *rely* on them for continuing your work. Just like a musician who needs to practice continually to keep up his skills, you will need to continue to apply for funding to keep your lab functioning.

Of course all of this constant need to find money becomes a major stress. This requires constant focus and searching for new grant opportunities at every opportunity can often take center stage. And as if it is not difficult enough obtaining government funding, you also become subject to all the whims of Congress, including budgets that never get settled leaving you anxiously waiting to hear and basically paralyzing your ability to do any new work or even plan effectively.

Of all the downsides to a career in biomedical research, I would have to say that this is probably the most significant one, since it is ever-present. You might have time periods of peace, but you always know that sometime in the not-too-distant future, you will once again have to go out and seek additional funds.

6. **Stresses of running a team and being a manager**. While research is definitely a team sport, running that team can be challenging at times. First, one has to pick your players. Hiring great individuals is not easy. You must first determine what position you are actually hiring for. While this may sound obvious, it is not always the case as you may find that you need one person to do several tasks (e.g., simple computer programming and running animal experiments) or you may find that the area of expertise you wish to hire someone is so specialized that finding a person is virtually impossible. Moreover, once you have a team in place, filling in additional people demands that they fit well into the group, both from a personality

and from an expertise perspective. Another major issue is turnover. When you hire people into most "standard" jobs, you hope and anticipating that they will stick around for at least 3–5 years. But that is often not the case in the realm of academic research. Many of the most talented young people who you may want to hire as a research assistant are usually looking for no more than 1–2 years experience after college and before graduate school to sow their research wild oats. And that year can go by very, very quickly. You may find yourself relying heavily on one of these people just to find them disappearing right when you need to submit a huge grant application.

There may be squabbles and disagreement and annoyance between members of a research group. Someone in the lab may feel that another individual is lazy or inefficient, while others work really hard but are not being recognized. Young love may develop between two coworkers that can lead to real complications if there is a falling out. Some people may be poor workers or problematical for some other reason. Current employment laws create such a layer of bureaucracy that trying to actually fire an ineffective employee can be remarkably difficult, especially if that person has been in the position for more than a few months.

7. **Future self-reflection**. The final point, and it is more of an existential one, is whether it is all worth it. When, many years hence, you finally decide that enough is enough and retire, you hope to feel that you really contributed in a meaningful way to the world. As I noted earlier, most of us are not expecting fame or even significant respect—we just would like to feel that we have done good work and have made some difference for the greater good of society, even if it was small. And if you had cared for patients and had done a reasonable job at it, you would have been receiving those rewards all along—knowing that perhaps you relieved someone's suffering or improved another person's health in a tangible way. And if you had taught and mentored, you would know that those people are now leading rich and fulfilling careers of their own. But research itself often simply has to stand up to time. Do people care really about it 10 years hence? Did it really change anything in any real way? Did it become an integral part of the canon a stepping-stone to bigger things? Or did it get cast into the junk heap, the work proving to be nothing more than a mere side note with no relevance or meaning.

It is the idea that one could struggle so hard for so long and ultimately fail that is so painful. Of course, there is one way to mitigate this: don't work your entire life on just one concept or hypothesis—spread out your ideas, pursue different areas of research, and don't be afraid to change paths. Adopt new technologies and theories into your work as you go along. All of these may help. And of course you will probably be doing more than just research. You will undoubtedly teach and mentor and perhaps you will also take on important administrative roles within your institution.

But in the end, as you sit in your reclining chair, drinking your nice glass of merlot watching the sun slowly descend over the horizon and the sky turn its spectral colors, hopefully in a pleasant tropical place, wouldn't it be wonderful to feel good about all you had achieved in those 40 or 50 years in which you struggled so hard? Unfortunately, there is no way to know if you will be so lucky.

Chapter 4
One Degree of Separation

Unlike driving a car, flying a plane, or practicing law or medicine, you don't actually *need* a degree to pursue biomedical research. There is no governing body that will only issue a license to conduct biomedical research to card-carrying PhDs or MDs from an accredited program in the United States. In fact, there are, technically, no restrictions whatsoever, and strictly speaking you don't need even need any kind of degree to pursue clinical research on human subjects, although you may need to work with a licensed medical doctor. You don't even need a graduate degree or for that matter an undergraduate degree. It is worthwhile to consider that some of the greatest researchers of the nineteenth century never even finished college (e.g., Michael Faraday of electricity fame and Gregor Mendel of basic genetics), though admittedly that would be pretty tough today given the huge amount of scientific knowledge out there. So if the research bug has bitten you, you shouldn't necessarily restrict yourself to any one type of degree. And if you have already finished your training, there is no need to go back and get another degree—you simply don't need it. And yet these stamps of approval, offered by venerable institutions, seem to hold a special power over us.

While I personally took a pretty straight and narrow path, going directly from college to medical school and graduating with an MD, I was repeatedly torn both before, during, and for some time after finishing as to whether I should have attended graduate school for a PhD instead of an MD, whether I should have obtained a PhD along with an MD as part of a combined program, or whether I should have returned to school after my MD and residency to become "fully qualified" to do serious research with a PhD. I, frankly, seriously considered leaving medical school on several occasions, especially during my first and second years, feeling that I was learning a trade rather than science and that it would be challenging if not impossible to do serious research with a mere MD, even though some of my mentors assured me otherwise.

To complicate matters further, MDs and PhDs are not the only "terminal" degrees out there. There are other degree possibilities too: MPHs, Master of Medicine, along with a litany of others. In fact, with every passing decade, it seems

© Springer Science+Business Media New York 2016
S.B. Rutkove, *Biomedical Research: An Insider's Guide*,
DOI 10.1007/978-1-4939-3655-7_4

that there are more and more degree types that are created to serve an ever-increasing need to provide documentation of one's knowledge and skill set. All of these choices make for an ever more complicated landscape, where it is very, very difficult to know exactly what kind of imprimatur you need to succeed in biomedical research.

Relax. Let me start by putting your mind at ease: it probably makes less difference than you think. If you really want to do research, the degree is definitely secondary to having the brains, perseverance, and know-how than the actual degree. I find it useful to always recall what the Wizard of Oz told the Scarecrow after revealing his true self from behind the curtain: "Back where I come from, we have universities, seats of great learning, where men go to become great thinkers. And when they come out, they think deep thoughts and with no more brains than you have. But they have one thing you haven't got: a diploma." And honestly, the diploma that hangs on your wall does not automatically confer the ability to do great research. I've seen plenty of people with those degrees who do not have the wherewithal to pursue science or the gumption to undertake a career in discovery. But, I must admit, it is a testament of a sort that you should at least be capable of it. Let's review a few of them here:

PhD. We generally think of the PhD as the "serious" research degree and to a large extent it is. If you choose to obtain a PhD, you are basically saying that you want to become an expert in a discipline and that you are going to spend your time studying that area and potentially teaching it to others. A PhD demands a thesis that in turn requires a serious, prolonged research effort that will teach you a great deal about doing creative investigative work that will serve you well in the long run. You will learn firsthand the challenges of collecting data, how experiments often don't go as planned, how minor changes in protocol can cause unexpected findings, and how absolutely complicated doing anything well really is. You will see how hard it is to write a well-formulated research paper and the challenges of getting acceptance into a prestigious journal. You will learn how to write a thesis and to defend it, understanding that every study is full of flaws and limitations. You will learn the importance of collaboration and the grant application process, either by observing your mentor go through it or perhaps pursuing it yourself. And you will see how people have differences of opinion and how those differences are handled, either through considered and thoughtful scientific discourse or outright, primal hostility.

Once you have survived the challenges of your PhD, you will likely then take one or more postdoctoral positions where you may spend potentially upward of 5–7 additional years in study and training, further honing your skill set as you begin to apply for teaching or research positions in universities. Or perhaps you will see the challenges of supporting a career in research and decide to go into industry instead.

Now, while we often think of PhDs as doing "basic" research, in fact many PhDs do very translational or even clinical work. There is nothing that precludes them from doing so, though they may need some assistance from an MD or registered nurse or similar depending on exactly what they are doing. So that in itself should not be used as a determining factor as to degree choice.

One major advantage of a PhD over an MD is that it allows you to delve very, very deeply into one area, developing you into a true expert in that discipline. We will discuss the 10,000 hours rule later, of which you may be aware, but there can be no question that you will have spent far more than 10,000 hours becoming truly all-knowing about one specific area and the methods that you will need to pursue questions relevant to it. Another major advantage is that you won't have clinical responsibilities distracting you, which is inevitable for MDs. However, you may have other distractions, such as teaching or committee work, which can also become time-consuming. And, at any rate, even with an MD, you may be required to do considerable teaching as well.

MD. An MD is definitely a professional degree—it does not confer with it the immediate gravitas of PhD in terms of research credentials. You can obtain an MD from a top-notch medical school and come out not knowing the first thing about research, basic or clinical for that matter. You can go through your residency and fellowships and go off and practice medicine or surgery, never having stepped one time into a laboratory. Turning an MD into a research degree requires applied effort on the part of the MD candidate or recipient. It could mean taking additional courses, working in the basic lab alongside postdocs and graduate students or it could mean partaking in clinical research opportunities during and after medical school and residency. Fortunately, there are many occasions to pursue this, and as long as one keeps a lookout for them, they are readily available. But it will require extra time at some point in one's career.

There are definitely disadvantages to an MD if you are mainly interested in pursuing research in the biomedical field and not practicing medicine. You will waste time doing things that are completely irrelevant, from learning about correct billing practices and documentation to learning subspecialties of medicine with which you will want little to do in the future and which you will have to force yourself to enjoy. Another huge issue is the cost. A medical education is extremely expensive and only increases year after year. Currently, a 4-year medical education at a private medical school (in 2015) is more than $280,000. Compare that to a PhD where you may accrue relatively little debt, paying off your years of education by helping out as a teaching assistant or through other fellowships. Obtaining an MD may mean that you'll be so saddled with debt that when you finish you may simply give up on the idea of doing research at all and decide to go into lucrative practice in a relatively well-paid procedural subspecialty. While you may ultimately earn considerably more as an MD as compared to a PhD in the United States, that advantage may not seem self-evident as you finish, burdened with your huge debt. Thus, if you are interested in pursuing an MD and want to do research, you will have to carefully consider your options if you are to make it work.

On the other hand, the MD definitely confers certain advantages (and as an MD myself, please recognize my biases here). The first and perhaps largest advantage is that it provides a powerful contextual understanding of the research that you will be doing that may not be apparent to someone with a PhD. As an MD, one constantly sees the potential final, practical application of what is being developed. This gives one a deep understanding of what is important from a clinical standpoint and what is not. PhDs may find themselves struggling to figure out what direction to go in or the clinical application of what they doing. This becomes especially important when writing grant applications. An MD with experience can see and understand the application of what is being pursued. While a PhD can do so similarly, it is often not so easy. Having sat on many review committees, I can say that many grant applications simply miss the point since the writer is not quite sure what he is after in terms of long-term outcome, somehow getting lost in the details of the science and not their long-term relevance to health. Another obvious advantage is that it confers on you the ability to generate salary outside of research dollars. If Congress is in a cost-cutting mode and NIH gets hit, grant funding can be tough to come by. As an MD, you will still be able to earn income and feed the family, reducing the amount of effort you have dedicated to research and instead focusing on clinical care. An MD also means you'll potentially have other sources of philanthropy to help you through the tough times, since you may have helped one or two grateful (and wealthy) patients. So, despite the painful upfront cost of an MD, there are potential returns down the road.

MD-PhD. I think few titles sound more impressive than "MD-PhD." Not only have you achieved the approval to practice medicine, but you also have achieved a PhD, the ultimate evidence that you are now fully equipped to pursue biomedical research. You may need to downplay the fact that you are already finding yourself needing reading glasses at the same time you have landed your first real, adult, salaried job. It can also be especially painful at college reunions when one of your roommates tells you he has been successfully practicing law for nearly two decades and another is considering early retirement after launching a successful start-up while you are still living in a cramped apartment with partying college kids all around you.

I am not trying to criticize MD-PhD programs. In fact, they can be very valuable. Some programs still allow you to obtain the two degrees and accrue no medical debt whatsoever. You will learn everything you know to be a practicing MD and also all the serious science necessary to be an outstanding "bench" researcher. But it is a huge time commitment, and when one signs up for such a program, for example, during your senior year of college, you may not really be thinking about the long-term consequences of such a choice. If you are an MD and really want to do research when you are done, there are plenty of opportunities to learn the skills that you need without a PhD. And if you have finished your PhD and realize that you really wanted to be more clinically oriented, you can always go back and get the MD. But I think it is a challenge for a person to be in college and make a decision that will basically control potentially the next two decades of her life.

As an aside, I think time-wise, the choice between MD and PhD is approximately a wash. An MD is generally 4 years; if you add in 4 years of residency and another 2–3 years of fellowship, especially if you are considering a research fellowship, you are looking at maybe 10–11 years of postcollege education/training. For a PhD that may take 5 years plus another 6 years of postdoctoral time, you are again at 11 years. For an MD-PhD, you are looking at 4 years of medical school, 4 years of PhD-dom, and then another 5–7 years of research fellowships/residency/postdocs, and you are looking at maybe 15–16 years postcollege education/training.

Additional degrees. As I noted earlier, there are many other degree opportunities out there that may enhance your stature or, more importantly, give you additional education to help you do better research. One of the more popular is the Master of Public Health degree. With some extra course work, some medical schools award these along with the MD. Depending on your interests, these can be useful; they will certainly give you some additional biostatistical training, which may be helpful regardless of what you end up focusing on as a researcher. But in the end, I think the most important thing is not the diploma, it is the experience. The scarecrow never went to school, but he was definitely the wisest of Dorothy's friends.

Summary. For many people reading this book, your choice of degree may already be yesterday's news. You have already committed to a PhD program or perhaps you are finishing your internal medical residency or are already junior faculty somewhere. So my point here is not to make you second guess a very old decision. No one solution fits everybody's needs, and many extraneous factors may come to bear, including whether you will be burdened with large medical school debts or whether you are wanting to start a family sooner than later or simply cannot envision yourself being a student until middle age. My bottom line is that if you really want to pursue research, the type of degree that you plan to pursue or already have obtained will suit you just fine. It is the ongoing work, perseverance, creativity, determination, and smarts that will ultimately help you succeed, not the framed pieces of paper hanging on your wall.

Chapter 5
Choosing and Working with a Mentor

Identifying a mentor. The purpose of this chapter is to help you better understand what makes a good mentor—not only to help you find one early in your career but also to help you as your mentoring duties increase over the years. Of course, there are no absolutes or specific recipes for success. To a great extent, finding a good mentor is very much luck of the draw. You can't guarantee that there will be someone at your institution in your particular field sufficiently skilled to help you along your way. Similarly, it is also very possible to launch a successful career without a mentor being deeply involved in your work. However, I would say that it is pretty much impossible to start a successful research career entirely on your own or just by reading a book (yes, even this one!). On the other hand, it is very possible to succeed with just some gentle assistance and direction from senior colleagues. For example, one major challenge is identifying a research niche without any outside direction or guidance, as will be discussed in a later chapter. At the very least, a mentor can help you identify a potential place to "plant your flag" and start your work. At the very most, they can become a lifelong friend and colleague with whom you will work for years or decades to come, whether or not you are still at the same institution or across the country from one another.

Mentors really come in all forms, and a person who is a terrific mentor to one newbie investigator maybe a poor fit for another. For example, some mentors are deeply involved and enjoy carefully managing the research that their mentees are pursuing; others are very much hands off, allowing the young researcher a remarkable amount of freedom to explore their own ideas. While this latter approach may sound appealing, it also means allowing them to potentially waste months going off on useless research tangents.

In point of fact, most people choose their research niche based on a specific mentor rather than finding a mentor in a specific research niche. That person is likely someone you may have met in medical school, residency, or perhaps in a graduate program. Perhaps it is your clinical fellowship director, an attending you worked with during a month of consult rounds, or perhaps a researcher in the department you have reached out to after a conference. Regardless of the specifics, it is pretty

© Springer Science+Business Media New York 2016
S.B. Rutkove, *Biomedical Research: An Insider's Guide*,
DOI 10.1007/978-1-4939-3655-7_5

common that this person will be someone located nearby. Occasionally, you may seek someone out far away that you think may be very relevant to your career, especially if you are perhaps planning to move somewhere else. You'll know that this person will be able to serve as a mentor because they have a variety of specific characteristics including the fact that they do research in which you are interested, they are communicative, and they have expressed a need to help young people interested in pursuing a research career.

Regardless of how you meet, there are some definite characteristics to look for in a mentor. Hopefully, you will be able to determine whether this person has at least some of the prerequisite requirements to serve as a mentor simply by getting to know him superficially both directly and indirectly through friends, or other mentees. In fact, there is no more valuable way of learning whether this person has the potential of serving as a great mentor than by obtaining opinions from others who have worked with him.

I now provide a brief list of a few characteristics that I think most outstanding mentors share in common while recognizing that mentors can vary dramatically in their characteristics and most will only have a subset of these.

1. **Communicativeness**. Being taciturn is definitely not a quality you are looking for in a mentor. A person who is friendly and well spoken is likely to be someone you can be sure will run an effective team and can serve to provide you with ongoing feedback and ideas. On the other hand, an especially loquacious individual may also be challenging to work with. So make sure you find someone who is both well spoken and a good listener.

2. **Open-mindedness**. This can be a little tricky to judge from the outside, but generally people who are successful in research are fairly open-minded about what is of interest to them. They are willing to entertain ideas somewhat outside their specific area of interest and determine whether it is plausible and worth pursuing. Perhaps the specific idea suggested is on the right track, but is not perfect—and they will be able to tell you that. A good mentor should be able to recognize the value in an idea and modify as needed to make it doable and successful. A mentor that is obsessively entrenched in one area of research to the exclusion of all others may not be the best choice.

3. **Open and forthright**. One thing you definitely do not want in a mentor is someone who plays everything close to the chest. A mentor should be open and honest and tell you his/her concerns and ideas. People who are very cautious about talking about their work or discussing openly about new ideas or the interpretation of data or where their grant money is coming from should be viewed with considerable skepticism. There really is never anything to hide, and I believe teaching young investigators the importance of generosity and openness in thought and action is critical to their someday becoming outstanding mentors themselves.

4. **A people person**. Part of being communicative means also working effectively with others and honestly enjoying the role of helping run and organize a research effort. For the most part, the medical field does tend to weed out real loners, but some people who on the surface are fairly communicative are actually fairly antisocial to the point of being unpleasant to work with. You can usually identify

these people because they are not well liked. You don't have to be a party animal to be a researcher, but the idea of enjoying or at least tolerating the company of others is definitely a prerequisite to being a decent mentor.

5. **Avoid "difficult" people**. No matter how fascinating an area of research someone is pursuing, always avoid someone who is generally considered "difficult" or "temperamental." It is almost never worth the agony—and I guarantee you that it will be agony—of aligning yourself with somebody everyone knows is difficult or impossible to work with just to enter a specific area of research that is of interest to you. And that means even if that person is famous or incredibly well respected within their field. Think of your day-to-day sanity, as it may be a long relationship.

6. **Being willing to put your interests first**. This is another aspect that can be tough to determine, but a good mentor shouldn't be excessively focused about getting herself into the limelight. She should be looking out and thinking ahead for you. How is a grant application going to help you? What kind of papers would you need to strengthen your CV? How can you identify an area of research that is aligned with, but clearly distinct from, her work? And what opportunities are there for you to present your research at conferences or to give talks? You will not know of all the possible venues to help your own career develop, and a mentor who can keep those things in mind, constantly being on the lookout for you, especially in your early years, is definitely someone to align yourself with.

7. **Not a micromanager but not an absentee landlord**. The best mentors keep an eye on the work going on, give regular direction, try to identify problems before they arise, and take a step back when they see things are going well. But they are not traveling 364 days a year or routinely unavailable to answer questions. For good mentorship, there has to be some regular back and forth in person. Regular research meetings, a brief stopping by the lab bench or your desk, or a friendly chat over a cup of coffee can make the world of difference in developing and sustaining an effective working relationship.

8. **Look for an open-door policy**. Mentors should be readily available to answer questions or provide advice on an as-needed basis. If you are finding yourself lost or confused, you should be able to interrupt them and ask for assistance. Doing so should never bring trepidation or the expectation of a snide or annoyed comment. A good mentor should be willing to answer questions, consider alternative points of view, or simply be around to assuage anxiety over complicated data sets, reprimands from institutional review boards, papers that don't seem to want to hold together, or challenging career decisions.

9. **Avoid the prison sentence mentality**. Some mentors have a difficult time "letting go" of their advisees. They have no choice ultimately, but they can make life surprisingly difficult—for example, by not being willing to write a strong letter of recommendation for a new position or sequestering you away so you don't have opportunities to meet and become part of the greater research community. Fortunately, such people are relatively few and are readily identifiable because most of the people working for them wear forlorn and depressed expressions.

10. **Would you like to be a colleague with this person?** The truth is that many times you are not looking to leave the institution in which you have been working.

In fact, if you have settled in an area and are starting a family, you may be especially loath to pack up and ship out across country. For that reason, it is good to think practically from the outside. Is this mentor someone I can actually continue to work with for years to come? You'll know in part because she should have been treating you as a colleague from day one, rather than just as a student or a gopher. If that is the case, then it may make a lot of sense to try to be thinking long term. If you feel that this person is looking for someone like you to become a colleague, this can be the best situation. And it is also evidence that this person could serve as a terrific mentor in the near term, whether you end up staying put or not.

Working with a mentor. Like choosing a good mentor, there are no strict rules whatsoever to help guide you. Most mentor-mentee relationships also morph over time to become increasingly collegial and less hierarchical. You may find that in the early days you need to meet with your mentor very regularly to obtain guidance on a project or that you are exchanging emails several times a day as you are working on a grant application. And there may be other times that you are pretty much on your own—perhaps after you have worked out details of a protocol and are in data-collection mode. At these times, you may find yourself providing only brief updates at research group meetings or perhaps just every couple of weeks during one-on-one sessions.

A good mentor, however, should always make herself available to discuss concerns or questions or to entertain new ideas or directions. And you will both discover each other's working habits and how to most effectively collaborate. Perhaps the mentor does much of his work in the early morning hours, while the mentee works through things later in the afternoon or evening. Or perhaps you will find that communication is the smoothest if questions are in writing. Whatever the details, these things generally evolve over time, as the course of the workload ebbs and flows and people discover each other's idiosyncrasies, likes, and dislikes.

Becoming a mentor yourself. Perhaps there is no better way of understanding how to work with a mentor than becoming one yourself. And the truth is that opportunities for mentoring, at least in a limited fashion, often start surprisingly early in your career. As a graduate student, you may find yourself mentoring undergraduates. As a postdoctoral associate, you may find yourself mentoring graduate students and undergraduates. As a medical resident, you'll find yourself mentoring medical students. Essentially the interactions are endless. Some are short lived and others much more enduring, but the approaches you take and the thinking processes you engage in, as you try empathize and see the world from their perspective, are great chances to practice the skills of good mentorship. It is a process that will continue throughout your life. In short, you should always seek opportunities to mentor—not only because it will help hone your mentoring skill set but also because it will allow you to more effectively work with your own mentors.

Summary. There are no strict rules as to what makes a good mentor. But you will usually know it because the person will be generally well liked by others in the institution, have a group of contented people under his guidance, and still be successful in terms of recognition and achievements within his field.

Finally, it is worth pointing out that many of us intermittently seek the advice of mentors or colleagues, many years later, even when we are fully "grown up." There is nothing wrong or embarrassing about going back to an old teacher and asking for their solemn input. Professional musicians do this all the time. Years after they have finished studying and launched a successful career, they may find themselves seeking advice as to how to solve a new problem or interpret a difficult piece or to make fine adjustments to their technique that has gradually morphed into relative disarray. Not only do such consultations help the mentee, but they also make the mentor feel good that she can still contribute in a meaningful way to the further success of someone who has already achieved recognition on their own.

Chapter 6
Identifying a Research Niche That You Can Call Your Own

Without a doubt, one of the greatest challenges as you approach a career in medical research, and for that matter, in all forms of research, is identifying a specific area of study to pursue. As a graduate or medical student just starting out, one is buffeted with an immense amount of information and data. And many of us find that there are many areas of research that seem potentially fascinating and that there is an endless wealth of possible directions in which to go. The sky's the limit.

But as one progresses through the educational process, it also starts becoming clearer that things are not quite so simple. In fact, many areas are very thoroughly researched, whereas others seem of dubious value. Soon the student goes from feeling that there is a plethora of potential directions to believing that things are relatively constrained. What kind of research can I pursue that will really make a difference, she may ask? What is genuinely interesting and that could fulfill many years of pursuit? Graduate students generally have an easier time with this since they can stark seeking out advisors from an early time and can become interested in the work going on in a specific lab. But undergraduate and medical students, residents, and clinical fellows have a decidedly more difficult time. I think this is, in part, due to medical school's teaching science more as a fait accompli rather than a work that is in continual progress. From the school's point of view, the research is over, and now all you have to do is to learn the rules to be a good practicing physician

Finding a specific area of research. In my own experience, it is very rare for someone to have already identified a specific area of research entirely on his own. In fact, when people have approached me with fully formed ideas that they would like my assistance in pursuing, I am usual fairly skeptical, since most have not fully vetted the idea or understand its context. The truth is that it takes years of experience in a discipline to really understand fully what is important and what is not important, what directions are likely to be promising and what are more likely to be dead ends, and what ideas are doable and what are simply unrealistic, either from a funding or scientific standpoint.

For this reason, once you identify a general field of interest to you, it is pretty typical that a research mentor working in that field will help guide you to a specific

© Springer Science+Business Media New York 2016
S.B. Rutkove, *Biomedical Research: An Insider's Guide*,
DOI 10.1007/978-1-4939-3655-7_6

project that has the potential for further expansion and development. Sometimes such projects will end quickly in frustration, but a good mentor will generally see opportunities, whereas a more junior individual may not appreciate the potential value of a new line of research. In fact, most projects may seem rather dull when you are first introduced to them; but as you become fully immersed in the work, they may start to appear remarkably interesting and full of promise, as you become aware of an array of intriguing and exciting nuances to the work.

Of course there may areas of research in which you will have no interest no matter how deeply immersed in them you become. If you go into cardiology in order to better understand electrophysiologic testing and treatment, you may find the idea of pursuing new measures for detecting ischemic myocardial damage as entirely banal, perhaps. And even after spending some time learning the finer points of enzyme assays and cardiac imaging modalities, you may still not feel content if your first love really was electrophysiologic testing. Similarly, if you are pursuing a PhD in immunology and are specifically interested in understanding the concepts behind the development of lupus erythematosis and the associated kidney disease, you may not find it very interesting to study the mechanisms atopic rhinitis (allergic runny nose) just because it is a topic vaguely within the field of immunology. It may simply not seem sufficiently important. Ultimately, it is the perceived significance of a subject and the science underlying the topic that will drive you. If you find the significance uninteresting/unimportant and the science decidedly out of your area of interest, no matter how much you convince yourself otherwise, you will probably not enjoy it. Or perhaps you simply don't have a knack for the subject matter. Regardless of the reason, you should not feel compelled to pursue something just because a potential mentor seems like a nice guy and has been trying to sell you on a project.

But also don't forget that over a lifetime of work, a person's research focus may change and that is perfectly fine. While you may at first be convinced what you are working on is incredibly worthwhile, you may discover that an aligned field is actually far richer and far more deserving of your attention and that you need to jump ship. Or, more likely, one thing leads to another, and your line of work gradually transforms from the study of A to the study of H or I. And that is a natural progression. So just because you decide to pursue one area of interest when you are 25 does not mean you will still be committed when you are 75, though that always is possible, of course.

Identifying the specific questions of interest. Okay. So perhaps at this point, you have identified an area of potential interest and a mentor that you would like to work with. Perhaps she has already made some concrete suggestions as to a topic that *she* considers interesting and something you would be happy to pursue. But you want to come up with something on your own. Or perhaps you have already been working with a mentor and would like to define something separate and distinct that you would like to pursue, but you have not yet identified an exact question to ask. Or perhaps you don't have a mentor and are just struggling to come up with some interesting question. Here are some general thoughts as to how to develop new research ideas that are doable and may have potential interest. These are not guaranteed recipes for success—but rather just a collection of concepts to consider.

Think big. When I was in medical school in New York in the 1980s, I would meet up with my girlfriend (now my wife of 25 years) who lived on the Upper West Side, and we'd stroll down Columbus Avenue. Somewhere around 75th street on the east side of the avenue was a store called *Think Big*. The store sold a variety of absurdly, ridiculously oversized items from huge tee shirts that several people could fit into and a pencil the size of a small tree. It was clearly a silly idea for a store, although it somehow managed to survive for several years; I never could figure out who would buy anything that the store peddled.

My bringing up this shop hits exactly at the point I am trying to get at. When I say, think big, I don't mean to propose a big project just for the novelty of creating a big project. Don't try to produce research that *seems* important; pursue work that *is* important. In other words, you don't need to study a disorder that affects billions of people (say osteoporosis in the elderly or mechanisms of obesity or malaria, although those all are important in their own right) or is so huge as to be virtually impossible to do. Rather, think big in terms of implications. For example, ask yourself, "If I figure out the answer to the question, what else might be impacted by it?" You can easily pursue a huge topic that actually is providing nothing more than filler material for other basic concepts. One of my friends refers to this as "interstitial research"—in other words research that only fills gaps in knowledge and is incremental in nature rather than "paradigm shifting," to borrow Thomas Kuhn's terminology. Kuhn developed the concept which has become something of a cliché in his book *The Structure of Scientific Revolutions*. In that work, he was not advocating for individual people necessarily to try to change science, but rather described how new ideas are generated and then become adopted. I admit that it is not easy to identify paradigm shifting ideas, but if you start out only asking small questions, you'll only pursue small goals, and the cumulative effect of your work will be relatively small. But by asking more challenging questions, you may actually achieve greater things. I often repeat John F. Kennedy's famous quotation, "We choose to go to the moon in this decade and do the other things, not because they are easy, but because they are hard." Don't be afraid to go places other people may not want to, even if the problems seem insurmountable.

Read widely. I think if I were to be able offer only one piece of advice to young investigators, it would be to read widely. If we each only read journals and articles and books in our own field of interest, no new ideas would virtually ever be generated. In fact, the only way to really hope to generate new ideas is to read well outside of your area of interest and outside of your comfort zone. You may not be able to identify a specific research niche, but it may make you start to understand other disciplines and how they could potentially impact your own. And I don't mean necessarily reading even in medicine or biomedical sciences. Reading history, other scientific endeavors, mathematics, and even fiction can generate ideas that at first may seem a little wacky or off the wall, but may end up having significance. For example, look at all the use of leeches to stimulate blood flow and decrease congestion in reattached limbs and organs. Leeches had been in fact used for millennia for medicinal bloodletting, and in the early nineteenth century, there was something of a leech mania that swept through Europe. However, as the nineteenth century came to a close, the use of leeches for medicinal purposes became increasingly uncommon, frowned upon, and eventually stopped altogether. It was not until the 1980s that some daring and well-read surgeons first began reinvestigating the use of this segmented worm to treat the vascular engorgement that occurs in a severed limb after it has been reattached. The results were so successful that most larger hospital pharmacies with trauma centers actively keep a supply of leeches available for treatment of reattached limbs and digits. Only in retrospect does this idea seem to be in any way intuitive.

Use your imagination and risk-taking. In short, we sometimes must let our imaginations run freely to come up with new ideas. There is definitely a dearth of teaching in medical school, PhD programs, and in postgraduate medical training on how to think imaginatively in science. To a great extent, many of us feel very much enslaved to the vast body of information out there, and it is to difficult for us to embrace the idea that research is anything more than digesting enough information such that you can now make your small contribution to an ever-enlarging field. In fact, much of our current day teaching culture focuses precisely on learning the canon. Perhaps this is to some extent the powerful influence that medicine has had on biomedical science and perhaps science in general. We are uncomfortable considering outlandish mechanisms, devices, or ideas since the scientific community has become so entrenched. We see ourselves as part of a large industrial team of sorts, each needing to do his or her own bit to help to push science and medicine one step further toward some ultimate culmination. There seems to almost be an implication that veering off from an established path may lead to failure and self-loathing.

Using your imagination does not mean creating nonsense or fiction. It means thinking about things in unconventional ways and not having the voice of your mentor, your colleagues, or your parents in your head discouraging you from thinking contrarily. The phrase "out of the box" is currently very popular, but most of us are not ready to embrace that idea wholeheartedly. That may be because we are also naturally afraid. Introducing unconventional ways of thinking is risky, and many of us who decide to go into medical research are not natural risk-takers. In fact, we are often risk avoidant, and that may be part of the problem. We are at some deep level afraid of being ignored or concerned about becoming a pariah. But honest work, even if it flies in the face of conventional wisdom, should never be considered foolish. Even if it ends up being wrong, it may introduce other ways of thinking or new ideas that may ultimately prove their value.

Ada Lovelace, the early nineteenth-century figure who, along with Charles Babbage, spent a great deal of time thinking about and then ultimately developing the first rudimentary mechanical computers, pondered a great deal about the human ability of creativity and originality. In one famous quotation, she posited, "What is imagination?" Her answer: "It is the combining faculty. It brings together things, facts, ideas conceptions, in new original, endless, ever-varying combinations ... It is that which penetrates into the unseen worlds around us, the worlds of Science."

Browse the Web widely. When the Internet and World Wide Web were first created, it was generally considered to be an index of sorts and that you would be able to browse titles of articles much as you would browse books on a bookshelf in a store. However, over time and with the development of powerful search engines, it became clear that the Internet was actually a remarkably effective tool to learn about a specific item of interest and related items. While it definitely remains possible to browse a list of unrelated items, whether it is at Amazon or an online educational site, we are usually automatically funneled into an area of apparent specific interest to us based on the terms we search. While this is great if you are interested in learning more about a specific topic, it doesn't afford an easy mechanism to browse, or at least the way we typically might think of doing it in a library or bookstore.

It is actually possible to browse effectively on the web, if you are willing to not constrain yourself to only one set of ideas, but to some extent that browsing must be self-generated. Google searches can lead to some unexpected hits that may be worth pursuing, but only if you combine two dissimilar ideas that may bring up new unexpected possibilities. Rather than trying to constantly hone further and further into one specific idea, we need to digest divergent and seemingly irrelevant data to come up with the most interesting and truly out-of-the-box ideas.

And now a short word of caution. It is pretty easy to take this out-of-the-box approach a little too freely and start moving off into the truly bizarre and untested. But I do not believe most of us need to be worried about that. We are well programmed to stay within the bounds of reason, almost to a fault.

Who is around who you can collaborate with in other disciplines? Another approach to coming up with new ideas is to consider who is in your community and with whom you can cross-pollinate ideas. Whether you are working at a smaller university in an isolated rural area or at a huge institution in a major metropolitan center, there are probably a variety of people with very, very different expertise from yours from which you may be able to draw. In other words, if you are just beginning to study glomerular diseases of the kidneys, don't reach across the aisle to someone studying the renal tubular acidosis. Reach far outside your realm, perhaps out of medicine entirely, if you hope to create really new work. Working with physicists, engineers, mathematicians, medicinal chemists, molecular biologists, and geneticists all may pay higher dividends; the work you will do will be inherently larger in scope and potentially of greater applicability and importance.

When you find these people, try to meet with them in person. Whereas the Internet and Skype to some extent obviate the need for proximity in research efforts, when forging new collaborations to explore truly novel directions, the ability to meet face-to-face over coffee and a white board can make a huge difference. There is no opportunity to be glancing off at your email every few minutes or to get distracted by people coming in and out of your office while you are talking on the phone—the body language and everything else that comes with face-to-face meetings is key. Plus it may be more than just the two of you. Perhaps there will be three or four, all bouncing ideas off one another. And if you do live in different towns or across the country, try to meet up at conferences or even plan a special trip out to the person to get the ball rolling.

The general concept, however, is that looking around your university, neighborhood, city, or region to see who is out there is a powerful way of working backward when it comes to identifying potential resources available to you to help generate new ideas. Is there a strong engineering school nearby? If so, maybe you can identify someone who has some good ideas for devices but really is unsure as to how apply them. Does your medical school have a strong pharmacology department/medicinal chemistry department? If so, maybe there is someone there who has a set of molecules they have been developing for one purpose but that you realize could be useful in your area of interest. Or perhaps there is an outstanding geneticist working in an area unrelated to yours who you think may be able to provide some novel insights into disease mechanisms that you are attempting to unravel.

And don't be afraid to reach out to these people sight unseen by email. They may be just as excited to hear unexpectedly from someone interested in working in a new area as you are in reaching out to them in the first place. I know that when I have been on the receiving end of a new query from somebody interested in working with me, I am always excited and flattered that they had reached out to me, even if we end up not being able to find a common question to pursue.

What resources are available to you, in terms of facilities, patients, etc. Another effective way of working backward is by seeing what resources are available at your institution, be it a university or hospital. In the clinical realm, this could be based on what population of patients are seen there. It is very challenging to start doing clinical research in a clinical area if your institution, for whatever reason, sees very few of those patients. Of course, for very common conditions such as hypertension, diabetes, heart disease, certain cancers, and many infectious conditions, every institution has plenty of patients to go around. But if you are thinking of studying rarer conditions, some medical centers mature into centers of excellence for the disease and patients tend to flock there — whether it is because the institution has received a large philanthropic gift or simply because at some point patients with one condition starting going there preferentially and that pattern has persisted over time.

For example, my institution has an affiliation with Joslin Diabetes Center, a world-renowned center for diabetes care. Not surprisingly, we have many patients with diabetes and diabetic complications, and so a number of years ago it dawned on me that it would be relatively easy to initiate studies in the field of diabetic neuropathy, since I had a huge patient population from which to recruit. I made some overtures to some of the people in that institution and soon we had several collaborations ongoing and we generated some interesting work. This led to two NIH grants (one R21 and one fellowship for my postdoc). A number of potential projects started developing from it, including a closer clinical collaboration. While my research interests eventually drifted into other areas, some of the collaboration that we fostered at the time persists, and I anticipate that other projects may eventually arise.

Other resources besides patient populations could include strong NIH-funded laboratory cores, special philanthropically created institutes, or special laboratory facilities found in few other places (e.g., super-MRI systems, hyperbaric oxygen chambers, cyclotrons, transcranial magnetic stimulation facilities, stem cell facilities, to name just a few). While it may be difficult to simply come up with an idea that utilizes these individual facilities, think about how they could impact your specific area of interest and then work backward from there.

What funding opportunities are out there? A final way of coming up with ideas is by working backward and letting the funding agencies call the shots. The federally funded research programs (via NIH, NSF, CDC, DoD, etc.), and to some extent foundations, not only have a number of standing grant opportunities but also solicit grants in certain areas of interest. These so-called requests for applications or RFAs typically focus on relatively specific questions that are of interest to the funding organizations. Such questions may be something that will then force you to reach outside your area of expertise to find collaborators in different areas to help you spearhead new work. And even if you do not end up applying for a specific RFA, possibly because you simply cannot collect all the preliminary data and other resources necessary to create a strong application, there is no reason you cannot apply at a later date, once you have reached that point. Applying for RFAs have their own sets of issues, namely, that there may be a couple of groups in the world specifically for whom the RFA was generated, and thus competition may be fierce. But still, it can serve as a source of ideas.

Don't give up on an idea prematurely. Once you have generated a promising idea, you'll find that it is pretty easy to talk yourself out of it. Perhaps you have unearthed earlier research that has studied something similar or the same basic premise incompletely. Or perhaps the whole project seems too daunting since it moves too far outside your area of expertise. But those are natural "morning-after" responses after you come up with an idea or new direction that sounds promising. For the first day, you are head over heels in love with your idea and the research question. The following day you feel chagrined about having have come up with it. In truth, most ideas are not fully fleshed out the first time around and everything feels daunting when you are just learning about it or starting new collaborations. The longer you stick with something though, the more you will feel comfortable with the unfamiliar concepts and ideas, which eventually leads to further inventions and ideas. So if a topic seems promising but you have uncertainties—that is natural. Try to stick with it nevertheless.

Summary. Nothing truly important can be achieved by only pursuing the tried and true. And while it is accurate to say that many reviewers when grading grants consider risk-taking research in a somewhat negative light, doing the opposite and simply performing incremental work on an already established idea is even worse. There are many ways of generating ideas, some achieved by working forward (reading widely outside your field, browsing the Internet) and others backward (finding collaborators or resources available to you in your area). Also, keep thinking big the whole time. And, most importantly, don't jettison an idea prematurely just because you discover that someone did something similar 20 years earlier. It may be that the earlier work only just scratched the surface and missed what was beneath: a rich vein of ore that could be successfully mined for decades to come.

Chapter 7
Useful Definitions

A research project versus a sustained research endeavor. One distinction I was introduced to early on in my career was the concept of a research project versus a sustained research endeavor. A research project describes a relatively circumscribed effort that attempts to answer a specific question. Research projects by and large have specific answers that will be identified and a definite timeline and expected outcome that need to be met. They, of course, can vary greatly in size and scope. A research project could include a simple retrospective chart review of patients in a single clinic or a pharmacokinetic study of a new drug in wild-type and diseased mice. Or a research project could be a 70-center trial with 1200 patients testing a new drug at three different doses. But regardless of scope, a specific question is asked with the aim of obtaining a goal-driven set of answers. Once it is over, that may be all there is to it, though inevitably there may be some follow-up studies.

A sustained research endeavor, in contrast, is something quite different. A sustained research endeavor is usually made up of a multitude of smaller research projects, but is driven toward testing of a more general hypothesis than a specific research question. There is an overarching theme underlying the research effort—but not a specific single outcome that will decide whether the research was successful or not. Importantly, such research efforts have to be more than simply descriptive efforts. "Fully describing the nature of idiopathic pulmonary fibrosis (IPF)" while challenging and certainly not a single project, since it could encompass animal disease models, human pathology, and a host of other mechanistic studies, is missing the one essential ingredient: a hypothesis. Instead, "environmental exposures in the pathogenesis of idiopathic pulmonary fibrosis" would represent a true research endeavor. There is an implied underlying hypothesis, namely, that exposure to certain environmental exposures may cause IPF. While the answer could still be potentially yes/no, the impact of toxins on pulmonary health and the mechanisms of these pathogens would likely be extremely complex. And the more you start thinking about the problem, the more other ideas become apparent; for example, is there a risk-dependent level of exposure or a certain time in people's lives when exposure is more likely to induce disease later in life? Perhaps one could even go further and

© Springer Science+Business Media New York 2016
S.B. Rutkove, *Biomedical Research: An Insider's Guide*,
DOI 10.1007/978-1-4939-3655-7_7

identify certain allergic pathogens and the concept that immunization could reduce the likelihood of developing IPF to those at highest risk. Or perhaps, certain mechanisms for reducing the likelihood of IPF can be identified such that drugs could be used to reduce the likelihood of the development of the condition in those most likely to develop the condition. The possibilities are endless. This is what identifies a sustained research endeavor versus a simple research project. A sustained research endeavor can represent a lifetime of work (or perhaps several lifetimes); a research project may take weeks, months, or even years to complete, but it has a well-defined beginning and end.

Throughout much of this book, when I discuss research, I do not make an effort to differentiate between sustained efforts and simple projects, using both terms interchangeably. But you should understand the difference from the outset since one can serve as the basis of entire career, while the other may represent nothing more than a few months of effort that are eventually relegated to the dustbin.

Investigator-initiated research versus industry-initiated research. Another important concept to understand is the basic distinction between "investigator-initiated research" and "industry-sponsored research." Investigator-initiated research refers to work that is entirely driven and developed by an academic investigator. This could be a PhD research scientist, an MD clinician, or perhaps an individual with a different degree, such as a physical therapist or speech/language specialist. Regardless of the specific qualifications of the individual, the work is conceived and spearheaded by a researcher in academia and that individual provides the energy to propel it forward.

This simple concept is in sharp contrast to work driven by a corporation. For example, a pharmaceutical company may want to perform a clinical trial of a drug in human subjects for the first time. Safety and efficacy data in animal models is promising, and after years of time and money, the company wants to test the drug in a specific population of people with a disease. However, the researchers are employed by a company, not a hospital or a clinic, and thus don't have access to such a group of people to study. Accordingly, they have to seek out academic partners with whom to do the work. Moreover, for the study to have scientific integrity, it needs to be controlled and run predominantly by people who are not part of the company. A strongly positive study funded and entirely controlled by a company may be greeted with skepticism or even downright disbelief. Perhaps even more to the point, such a study would likely not even be able to achieve basic institutional review board approval, given the conflicts of the people running it (more on this in later chapters). In contrast, a study that is funded by a large company but is run entirely by a group of relatively disinterested academic investigators will be held in much higher regard. If the study is small, it may be confined to just a single center; if it is very large, it could involve literally dozens of major medical centers around the world, especially if the disease is relatively uncommon and many patients are required. Usually, the company will identify one academic person as the overall principal investigator for the study. This person will be paid salary support for his or her work, but will not gain financially by the success or failure of the trial. The company will still remain very much involved in the study, from start to finish right through to publication, including the messaging that they want to promulgate when it has concluded, since the company's success or failure may depend on it. But the data integrity itself will be outside of their control.

Are you happy being in the infantry or would you rather be a general? Another broad idea to try to wrap your head around is whether you would rather be in the infantry or be a general. This military analogy, while useful, has some problems, even though it is used frequently. First, research is obviously not war, and being in the infantry does not mean you are going to have a much higher risk of suffering a nasty injury than your commander safely back at headquarters. Nor does it necessarily imply a hierarchy of power/rank—in the world of research, participating in clinical trials on the "front lines" is just as important and can be just as fulfilling as being behind the scenes designing them. However, the analogy is useful in that it highlights the fact that some individuals who want to do research would rather just have very specific, directed guidance, whereas others would rather be in the position of making up the rules themselves and figuring out tactics and strategies. And ultimately, if a study is successful, it will be the general, not the infantry, who will be able to take most of the credit. Though, alternatively, if a study fails, the general will also have to take the blame for it not working. Fortunately, however, unlike war, if you end up "losing" and having a negative study, there is no irreparable harm done to your career.

The analogy also falls apart in another basic way. Many investigators are not just a general or just an infantryman. Rather, they end up being infantry in some studies and generals in others. For example, if you are participating in a multicenter clinical trial being overseen by a colleague at another institution and being sponsored by a drug company, you will be serving as infantry in your capacity in that study. But perhaps you are similarly running an NIH-funded study of a drug in a related but different disease. Your colleague at the other institution is serving as your infantry and you are serving as the general. In short, there is no need for you to be one or the other. You can be both simultaneously in different studies. For example, as I write this section, I am a principal investigator in several studies of my design and a coinvestigator on others, where I am just helping to recruit patients and study animals.

It is important to recognize, however, that many researchers may not really want to ever do anything beyond, say, participating in trials. Why would this be of interest? Well, first, it offers the opportunity to participate in interesting work that is out of the ordinary and to help with a bigger effort that could potentially be important. You will end up with your name on a paper and this may ultimately help in your promotion at your institution. Moreover, it may actually help support your salary (funds brought in through a research contract may partially fund your salary/time). So while being solely infantry in a large study is not going to win you great glory, it can be fun, monetarily worthwhile, and ultimately important to moving the therapy for a disease forward. Without infantry, there could be no large-scale research. And by staying infantry, you will never have to deal with the substantial headaches of such things as obtaining an investigational new drug approval from the FDA. You will not be expected to write grants or run and organize endless conference calls or site visits or investigator meetings. There will be other annoyances to be sure—contracts and IRBs, for example—but they will be local issues to your institution and dealt with more easily.

I've been using as an example a physician participating in a multicenter clinical trial as someone in the infantry. However, this is only one example. If you are a PhD researcher and you are just not interested in pursuing endless grant applications and the uncertainties of funding, then there are "lab manger" positions that are potentially open to you, where you may be able to continue to pursue work and publish papers, but not feel constantly under the gun. You can also consider working in industry where there are also valuable opportunities. In many industry jobs, you actually can be very much an independent researcher although perhaps being subtly directed into certain areas (you could consider this being a "colonel" or "brigadier general"). You can also be a physician researcher helping out other investigators — perhaps taking part in a study in which your skill set is needed. One example would be a radiologist reading images in a new surgical or medical treatment study. In short, there are many, many ways to participate in research without having to be fully responsible from soup to nuts.

In summary, it is important to take stock of your own values and interests to make sure that whatever you do is consonant with your personality and interests. Of course, you are not committing to something unchangeable here. You can always go in one direction and later in life go in another. You can move from being a general to a soldier or a soldier to a general, and though the latter shift takes more work and sheer grit, it can be done.

10,000 hours. A final valuable concept to remember is that researchers are not born researchers — they develop. In Malcolm Gladwell's book *Outliers*, examples are provided of people who are very successful in their fields. What he shows is that most people who are really successful don't have special gifts or abilities. Although they are talented and capable in some fashion, a major component of their success is they have spent a remarkable amount of time and effort "priming the pump" as it were. They work and work and work — often for years, honing their skills and abilities, with little attention or recognition. Examples that Gladwell gives include the Beatles and Bill Gates. The Beatles performed in nightclubs in Hamburg, West Germany, at a furious pace from 1960 to 1962, achieving something approaching 10,000 hours of "practice." Bill Gates garnered hundreds of hours experience programming at the private high school he attended in the suburbs of Seattle. All of this repetition meant that both Gates and the Beatles obtained huge amounts of practice, allowing them to be highly skilled at the art even though they appeared on the world stage virtually out of nowhere. In fact, they had been incubating their skill sets for years before going public.

And the same holds true for scientific endeavors, but unlike the Beatles in Hamburg or Gates in a Seattle high school, your years of practice usually only come when you are already setting out on your own path. This is not something you can get from a book (yes, even this one). It takes an immense amount of practice to develop the instincts to help you write really strong grants and research papers, know which lines of research are likely to be the most promising and which are best to jettison as they are unlikely to yield anything valuable. The same holds true for becoming a good interviewer to find the people you need to hire or how to work with grants officers at funding institutions and foundations. And the same can be said about working with institutional review boards or animal care and use committees to make sure that you are staying on top of issues and preventing things from going wrong. These are skill sets that only develop gradually over many years of experience. And even then, despite considerable practice and effort, even seasoned researchers mess up occasionally — it is inevitable. It is all simply too complex to do everything "right" all the time.

If you do the simple math, 10,000 hours at 40 hours per week at say 50 weeks a year = 5 years, of doing no work outside of research-oriented work. I think it is more likely to equate to 10 years when all is said done, simply because we are drawn in so many other directions. That is not an insubstantial investment of time. Ultimately those 10,000 hours will be accumulated through a variety of means: during your period of training with a mentor, during your first few years of independence, and your next few years of "mature" independence. I personally would say that it took me close to 15 years from the completion of my training to feel reasonably competent at research. But that is absolutely not to say that I am still not learning all the time.

But at some point, you will actually realize that you do actually know what is going on. I think that usually happens when people abruptly start turning to *you* for advice and you are increasingly unsure anyone can give you worthwhile advice anymore.

Summary. In this chapter, I have attempted to provide a broad overview of some basic concepts that are worth considering as you are thinking about embarking on a career in biomedical research. If there is anything I hope I have emphasized, it is that while the path is long and slow, there are many different and exciting paths from which to choose. One of the nicest things is that you don't have to stick to one plan throughout; as the world changes, science evolves, your home morphs, and your own work matures, you may find yourself drawn into a different direction from where you began. And that is absolutely fine. Those 10,000 hours you spent during your earlier years will continue to serve you well, whether you have moved into industry, have decided to at last become a general, or help others as they start off on their own careers.

Part II
Research Structures and Foundations

Chapter 8
The Institutional Review Board: Do's, Don'ts, and Nevers

To the uninitiated, the institutional review board, or IRB, can seem like a fearsome entity. In fact, with just a simple action, they can entirely close down a multimillion dollar, multisite research study. They can suspend the ability of an investigator to do any kind of human-related research for months or years. And somewhat less drastically, they can put you through a surprise, detailed audit. Simply put, the IRB can make your life very difficult. But the purpose of this chapter is to try to show that, in fact, IRBs are in general very reasonable. And what they do is actually good and necessary. Plus my main purpose in discussing IRBs is not to make you worry, but rather to provide some practical advice for working most effectively with them.

IRB history. The modern IRB really was spawned directly from the atrocities committed by the Nazis during World War II. In attempting to classify the horrific experimentation performed on human subjects in concentration camps, the Nuremburg Code was developed. The main component of the Code was the concept of voluntary consent as the cornerstone of all ethical experimentation, including the fact that the consent is given entirely without coercion, that the person giving it has the actual capacity to consent, and that there is a full understanding of the risks and benefits of the work. There is also an effort to minimize risk and to maximize the risk-to-benefit ratio and the capability of the volunteer to withdraw consent at any point. These initial concepts were then further developed by the World Medical Association's Declaration of Helsinki in 1964. Although the National Institutes of Health in the United States were already applying these rules by the late 1960s, it was not until 1974 that they were finally written into law in the National Research Act, which established the National Commission for the Protection of Human Subjects of Biomedical and Behavioral Research. Then, in 1978, the National Commission for the Protection of Human Subjects of Biomedical and Behavioral Research submitted its report entitled "The Belmont Report: Ethical Principles and Guidelines for the Protection of Human Subjects of Research." The Report, named for the Belmont Conference Center at the Smithsonian Institution, the initial venue for the discussions held by the committee, created the basic ethical principles underlying the acceptable conduct of research involving human subjects. These principles

© Springer Science+Business Media New York 2016
S.B. Rutkove, *Biomedical Research: An Insider's Guide,*
DOI 10.1007/978-1-4939-3655-7_8

included respect for persons, protecting subjects from harm and maximizing anticipated benefits, and ensuring that the benefits and burdens of research be distributed fairly. (NB There are a variety of excellent web pages that explain these ideas in great detail.)

Many additional revisions have been made to these basic concepts and laws over the years. But one of the biggest occurred in 1996 when the Health Improvement Protection and Portability Act (HIPAA) became law, although it did not start to become phased in until 2000. This complex set of laws instituted another layer of complexity/mission for IRBs, in that in addition to monitoring all research activities, they now were also charged with the duty of insuring the privacy of data from all research subjects.

Where do IRBs come from and who sits on them? Many researchers typically associate the IRB with a hospital and think of it as part of the hospital, and while it is true that most hospitals have their own IRBs, they really are functionally independent of the institution. While the physicians, nurses, statisticians, and others who make up the members of the IRB may be paid salary by the institution, the IRB must be an independent entity since it has the responsibility of ensuring that the hospital itself is fully protecting people participating in research. In addition to hospital personnel, the IRB also includes individuals outside of the hospital itself, including lay members of the community and clergy. An IRB must have a minimum of five individuals, including one scientist, one lay individual, and one person from outside the institution, but in practice, most IRBs have considerably more such that all areas of medical research are reasonably covered as protocols are reviewed. The IRB seeks experts who not only can judge that the proposed work will be performed safely but also that the work being proposed is worthwhile and the risk-to-benefit ratio is low enough as to ensure the research is really worth pursuing.

Another concept that people don't often appreciate is that there are also commercial IRBs. Weird as this may seem, human subject research can be performed in a variety of contexts. In fact, sometimes companies find themselves needing to test a new product or device on a group of people. In order to ensure that they are meeting the highest ethical codes, and especially if they are seeking FDA approval, it is critical that these studies are done with IRB approval. Like hospital- or academic center-based IRBs, these have similar structures, but rather than being supported by hospital, these are paid for by the companies who are requiring their services. However, for research being performed at a single hospital, the IRB involved is usually (though probably not universally) the hospital's own IRB.

More recently, however, the concept of a "central IRB" has been created to help simplify the enrollment in a complex multi-institutional study. In fact, NIH/NINDS has recently developed this concept as part of their NeuroNEXT initiative. A single central IRB approves a study to be performed at 25 different medical centers across the United States. Unfortunately, this wonderful concept is not without its own challenges—as each institution has to have a separate agreement (a so-called reliance agreement) to ensure the legitimacy of the central IRB for all studies. However, once such an agreement is in place, all research can be performed using the central IRB mechanism. Hopefully, such efforts will take on wider use over the coming years as it offers the promise of shortening approval times and speeding research, not to mention greatly reducing the number of person-hours spent reviewing and revising protocols.

The IRBs: unstated realities. First, it is safe to say that the nature and structure and responsibilities of the IRB are forever changing. Don't be misled into thinking that things are static. They aren't, nor have they ever been. What you read here today may be different within a few years. One study that is approved by the same committee today will not be allowed next year. Regulations only seem to get more complex and the rules more challenging to understand every year. I suppose one way of thinking about this is that it has only been 40 years since IRBs were even introduced, and it is natural that a certain maturation and evolution of the process will occur for years to come and that at some point, IRBs will reach a relatively steady state without additional modifications. It's possible that point has already arrived, but I doubt it. At my institution, back when I started pursuing clinical research in the mid-1990s, there were about seven or eight different short subsections to the applications, going through letter I in the alphabet (each section having its own letter). Today, there are 19 sections extending through letter S.

The unfortunate aspect of this, in my view, is that legal/compliance necessities have taken reign over common sense. For example, current day informed consent forms, for even the most simple of studies, are a dozen-page long. (I was recently cleaning out my old files and came across an IRB-approved consent form from 1995. It was just two-pages long.) While theoretically written for people with no greater than a sixth-grade education, they require monumental stamina to get through. Virtually no subject participating in a trial will read one cover to cover nor will he likely fully understand the implications, unless he is a lawyer (and I will say that I've had a few lawyers as research participants and even they find these things inscrutable). From a legal and ethical perspective, strictly speaking, everything is being covered, but it is not clear how much the participants are really digesting. I do hope that over the coming decades, we will see efforts made to simplify the informed consent forms such that the legal mumbo jumbo can be reduced to the fine print and the essence of the study captured in a short, clear explanation of risks, benefits, and what the subject should actually expect to experience as part of the study.

All IRBs are not the same. One of the strangest aspects of IRBs is their variability. This variability is the most obvious when you are putting together a multi-institutional study that is being reviewed by several IRBs. One IRB may be very critical about one aspect of a study and another remarkably loose about it but concerned about another point that the first IRB did not have an issue with. Some will request minor changes. Others will demand multiple changes. And still others will become focused on one point that will seem to doom the study until it is clearly explained by the investigator directly to the IRB. For example, one area in which I have observed remarkable inconsistency and frank misunderstanding is with experimental medical devices, my specific area of research. The rules are complex, but one thing is clear: you do not have to have an investigational device exemption from the Food and Drug Administration (a type of approval from the FDA that you can do research with an experimental device) unless the device is deemed as "significant" risk by the IRB itself. So if you have a very safe device (e.g., a new pulse monitor) and you want to include it in a research study, you don't need to go to the FDA to first get approval to include it in a study. But some IRBs do not understand this fine point, especially since it doesn't arise that often.

The IRB application. To make matters still worse, there is no universal standard IRB application. Every IRB has it own set of forms. But you will quickly get used to the nuisances of those at your institution (though the forms are forever being revised). It may seem daunting at first, but most of the questions are fairly straight-forward and most IRBs have personnel to help you and answer those questions that are more challenging. The good news is that if your study entails only minimal risk, you may be able to be able to submit your IRB as "expedited" which requires fewer details.

There are also exemptions to research that are worth pursuing, but you should do this through your institution. You pretty much should not be doing research at your institution without some form of IRB approval ... even if you think it is exempt, you should first get an official exemption from your IRB before proceeding.

After you submit your application, you will likely also need to present to the entire IRB. This is usually a bit of a formality, but it can be daunting since you may find yourself attempting to explain a complex study to a couple dozen people. And they may ask you unexpected questions that you will find yourself unable to answer in any coherent way. Scary as these events may be, they are generally nothing to be excessively concerned about—they are just part of the process. And if you have trouble answering some questions, there will be plenty of opportunities to provide clarification and additional answers down the road.

Multi-institutional studies. Multi-institutional studies are complicated and require considerable effort and data coordination, and I would strongly advise any would-be clinical researcher to first submit a single-institution IRB before consider-ing running a multisite study. Most multi-institutional studies with which I have been involved have used a data-coordinating center with several full-time employ-ees to help run the show. The principal investigators and coinvestigators all become secondary players, with the data-coordinating team really taking the lead. Of course, if you are reading this book, you are probably not running these kinds of studies—at least not yet. I have run one multisite study on a shoestring budget. It was doable, but it was really only through the kindness and generosity of my colleagues at insti-tutions from Boston to Miami that made it possible. And the data monitoring was really not what it should have been. The bottom line is that if you are going to pur-sue a multisite study (say with more than three sites collecting data), be prepared for a Herculean effort for which you will need proper funding if you hope to do it right.

Protocol violations and deviations. Almost inevitably in every study, you will have protocol violations or deviations. These are nuisances—they may require some additional paperwork—but they are easily manageable. I've had numerous small ones—inadvertently consenting someone with an expired consent form, inadver-tently recruiting a person a second time for a study when they were only supposed to have a single visit (they never told us they had already participated a couple of years earlier), or inadvertently leaving out a test the person was supposed to have.

The purpose of reporting deviations and violations is to make sure you are doing things appropriately and are playing by the rules. Unless you or one of your staff has done something truly grievous, such deviations and violations are pretty much a matter of course and should be dealt with expeditiously as soon as they are identified.

Audits. As a researcher involved in clinical research, one of the most frightening events you may find yourself facing is an audit. And audit means that designated individuals from the IRB will descend upon your research area and start reviewing all of your documents—study records, both paper and computer—to determine whether you have been fully compliant with the protocols that you have created and with IRB, state, and federal mandates and policies. The goal is to find errors and correct them and if necessary to take any actions necessary to ensure that future errors do not happen. And remember, the IRB is not doing this just because they want to "get you" or "entrap" you; they are mandated to ensure the work they are doing is up to federal guidelines, since the IRBs themselves are monitored. Accordingly, don't shoot the messenger. They are doing what they are mandated to do: provide oversight to clinical research activities at an institution. And an audit is a regular part of that process.

There are two types of IRB audits: for-cause (also called directed) and not-for-cause (also called periodic or routine). The latter types of audits are simply a means for ensuring that the research being completed is up to high standards and that research subjects are not being put at additional risk for any reason and are being consented in a fair and noncoercive manner. Someone from the IRB will visit your lab and go through all your records in great detail, a process that can take several weeks to complete. He will also ask for access to all of your computer records and any online databases for their review, attempting to determine if there are any inconsistencies in the number of people consented, who consented, which of the staff did the procedures, and where were any adverse events or other problems noted. And if any patients did drop out from the study, they will want to understand why that happened and whether it was well documented. Not-for-cause audits are not meant to be punitive or harsh; they are simply checking to see if you are doing an honest job. If you are, and there are a few mistakes here and there, you will be asked to correct them, usually with protocol deviation forms and several amendments, and it will be over. It will also be educational for you and your team. But if there are some bigger issues, especially any that are perceived to increase patient risk, or procedures being performed that are not clearly stated in the protocol, that can become a problem too and you could find yourself now in a second directed audit.

For-cause or directed audits are initiated when an issue is brought to the IRB's attention by a patient, family member, caregiver, a member of the research team, another whistle-blower, or, rarely, the PI himself. Or perhaps they are initiated by a not-for-cause audit that raised a number of red flags. These audits are another matter entirely. The initiation of such an audit could mean that the study is put on immediate suspension and all other research protocols under the PI guidance may be similarly audited and possibly suspended until the audit is complete. This is especially true if there is an indication that the study violations are putting subjects at increased risk, that procedures are being performed that were not approved, individuals are being enrolled without undergoing proper consent, or if people are being enrolled who do not meet proper inclusion-exclusion criteria. It is important to remember that just because someone complains and a for-cause audit is initiated, it does not necessarily mean you have done anything wrong. However, IRB's main interest is in protecting the rights of the human subjects who are enrolled in studies, and so to some extent, you as PI will be considered guilty until proven innocent.

Fortunately, if you do follow the rules, are careful about managing your research team and are not simply an absentee landlord in ongoing studies, and have been honest all along about any study deviations or violations that have occurred, you will probably never be subjected to one of these audits, and even if you are, you will pass without any major trauma.

Other Useful Tidbits About Working with IRBs and Preparing IRB Applications

1. **Don't sacrifice your integrity**. At many points in this book, I will repeat the same advice: Don't lie, don't obfuscate, and don't deceive. If you have made an honest study violation, simply report it, try to ensure it does not happen again, and move on. If there has been a bigger systematic problem with your study—say you have inadvertently done something that was not part of the protocol—then it is better that you come clean and make the corrections as soon as you discover it. On the other hand, I would say that this can be taken to an extreme extent, so don't start creating problems when there really aren't any. If you are unsure of whether you should be concerned about something going on in the study but are hesitant to bring it up to the IRB, talk to a few colleagues who will have a clearer big picture view than you. And after all that, you are still unsure, it is better to bring the IRB up to speed than trying to sweep dirt under the rug.

2. **Don't straightjacket yourself with an overly detailed protocol description**. Oh, I so wish someone had told me this idea when I first started doing research! If you are creating a research study on your own, you will need to list a group of procedures that you will be doing. While you do need to list them, the more detail you give, the more you are making it necessary for you to submit amendments for every little change you make going forward. Here is an example of what I am saying. If you were to write a protocol that said the following "After changing into a gown, we will perform the following tasks in this order: (1) measurement of pulse at the right wrist, (2) measurement of blood pressure at the right arm, (3) body weight using a standing scale, and (4) oral temperature with a digital thermometer." But what if the person is missing a right arm? What if the oral thermometer is broken and you need to measure ear temperature? And what if you accidentally did the weight first on the way from the waiting room into the office? Strictly speaking, all of these would require you to complete deviation and violation forms. So, a much

better would say "The following measurements will be obtained: pulse, blood pressure, body weight, and temperature." Now you are free to measure these in any way, in any order, and with any device. This is a very simple example, but you probably get the idea: keep it simple, keep it flexible, and don't give unnecessary details when you don't have to.

3. **Be kind to your subjects and make sure they get reimbursed for their participation quickly**. Happy participants will not complain. Unhappy ones can complain to the IRB about your or your team's behavior. You don't want your IRB chairperson calling you because you insulted a patient or your staff was not sufficiently polite. And, if they are going to be reimbursed for their time and travel, just make sure it is done promptly. Fortunately, if there are complaints, such as slow payment, they usually complain to my team rather than the IRB and we are able to address the problem in short order.

4. **Stay on good terms with the IRB members and their office staff**. I wouldn't say go out of the way to befriend them, but knowing the people who will be reviewing your application does make life a little easier—they will at least be polite to you when you present to all of them. If there are concerns down the road, they will try to deal with things one-on-one before getting excessively bureaucratic. Familiarity never hurts. And obviously, try to avoid antagonizing the IRB members or office staff. That will serve nobody well.

Summary. It is easy to get frustrated with IRBs. Sometimes their decisions seem to be made out of ignorance or are just entirely arbitrary. But they are charged with a very challenging task and the legal rules put them in a complex position. They need to make sure everything is being done appropriately, often with limited resources and personnel. The last thing anyone wants is the Department of Health and Human Services shutting down all research at your institution. And that is a real possibility if things go really wrong. The IRB tries to do the right thing. If and when you come into conflict with them for any reason, just remember that your job should be to help them come to a satisfactory conclusion as soon as possible and to be as least obstructionist as possible. It will make everything easier for you in the long run.

Chapter 9
Animal Care and Use Committees

Beyond the obvious distinction that Institutional Animal Care and Use Committees (IACUCs) deal with animal ethical concerns and institutional review boards deal with human ethical issues, there are some other major important differences as well. IRBs generally are focused on protocol approval and for the most part rely on the investigators to self-report all serious adverse events, protocol violations, and deviations. While there are IRB audits, as noted above, these are performed only intermittently and not in a predetermined fashion. In the world of animal research, however, the committee and the animal research facility staff will be keeping an eye on your activities to ensure that you are doing what you said you would do in the protocol, i.e., not cheating. This means that your lab and research will be policed; this includes semiannual unannounced inspections as well as intermittent announced inspections. Moreover, the animals that that are being housed in the animal facility will be inspected and you will be notified if there are problems that need to be addressed. So while I think there is the general sense that dealing with IRBs is "tougher" since they are overseeing human research, IACUCs can be more challenging in some sense because they are monitoring your animals and procedures on a regular basis and bringing up issues that could go unrecognized by an IRB since they do not routinely have any form of surveillance. From my own experience, it has been more frequent for me to have a delightful Caribbean vacation unexpectedly interrupted with a concerned email from IACUC than from the IRB (this is why one should not check one's email when on vacation, by the way).

Although I think many researchers do not pursue both animal and human research as I do, it is interesting to compare the two types—which I do in the following table (Table 9.1). One of other huge differences between IRBs and IACUCs is that IACUCs don't care about the animal tissues once the animal is sacrificed. Their only concern is with the humane and proper treatment of live animals. IRBs, however, also have to ensure that all material obtained from human subjects is dealt with appropriately during the study and after, even if the patient has passed away.

© Springer Science+Business Media New York 2016
S.B. Rutkove, *Biomedical Research: An Insider's Guide*,
DOI 10.1007/978-1-4939-3655-7_9

Table 9.1 Comparison between IRBs and IACUCs

IRBs	IACUCs
Deal with humans	Deal with animals
Minimal ongoing monitoring	Ongoing monitoring
Yearly protocol renewal necessary	Yearly protocol renewal necessary
Protocols are not time limited—you can renew a protocol indefinitely	Protocols are time limited to 3 years; an entirely new application must be submitted at that time if you wish to continue your research
Have the power to suspend all research	Have the power to suspend all research
Are run independently from the institution	Are run independently from the institution
Report to HHS/FDA	Report to NIH Office of Laboratory Animal Welfare (OLAW)
No specific literature search requirement needed for application (though you will have to supply scientific rationale)	Applications require documented literature search showing that the work has not been performed previously
Responsible for tissue/products obtained from human subjects, alive or deceased	Only concern is for proper care of live animals; after death, not in their jurisdiction
Amendments submitted only occasionally since the basic goals and procedures of a study are relatively stable	Frequent submission of amendments since most animal research is fairly flexible, with constantly changing goals

History of Animal Use in Research and the Development of Oversight Committees Perhaps one of the oddest facts in the history of biomedical research is that codified law covering the misuse of animals for research purposes predates the laws over misuse of human beings by more than a century. Indeed, the first such law was passed in England in 1822 followed by the more comprehensive Cruelty to Animals Act in 1876, the latter specifically attempting to regulate animal experimentation. In America, the American Society for the Prevention of Cruelty to Animals was founded in the 1860s, as well as the American Anti-Vivisection Society founded in 1883. However, unlike England, these sentiments were not codified into law for more than 80 years. And don't forget that in human research, these issues really did not start coming to the fore until after World War II and not in a truly comprehensive way not until the 1970s.

In the United States, prior to the 1960s, many institutions had their own animal use oversight committees, but there was a great deal of inconsistency between policies. In 1961, a group of investigators joined forces and created the Animal Care Panel and in 1963 published *The Guide for the Care and Use of Laboratory Animals*. The panel then created an oversight committee that is today known as the Association for the Assessment and Accreditation of Laboratory Animal Care International (AAALAC). The federal government came into the act a few years later after a series of disturbing articles were published in *Life* magazine about the mistreatment of animal laboratory animals, and in 1966, the Animal Welfare Act became law, in which the US Department of Agriculture took over broad responsibility for this effort. In 1971, the Animal Welfare Act was further revised to include certification of hospitals that abided by AAALAC rules or had an independent oversight committee at the institution. In 1979, the Public Health Service via the National Institutes of Health took over the responsibility and established the need for an independent committee at each institution, generalizing their jurisdiction to all vertebrate animals, with the term IACUC introduced in additional legislation in 1986. The IACUC was to be constructed of a minimum of four individuals including a veterinarian, a practicing scientist experienced in animal research, an individual with no scientific interest in animal use, and a final individual with no connection to the institution outside of their role on the committee. The IACUC itself reports to the Office of Laboratory Animal Welfare (OLAW) at NIH. The IACUC and institution are thus responsible directly for their oversight activities of individual investigator laboratories as well as for the maintenance and care of animals within their facilities.

What the IACUC Does The main purpose of an IACUC is to ensure that you are performing experiments that are necessary, that you are not utilizing unnecessary numbers of animals, that there is no less-sentient species available for use, and that any animal suffering is minimized or eliminated. You will see that absent from this list is ensuring that the laboratory animals are otherwise allowed to live out their lives to old age. In fact, the IACUC and animal facilities do not prevent or discourage the euthanization of animals (also described as "sacrifice"); however, they want to keep animal usage limited to only the number of animals necessary to answer a scientific question. But if an experiment is not working and you want to end it early, there is no penalty for stopping and simply euthanizing all the animals approved for the protocol. This concept is especially obvious when looking at breeding animals for a specific strain. For example, if you were breeding up animals with a recessive mutation, you may want to keep only 25 % (or perhaps 50 % if you need controls) and euthanize the rest.

Completing an Animal Protocol Animal protocols, like human subject protocols, can at first seem daunting when you set out to complete one. But in fact, they are broken down into straightforward sections that are not all that challenging to deal with one at a time. You will need to start by clarifying the training of the individuals involved and then an overview of the scientific necessity of the work, followed by a detailed description of the experimental plan, justifying the number of animals (this justification is usually not as intense or as closely questioned as that for an IRB, since it is often difficult to predict the exact number of animals you may need when starting a study), methods for prevention and relief of suffering, plans for euthanasia, and a detailed description of all substances utilized in the study. An important part of every protocol involving anything beyond the most limited of procedures is to do a literature search and documenting that the search indicates that there is no other approach for doing the studies, i.e., one that does not involve the use of animals (e.g., computer modeling) or the application of cell culture or a less-sentient species (e.g., invertebrate versus vertebrate).

After your protocol is approved, you will need to submit amendments for any minor alteration in the study. These are usually quick and simple to do, unless you are planning on a new complicated procedure, increasing the number of requested animals beyond 20 % of the initially approved amount, or introducing a new species to study.

Larger Animals and Nonhuman Primate Research I am not going to get into a detailed discussion here about dealing with nonhuman primates or large animals. These are special circumstances that most early-stage investigators would only be involved in only if they were part of a much larger research effort. Usually, you will have a very supportive complex structure around these kinds of studies to ensure that you are fully trained. My only comment on this front is that when you start to move to larger animals, additional certifications are necessary. In addition, the precautions involved in nonhuman primate work are immense given the potential for diseases to spread from such animals to humans and vice versa and ethically complex and delicate nature of the work. Fortunately, greater than 90 % of all animal work performed in the United States is completed using standard small animal laboratory species, namely, mice and rats.

Practical Suggestions for Working with Your Animal Facility and IACUC

Like IRBs, you know things are going perfectly fine when the IACUC is silently in the background, and the only time you find yourself dealing with them is when you are submitting a protocol or an amendment. But unlike the IRB, since they are obligated to perform unannounced biannual inspections of the lab, you may get an unexpected email that something was found amiss in your lab or that a group of animals in the facility appear to be in poor health and could be suffering. They want to ensure that you are doing procedures correctly and that none of your compounds are expired or your experimental procedures have gone off in a new, unapproved direction. So keeping these things in order and ensuring that you are constantly submitting amendments will help avoid any problems on that front. Indeed, unlike human protocols, in animal work you may easily find yourself submitting amendments quite frequently to alter standard procedures or adding new drugs. Animal work generally changes a lot more rapidly than human studies.

If you do receive a warning or reprimand, which usually occurs because something is found amiss in your animal care, first remember that they are under obligation to keep an eye on your work and the IACUC and animal facilities themselves are being audited and have to report to the AALAC and OLAW; they need to ensure that your infraction does not endanger the wider scope of research at the institution and bring the entire IACUC and animal facility under investigation. You would not be too happy if you found out that your entire research program was abruptly suspended not because of anything you did but because of a major transgression by another investigator that the IACUC had turned a blind eye to. So generally, when something is found amiss in the lab, which will always happen, quickly respond and correct the problem and document in writing that it has been corrected, and if necessary, also describe any steps that you can take to ensure that it does not happen again.

Another good idea is to always speak with your veterinarian ahead of time regarding questions about a new protocol or animal species that you are going to study. This person is hired by the institution to help oversee animal care and she is usually more than happy to help guide you in your efforts and provide advice as you prepare a protocol for submission or consider a new set of experiments. Talking things through ahead of time can save you a lot of time and effort going back and forth on protocol amendments that may end up being unacceptable for one reason or another.

Also, from practical experience, it is a good idea to review your protocol every so often to ensure that it is actually reflecting what you are doing. Procedures sometimes morph gradually over time, and before you know it, you may be doing something slightly different than you had included in your protocol; if that is the case, submit an amendment and make sure you have it covered. There is no amendment that is too small. But, as with IRB submissions, if you word your initial submission carefully and find a happy medium between excessive specificity and excessive vagueness, you can stay true to the letter of the document but still give yourself, your research staff, and your experiments at least a little flexibility.

Conducting Outstanding Animal Work

OK. Enough about rules and logistics of working with the IACUC and animal facility. What about actually doing top-notch animal research? Well, summarizing how to go about this in a few paragraphs is not easy, in part because animal research can take so many different forms and many of the issues relate to scientific research in general. But there are a couple of specific issues that have really risen to the surface over the past few years. One of these is the need for blinding and using sufficient numbers of animals.

Blinding. Blinding refers to the process of ensuring the researchers performing the experiments are unaware as to which group an animal is in or what treatment an animal is receiving—and thus helping keep the measurements and other outcomes completely unbiased. Unlike human clinical drug research, which usually demands such blinding, many animal researchers are unused to putting in place the same rigorous safeguards. Blinding must be done carefully and almost always involves the use of two researchers to ensure that it is done correctly. The challenge with blinding in animal research is that it can slow things down dramatically, since you may not know when to end an experiment. However, like clinical studies, monitoring of the data by the unblinded person can ensure that a study can be ended appropriately. Also, blinding is not necessarily always valuable. Very early on in a study, it may make sense to perform tests in an unblinded fashion, and then only when you are really understand what you are trying to do, repeat the study fully blinded.

Animal numbers. Another tendency is to use tiny numbers of animals in studies, for example, five or six animals in a given cohort. Again for preliminary work, such numbers may be entirely reasonable both to help nail down your procedures and also to assist in demonstrating the effect or answer you are looking for. Moreover, you may not really know how many animals you will need ultimately to prove your point statistically (i.e., to perform an adequate power analysis). However, once you have performed your initial set of experiments and have that data, it may make sense to now repeat the study in a blinded fashion with a larger number of animals to fully prove your point. Of course, all this depends on the type of research you are doing. If you are working on performing neuroanatomical studies, for example, you may only need to demonstrate a pathway in just a handful of animals.

One argument that can be made against performing studies with a larger number of animals is "if it is significant in five or six animals, it will only be more significant in 15 or 20 animals, so why bother?" Well first, replicating an experiment is always a good idea—just because it works the first time does not mean it will work the second time. Second, there is the issue of performing many experiments with small numbers of animals. Consider for a moment that you are performing 100 independent studies in your lab with just six animals (e.g., three per group). Statistically speaking, using a p of <0.05, and applying that value separately to each of the studies, 5 of those studies will be positive—i.e., will end up with a $p < 0.05$ (i.e., type 1 error). Since those studies were positive, you would be tempted to report those studies, whereas the 95 negative studies would not be. Yet, those studies do not prove anything, since probability demands that a certain percentage will show a significant difference. Given the tendency to report any positive results, there is a frequent flaw in overreporting false findings with small numbers, the results of which cannot be replicated.

A flip side issue with using small numbers of animals is underpowering studies. Just as you may overcall a treatment effect by performing many studies with small numbers of animals (type 1 error), using few animals may lead to your missing subtler, but still important treatment or other effects (type 2 error). Of course, utilizing 500 animals per group to discover a difference of 5% in drug efficacy is probably not going to be too exciting (such a small effect may be hardly interesting or important), so a larger sample size should be chosen keeping the relative value of the difference in mind.

Ongoing oversight within your lab. As a junior investigator, you will usually find yourself doing much of the hands-on work yourself. Gradually over time, you will begin to find yourself delegating more and more until the point where, you will be overseeing a small cadre of research assistants, graduate students, and postdocs who are doing the work. Of course, your funding will undoubtedly vary over time and at some points you may find yourself with a larger lab and other points with a smaller one. But regardless, you will have a constantly shifting group of assistants. It is always good to stay in contact with what is going on, through weekly or more frequent meetings and dropping in unexpectedly to see what is happening. And ensuring that when there are transitions—old employees leaving and new ones beginning—you are able to transfer as much knowledge as possible from one to the other before the old one departs. Reading protocols and emulating them are not always simple, as anyone who has tried to assemble a gas grill or a piece of Ikea furniture well knows. There is the concept of "tacit knowledge"—i.e., that knowledge that is generally very difficult to verbalize in a written protocol—for example, how to position an animal during a procedure or how long to mix a group of reagents. That information often ends up getting passed down from assistant to assistant verbally and visually, much like storytelling in ancient times. And those minor changes can often make the difference between successful experiment replication and unsuccessful replication, even in your own lab.

Summary. Performing animal research requires a considerably different mindset than human clinical research. The functioning of the IACUC is very different than that of the IRB and you will find yourself more regularly observed, which can be unnerving. But by adhering to the rules, talking with your institution's veterinarian and animal research facility people when you have questions ahead of time, most problems can be avoided. It can also save you a huge amount of wasted effort. Once you have approval for a protocol, animal experiments are often fast to perform and data can come in quickly; there is a tendency to overemphasize the positive and ignore the negative, which leads to an overreporting of positive results. While this makes for plenty of papers and perhaps faster promotion, you have to always be careful about performing top-notch science and repeating experiments to determine whether your initial findings hold true. And don't let your lab ever start running autonomously—keeping a vigilant eye on things and doing unexpected audits on your own can help ensure that quality of your science never starts to falter.

Chapter 10
Research Beyond Humans and Vertebrates

Many of my research efforts have focussed on developing new approaches for evaluating muscle and nerve disorders, and accordingly, most of the work has involved human subjects and animals (mostly mice and rats). However, a number of years ago, we began to seek out "analogues" or model media that would potentially substitute for performing measurements in people or animals. The goal here had not been to avoid doing human or animal-based research, but rather to attempt to answer some questions about how our methods worked—questions that were difficult to answer using live humans or animals *in vivo*. We played around with all sorts of materials—even, weirdly, balsa wood soaked in saline—but eventually decided to try something more obvious and far more relevant: steak. Or more specifically flank steak, since this cut of meat from a cow abdomen has relatively uniform thickness, is very flat, has relatively little fibrous tissue or other inclusions, and, perhaps most importantly, also has a very prominent primary muscle fiber orientation that is readily observable with the naked eye.

So I went to the nearby market, purchased a relatively fresh looking cut, brought it back to the clinical electromyography lab (at a time when no patients were around), and wheeled in our equipment. We laid out the steak on the examination table on a plastic sheet. After carefully shaping and cutting the flank steak to a near-perfect circle and marking angles relative to the major muscle fiber direction with a marker, we placed adhesive electrodes on the tissue and began performing measurements. The model worked remarkably well. We repeated the experiment a few times just to make sure our data were consistent and also played around with some other ideas (e.g., seeing what happened when we injected saline into it or macerated it lightly with a knife).

Of course the whole thing felt quite perverse. Our patient had turned literally into a piece of meat. And when we were done with the experiment, we took the steak, electrodes, and all, wrapped it up tightly in a plastic garbage bag and tossed it into the trash. (During a later steak experiment, one of the MIT graduate students with whom we were working insisted that this was a terrible waste. When we were done with the measurements, he removed the electrodes, cleaned off the marker ink, and

© Springer Science+Business Media New York 2016
S.B. Rutkove, *Biomedical Research: An Insider's Guide*,
DOI 10.1007/978-1-4939-3655-7_10

took the whole thing home with him to Cambridge. He marinated it over night before grilling it on his hibachi. He said it was delicious.)

These data were interesting and valuable to a number of our future studies. And we were even able to see it safely guide the study through to publication in a peer-reviewed journal, although we didn't call it flank steak, but rather rectus abdominis, its true anatomical name (See Tarulli et al. Electrical impedance in bovine skeletal muscle as a model for the study of neuromuscular disease. Physiological Measurement volume 27, page 1269).

My main reason for relating this anecdote is partly because I think it is kind of funny. But it also points out that there are many other types of research, some of which do not require any specific approval, since human subjects, animals, infectious particles, human materials, stem cells, or special agents (i.e., toxins) are not being utilized. I still recall throwing out that bag containing the steak, electrodes, and paper feeling decidedly uncomfortable. What would happen if an IRB or IACUC committee member caught me in the act? Won't some hospital officer call me out for misuse of the hospital trash facilities? The truth, of course, is that absolutely no one cared; it is completely outside the jurisdiction of the IRB or IACUC and I am quite certain that the hospital has no policies in place for the measurement of store-purchased steak or its disposal.

Of course, not all such research is without some kind of control. In this chapter, I will review some of these other types of research and the various policies and statutes that apply to them. But before going through each, it is worth pointing out that there is the concept of Good Laboratory Practice (GLP), and all institutions have a variety of guidelines and rules, from fire and safety to radioactive materials, etc., that need to be followed. I am not going to discuss those more general rules here, as they are easily obtainable online. My goal is simply to provide a brief overview of other types of work that fall outside the realm of human subject and vertebrate animal research that you may find yourself someday pursuing.

1. **Invertebrate animal research**. The rules regarding the use of invertebrates in animal research are quite variable and often nebulous. In the European Union, it is required to obtain approval for use of cephalopods (e.g., squid and octopus), but no other invertebrates. In the United States, no such specific rules exist and the IACUCs may or may not attempt to regulate or provide oversight for invertebrate work. You'll need to check in with your institution to understand their rules. Generally, the less sentient the species, the less likely anyone is going to care, even though it is likely true that many invertebrates also can experience pain and distress. There have been some recent calls to action for a formalized rule to protect invertebrates, but without a law or specific policy mandating this, most IACUCs and individual researchers are unlikely to concern themselves with it.

Depending on your research focus, there are some clear advantages to working with some types of invertebrates. For example, fruit fly work is extremely fast. Since the animals breed continuously, one is able to rapidly perform genetic modifications and see the results; with mice it would take weeks or months; with fruit flies, just days.

One limitation of course with invertebrate animal research is that it moves relatively far away from humans, and thus its relevance becomes more tenuous. Still, there have been fruit fly models of all sorts of diseases that have yielded valuable insights into pathology. And a Nobel prize was awarded to Eric Kandel for his pioneering work using the snail *aplysia* for understanding the mechanisms of memory development.

2. **Cell culture and other *in vitro* work**. Work involving cell culture and other *in vitro* systems (i.e., those in which cells or other biological material is placed in a self-contained artificial environment, such as a petri dish) does not in itself require approvals of any specific type. Thus, it is possible to work with non-pathogenic cell lines or other cultures without additional approvals. However, much cell culture work quickly veers into areas that do require additional oversight, from issues of biological safety (biological safety levels 2, 3, and 4), stem cells, and human tissues. It is beyond the scope of this book to delve into all the special concerns regarding these various categories of safety. However, suffice it to say that while the cell culture work does not inherently demand additional oversight, depending on what you do, you may very well be subject to a variety of regulations.

Policy issues aside, there are clear advantages to cell culture work and other *in vitro* systems that are worth considering, including speed of data collection and the ability to study many questions with surprising ease. Drugs or other treatments can be added to a system and the effects rapidly identified. Most fields from neurology to hematology to infectious disease to genetics all have work that can be achieved with remarkable efficiency *in vitro*. There are, however, also considerable challenges to such *in vitro* work, as well. In general, *in vitro* work is the most far removed from clinical application. And even though researchers can develop complex and impressive *in vivo* (i.e., within a living organism) systems attempting to mimic true biologic systems, they nevertheless remain only that: *in vitro* systems with questionable relevance to human disease. One example of *in vitro* systems ultimately failing and misleading researchers is in a study in one of the diseases in which I have a special interest, amyotrophic lateral sclerosis. Some excellent work by investigators at Johns Hopkins University and Columbia University, College of Physicians and Surgeons showed that the beta-lactam antibiotics, and especially ceftriaxone, provided impressive effects in slowing disease progression in brain slices prepared from rats with the genetic form of this disease. These data, supported by some additional mouse data, suggested that ceftriaxone could be a very powerful agent for slowing progression in ALS. These preliminary data were sufficient to encourage the creation of a large multicenter clinical trial of over 400 patients with ALS treated with ceftriaxone funded by the National Institutes of Health. A major complicating fact was that ceftriaxone could only be given intravenously, and thus all subjects had to have indwelling intravenous catheters placed. The drug also produced gallstones as a frequent side effect, forcing the study organizers to treat all subjects with ursadiol for gallstone prophylaxis. The fact that the study could be completed attests to the tenacity and determination of the study team and the dedication of the patients who participated. Nonetheless, when all was said and done, hundreds of patients, millions of dollars, and a great number of hours later, the study was negative. The drug had absolutely no effect on disease progression. Thus, while the initial report of a positive effect *in vitro* made for exciting news, including a letter published in the journal *Nature*, it was for naught.

I only relay this story because it speaks clearly to the fact that while what works in animals must be considered cautiously, what works in cell culture models must be considered with even more circumspection. Cell culture and other *in vitro* systems are great for many reasons, and when it comes to studying very basic mechanistic questions, it can be very fast and very effective. But the ultimate value of the results as regards drug efficacy and other more translational questions should be considered more skeptically. These issues should be recalled not only when considering pursuing cell culture work, but also when submitting research papers or grants that propose to pursue mainly *in vitro* work. Simply put, there is no free lunch.

3. **Computer or *in silico* modeling**. Computer modeling is another approach to research that can supply valuable and often relatively easily obtained data. Computer modeling is sometimes also referred to as "*in silico*" modeling, paralleling the concepts of *in vivo* and *in vitro* data collection. There are endless types of computer modeling ranging from epidemiological research to biophysical analyses, and I will not begin to attempt to summarize them here. Suffice it to say, that like *in vitro* modeling, *in silico* modeling can provide interesting data sets and results that have potential value. On the other hand, they are often very far removed from providing readily translational data. It is a good way of performing analyses, perhaps getting a relatively "easy" publication and providing useful data in a grant application. In my opinion, this approach is a great means to an end, but is in no way an end in itself. Still, I have used computer modeling in my own research to help guide development of technology and, in this particular application, it has been particularly valuable. But don't be "wowed" when you see the phrase "*in silico*" modeling. It is not as cool as it sounds.

4. **Large de-identified data sets and Internet research**. The Internet has created novel and remarkable opportunities for research that are far beyond the control of any IRB or governmental agency. The possibility for data analysis of entirely de-identified data sets is huge, and it remains possible to do all sorts of research that were unthinkable even just a few years ago. Moreover, multi-national de-identified data repositories are being created in diseases across the spectrum and these also create unique opportunities. But as with the *in silico* research discussed above, just because the data are there for the taking, does not mean it is simple to build a meaningful study around it. There have been many studies mining data sets in the hope of creating important new findings, such as biomarkers or epidemiological information; just because you can mine a set and say something new does not mean it is important or that it can turn into a sustained research endeavor capable of garnering grant support.

One new direction that also falls potentially in this realm is via the Patient Center Outcome Research Institute (PCORI), a non-profit, non-governmental research organization, which was authorized for creation by the Patient Protection and Affordable Care Act of 2010. The focus on patient-centered outcomes is an interesting opportunity that is likely to grow in the coming years. Some of the work here includes developing web-based or smart-phone-based technologies to assist with patient decision-making and evaluation of therapeutic effects. As with the digital fitness and health revolution continues, it is likely that we will see increasing opportunities to not only make new systems and products, but also to analyze the huge amounts of data that are being collected.

Summary: The purpose of this chapter was simply to review a variety of other research directions that one might find oneself drawn to in the biomedical sciences. These range from laboratory bench to epidemiological, each with its own sets of opportunities and challenges. Upon entering the biomedical research field, there is actually no real need to make a decision ahead of time or plan on confining yourself to just one type of research. In point of fact, spanning different types of research can be quite fun and provide a pleasant variety to your work. And the distinct platforms can sometimes feed into one another, improving and extending the importance of the work you are doing. So remain flexible and don't be afraid of shifting gears into an area with which you have less familiarity. It is likely that within a relatively short period of time, you can become well-versed in that as well.

Chapter 11
Hiring Research Staff

When entering upon the world of research, the last thing you will probably be thinking about is hiring research staff. Most of us are pretty used to sitting in the trenches and doing virtually all of the heavy lifting ourselves, from idea generation to data collection right down to submitting a paper for review and then handling the revisions. However, a strong research team that is managed effectively can greatly extend your capabilities. Not only can the members of such a team do the tasks you *know* need to get done, but if they are of high quality, they will also come up with their own ideas and suggestions that may lead to new directions in your research. Of course, how much of that can be achieved depends on their role in your team. A post-doc is going to be able to help you a lot more than a newly minted research assistant; on the other hand, the research assistant will simply usually do as he or she is told, while a post-doc may need to be reigned in to make sure he stays focussed on the work at hand and not veer off into other directions or start focussing on long-term future career goals only.

An important corollary to the idea behind hiring people is that you will need to give up some responsibility. For many of us trained as physicians or researchers, this seems almost antithetical. For example, you may feel that you need to know all the details of every process from how to use a database to knowing which URL in the hospital's website has all the IRB forms available for download. Or in the animal realm, this could include all the details about performing every procedure your lab does. But that, of course, completely defeats the purpose of having a team. The point of hiring a team is to be able to delegate—specifically to cast aside the need to know everything about every aspect of a study. For a novice researcher just starting to run a team, there is a natural inclination to feel that you need to understand every aspect of the research going on—that somehow you are being remiss if you don't know the specific details of the work that is ongoing or how they are doing it—but that is neither feasible nor desirable. Naturally, you don't want to be so uninvolved that you don't know what is going on (that can land you in hot water too), but loos-

© Springer Science+Business Media New York 2016
S.B. Rutkove, *Biomedical Research: An Insider's Guide*,
DOI 10.1007/978-1-4939-3655-7_11

ening up the reigns and letting your team figure out things on their own and report back to you on their progress is a critical step if you are going to have and run a productive research operation.

Hiring your first assistant to help you with data collection or paper work related to the IRB or IACUC can seem like a dream come true. And their use may be entirely pre-identified—i.e., you know you need them to help collect data in a specific study and interact with patients or perhaps take care of animals. But as your research matures, you may find yourself seeking people with specific skill sets and interests to perform a variety of tasks, some of which you may not be sure of at the time of hiring.

Having been running a reasonably successful research operation for nearly two decades, I have learned a few things are that I will itemize here. These were concepts that I so, so wish someone had told me when I had first started out looking for good team members.

Rule #1: *Honesty is key*. This may seem totally obvious, but determining whether a given person is honest is not easy. Usually it is the little things that give it away. Exaggerations or inconsistencies in their past work should make you wonder whether the person is being entirely square with you. Since you will be delegating a great deal of responsibility to this person, you need to know that, although they may make mistakes, they will honestly tell you when that happens. Any hint of any kind of subterfuge should be an immediate reason to not consider that person for a position. Though you do have to be a little careful—when people are interviewing, they will try to play up their skills and capabilities a bit—clear distortions of the truth cannot be ignored. So, the best way to figure this out is to probe them on their skill sets and experience. No person will have the ideal set of experiences or knowledge that you need, so push them into areas where you know they can't possibly answer "yes." If you find them circling the answer or simply not willing to say "No, I have no experience with that" or "I don't know how to do that," you should proceed cautiously. Of all the characteristics I list here, I think this is by far and away the most important.

Rule #2: *Always interview*. While interviews are definitely the norm, occasionally you may find yourself in a position of potentially hiring someone who you have not actually met or even spoken to, especially if they are a neighbor's friend or someone with a stellar resume who lives at a distance but is planning to move to your town. In the "old days" if this situation arose, I would at the very last have a phone conversation, although this was far from ideal since all the important aspects of body language and eye contact are lost. Fortunately, now Skype and other over-the-web programs are available to allow you to interview someone regardless of where they live and actually see them and interact with them. This approach is certainly not ideal, but I have now successfully hired several people with only Skype interviewing, and I have to say that it works quite well. One gets familiar with the challenges of using it (the fact that you can't exactly look in each other's eyes) and trying to extract what you need. But if the person is serious, they will dress for their Skype interview just as nicely as if they were coming to your office in person. And they will interact with you in a polite and courteous manner as if you had just asked them to come and sit down.

Rule #3: *Dress matters.* While I run a pretty loose ship when it comes to how my research staff dresses for work (for example, unless they are dealing with patients, jeans and T-shirts are fine), I do expect someone coming for an interview to dress appropriately. A disregard for the formality of an interview tells you that the person may not understand the importance of following norms and rules. And while I love to be iconoclastic and idiosyncratic in much of what I do and respect others who do the same, an interview is a time to relegate yourself to tradition and norms and not make a statement about your "uniqueness."

Rule #4: *Attitude.* This can be challenging to determine, but a major task when hiring anyone is to understand why he is looking at your job and what he is hoping to get out of it. While I think hiring people with a good sense of self is important, hiring someone who is overly self-involved should be a non-starter. I can't tell you how many people I have interviewed who slowly make it clear to me that they are more interested in understanding what they are going to get out of a job than whether they are capable of providing you with the services that you need. Of course, people should choose jobs that will benefit their long-term career goals—and virtually all people you will be hiring will not considering it as their final job. Usually they will be relatively young with a long career ahead of them. But during the interview process, what they are going to get out of the job should be implicit rather than a direct part of the conversation. If they find the details of the job are not to their liking, that should be a conclusion they reach quietly and on their own. You should not be pushed to do their bidding and reshape the job along the lines of what they would ideally like and not what you need.

Rule #5: *Know what you are looking for.* This can be tough when you are first starting out as a principal investigator since it may not be obvious—all you may know is that you need help and lots of it since you are drowning in work of every conceivable kind. But as your research endeavor grows, you may find that you need someone who is going to be helping to collect data from patients or working with animals in the lab or perhaps simply organizing and maintaining your database. Regardless of the details, make sure you know why you are hiring and what skill set you need. Try to define it as carefully as you can—make a list of everything you envision on their working; this will help you identify the individual with the right set of skills. And generally, if you do have more than 1 or 2 people working for you, it will be important that they are at least aware of each other's duties so if one is out for a period of time, they can successfully cover for each other to some extent.

But some potential assistants will be hoping to work with animals while others will just want to focus on human work and others may feel very happy about going back and forth between. It is very important to understand not just what someone can do but what he or she wants to do. Making someone work with animals who is ethically opposed to animal research or who finds it just unappealing is not someone you may want to hire even if they will only be doing animal work occasionally. I find the interview process a great time to really understand their interests, so it is important to push them on these kinds of questions. Again, they may feel tentative about telling you their true feelings, but it is really important that you learn about them before they join your team, not after.

Rule #6: *Never feel desperate*. There have been times when I've had a new project or I'm looking for someone with a very specific skill set where I feel like I have to get the position filled immediately. And then if I interview someone for the position who seems like they will fit the bill but are not great, I feel compelled to hire them immediately. But that is a mistake—you should never feel compelled to hire anyone, even if it seems like your whole research operation may come to a grinding halt for a time. If you start to feel that you should hire the person simply because they are "good enough," you should always stop yourself.

This is not without undue complications. As I mentioned earlier, that tacit knowledge that one researcher learns over time and shares with a new team member is critical to the smooth running of a lab. I have had some unexpected gaps in my hiring, and when the new person started working for me, they had to learn a great deal from scratch. While this definitely wastes time, in the end it is a better waste of time to hire a great researcher who can figure out the way on their own for a few months than to hire your "desperate choice" and suffer with ineptitude for years to come.

Rule #7: *Starting hiring early*. One of the worst mistakes I've made over the years is to not hire people early enough. In fact, you can never start too early. This definitely helps avoid the problem described in Rule #6. At my institution, it can take a couple of weeks between first submitting the request for hiring and the point that the advertisement is posted on the web. And then the interview process can take a while longer plus you have to wait for references even after you have made your decision. It can easily be 6 weeks between when you first realize you need to post a job and when you are prepared to potentially make a job offer. And if you wait too long, you may find yourself in a predicament where one of your team is leaving to go off to school and the new person won't be able to start for several weeks. Thus, I usually try to aim for a minimum 2-week overlap period between a departing research assistant and the new one who is starting. Three weeks is even better, but 4 is usually unnecessarily long, but it does depend to some extent on the new assistant's pre-existing skill set and the tasks that will be assigned to her.

Rule #8: *Don't expect more than a 2-year commitment*. A research group may consist of a collection of people at different levels of training: research assistants, post-docs, nurses, graduate students, research coordinators, junior faculty, and perhaps a lab director. Each person will have his or her own unique timeline. Post-docs generally may plan for at least 2 years and possibly much longer. Others, such as a study coordinator or nurse may be looking for a quasi-permanent job. On the other hand, most research assistants are only passing through: some will only be taking off 1 year between college and graduate school to get some more experience. Others may be reconsidering long-term career options and taking post-baccalaureate classes perhaps with a plan to apply to medical school or graduate school. Some may just really not be sure about what they want and simply want to get their feet wet with some experience.

I generally attempt to hire people who have a 2-year time line. This usually consists of people freshly graduated from college but also those who see a clear end to their tenure with you in sight. I have also taken plenty of people who have stayed for only 1 year, and this has generally worked out satisfactorily, although it usually takes people about 3 months to get fully up to speed and during the last 3 months they are already thinking about what comes next and not their job—hence you might get only 6–7 months of focussed, strong work from them. Moreover, these people are usually taking substantial time off to interview for schools, so you kind of lose out from that perspective as well. And then, you find yourself back in interview mode earlier than you would like. So if you can find someone with a 2-year timeline and you can usually be pretty sure about this since they are still needing to complete some outside course work or testing prior to being able to apply to graduate school, that is usually the best option.

It is also worth noting that you really can't get people to commit to anything. I have had research assistants who bailed on me after just 1 year when other good opportunities arose, after stating quite firmly, that they would definitely not plan on leaving until the following year. But that goes back to the honesty question as well. If these people probably had been more honest, they would have told me up front they could not commit definitely to 2 years. Of course, we sometimes even lie to ourselves without knowing it.

Rule #9: *Where to advertise*. I still struggle with this. I have found terrific people through a variety of means. My hospital advertises and although most of the respondents to a job advertisement do not have the qualifications I am looking for, there are usually a small subset of applications that come through in which the applicants are a great match. I have also, however, taken to advertising at local colleges, through word of mouth, and even on Craig's list at various times. There are also plenty of other job websites, but at this point, my general view is that if you advertise early enough and are patient, you can probably just work through your institution and leave it at that. It certainly makes life easier to let the human resources people do some of the ground work than your having to do it all yourself.

Rule #10: *Always review references*. This is a simple rule. As a matter of course, your institution will probably demand that there are at least two references in place before having the opportunity to hire someone. The references can be very telling since they usually provide real-world input on the effectiveness of the potential employee. People with stellar references generally are going to perform at least satisfactorily, though there are certainly no guarantees, since many people will try to say nice things about a person who has previously worked for them. But people with poor-to-mediocre comments are almost certainly not going to be great—it takes a lot for a person to be critical so any negative comments should be taken very seriously. I have turned back at least a couple of people based on their references and in one situation, my hospital actually barred me from hiring someone because their references were so poor. I was annoyed at the time because I thought he was actually a great fit for the position, but it was probably for the best.

Rule #11: *Hiring of post-docs is a special situation*. Hiring a post-doc is often a big undertaking, since she may be someone who will be in your lab for years to come and may really help move your work forward in a variety of important ways. Now when you are thinking of hiring a research assistant, you generally know what you need: people to help complete the day-to-day tasks of biomedical research from helping recruit patients to running gel electrophoresis. But when it comes to hiring a high-level employee such as a post-doc, it is very much another story. Here you are likely looking to hire someone with a very specific expertise. And these people are generally going to be of a very different ilk than someone fresh out of college. You will also have a much greater responsibility in terms of seeing them through to their next level of career advancement—hopefully a faculty position somewhere or perhaps just a second post-doc position. It is true that many post-docs join labs and can stay there for 5 or even 6 or 7 years, so the long-term nature of the relationship and the associated commitment should not be understated. Of course, strong post-docs will be able to participate actively in the lab's research, hopefully pushing the envelope and direction of the lab in a positive way. But these hires are big commitments and making sure that both you and your prospective new employee are both on the same page from the get-go is really important.

Some post-docs, however, will not be as comfortable in the transition from graduate student to independent laboratory researcher and will not move forward without having clear directions on a daily or weekly basis, even though they are entirely capable of pursuing this. Sorting that out up front (that is, before they are hired) can be very challenging. It may be that you don't care, or perhaps you'd prefer somebody serving in the role as basically a lab manager. And that is fine—it is just good to know up front. This is where interviews and references and reading between the lines can make a huge difference.

Rule #12: *Hiring lab managers, study coordinators, and other "permanent employees" should also not be taken lightly*. A good nurse manager for a study or lab manager can make your life much better, since they can help oversee critical aspects of your research group's organization and day-to-day operations, while leaving you to deal with some of the bigger issues—i.e., paper and grant writing. However, such people are generally not cheap and they are also looking for long-term job stability, something an entirely grant-supported enterprise simply cannot often promise. Usually, these people are most easily hired if you have some kind of institutional support or there is another guaranteed source of funding for the long term, such as a large philanthropic gift earmarked for this purpose. Another mechanism for achieving this is by having a number of industry-sponsored clinical trials in which you can set up a clinical-trials machine of sorts that can be self-perpetuating. But for smaller labs, these people are not inexpensive and you will have considerable responsibility ensuring that their position remains viable for a long time to come.

Rule #13: *They are not your employee until they actually show up for work the first day*. So you may go through the entire hiring process, have found a person who looks great on paper, is amazing at the interview, and happily accepts the position you have offered, only to discover that when they are due to show up for their first employee health screening, they are nowhere to be found. And perhaps later that day you will receive an email saying that they unexpectedly had something come up—another opportunity or a sick family member that requires their returning home—and thus have to unexpectedly and belatedly turn down the position. They are so sorry, etc., etc.

These situations arise more often than any of us would like. There may, in fact, be unexpected personal circumstances which arise may prevent a new hire from actually joining your lab. However, more often than not, a person interviewing is looking at a number of jobs simultaneously, and each job application process will have a slightly different schedule in terms of when an offer will be made and when the new employee is anticipated to start. You can't necessarily blame someone for accepting what in his view is the second best job since he is not sure he is going to be offered the one he wants most. And then when, at the last minute, that coveted job becomes available, how can he say no? While honesty is usually the best policy, many interviewees, are often pretty new to this entire process and have a tough time negotiating some of its intricacies, so it is not unusual for such last minute betrayals to happen. My philosophy in dealing with this is pretty simple: I do not believe someone is actually going to come work for me until the moment they step through the door on the first day. Of course, I can't keep searching for a "back-up" during the interregnum between the hiring date and start date—my institution wouldn't really allow that and it is very time consuming—but I don't feel like the whole hiring affair is settled until the person actually shows up for his first day of work.

Generally, however, if they do show up on time, it means that they are really going to stay. I have never had anyone show up day 1 only to disappear on day 2, 3, or 60.

Rule #14. *During the interview process, ensure that the potential new employee meets with other members of your team without you around.* Again, this may seem obvious, but it is critical that a prospective new member of your team get an opportunity to meet with their future peers and colleagues. Your team can then report back to you and let you know if they feel good about the person and would want to work with him. It is sometimes a little challenging to get people who are not used to casting summary judgments on people to actually provide a useful opinion, but a simple thumb's up or thumb's down is all that you really need. Plus it really helps to empower your team. On at least two or three occasions, my research team's input has unquestionably prevented me from making a poor hiring decision.

Other special categories of employees: Other categories of employees are also worth a brief mention since each brings along its own unique set of benefits and challenges.

Graduate students. If you are linked closely with a university, you may find yourself in the position of having a steady stream of PhD graduate students working in your lab and your being their thesis advisor. Graduate students can be a challenging group of employees since they have a very specific set of requirements that they are looking to complete in a pre-defined time period (or at least an approximately predefined period of time if they are seeking a PhD). Ensuring that their project is distinct and can be effectively cordoned off from other aspects of your lab's work becomes paramount, since a driving factor will be to ensure that they have a coherent and defendable thesis when all is said and done. So not only is defining their specific projects critical, but a graduate student's individual attitudes and interests must play into that as well. There needs to be a great deal of give and take between the student and the mentor in order for both to succeed. This is probably not as true in the world of post-docs, who may already have their own agendas or are willing to subjugate their individual wills for the greater good of the lab, or research assistants who simply are supposed to do what they are told. Thus, like any category of researcher, graduate students demand a specific type of effort from the principal investigator, the exact nature of which will vary greatly with the student's independence, drive, and creativity.

Undergraduate researchers. You may also have the opportunity to work with people who are not specifically seeking a science degree but want experience in the lab. If you are working in a university, you may have a steady stream of undergraduate students knocking at your door looking to gather some research experience. While such students are not fully formed in terms of providing outstanding research help the moment they are hired, within a short time, many of these people can become highly valuable in running simple experiments or performing other useful tasks around the lab. Plus they are usually cost free, which is a huge bonus for a lab. The only major downside to most undergraduate researchers is that they have a variety of other ongoing commitments, whether it is taking additional courses, having a busy social life and other extracurricular activities, or focussing on studying for the MCAT or the GRE.

Other undergraduate research programs are also available. I know my lab has benefited tremendously from a co-op program connected to Northeastern University here in Boston. Students are required to take 2–3 semesters during college to actually work in a job. These students for the most part serve as research assistants, but their focus is on learning and getting the experience of seeing how the real world operates a year or two earlier than is typical without making any kind of huge long-term commitment. I would strongly encourage working with such a program if available. It ends up being a win–win for all, not only because the students learn and your lab benefits, but also because since they are at a university and in a defined program, they are relatively inexpensive to hire: their wages are lower and the university provides health insurance coverage. About the only downside is that their time is usually limited to only a semester + a summer (about 9 months at most).

Medical student researchers. Medical students are being increasingly encouraged to take time off from their 4-year intense curriculum training to become doctors by pursuing a year of research. For someone who is doing this because they have a real love of research, nothing could be better. These individuals have a long-term vision about seeing themselves as a clinician-researcher or perhaps just a researcher and are looking to follow in your footsteps. They will try to squeeze every moment of value out their time in the lab without other commitments and it can be remarkably productive. About the only challenge with them is that you need funds to support their work, but there are many opportunities available to help underwrite salary/tuition—usually through the university or medical school or through foundations, such as the Howard Hughes Medical Institute.

High school students. I have brought on high school students for 6–10 weeks of the summer for years now through a connection with a neighboring school. These students are brought in as interns and thus no salary is expected. Given their limited skill set, at most they can usually offer only limited help with data analysis or simple experimental tasks. While they are usually very pleasant to work with, being both enthusiastic and energetic, their benefits to the lab are generally rather modest. Compounding their limited time and experience is the fact that most of these people are minors, further restricting their ability to perform activities without parent consent or additional oversight. So you should mainly consider your hiring such high-school students as a little payback to society—you will probably not get much out of it, but they will be unalterably affected by their experience. The one additional positive of having them in the lab is that it gives your research assistants an opportunity to work in a mentoring/teaching role, and this is something that most enjoy considerably.

Volunteers. There was a time when you could easily bring on a volunteer and have him do work as if he was one of your lab members. These people, usually seeking some experience after having arrived in the United States from a foreign land, may have been looking for someone to write a recommendation or to get any kind of work experience that could ultimately lead to real, paid position.

For the most part, those days are gone. Federal laws prohibit your bringing on someone who is supposed to be paid (i.e., as a research assistant) and calling them a volunteer and not paying them. Nowadays, at best, a volunteer can do work that you might not ordinarily need for the lab—perhaps outreach to a community group—say the elderly or underserved.

To be honest, this is probably for the best. Having brought on a few volunteers in the past, I was usually not satisfied with their performance (though there were exceptions). Without a formal contract and no sense of obligation or commitment to the lab, their work was generally of mediocre quality and their reliability (i.e., actually showing up most days) even less so. And I can understand this. It is frankly demeaning to be working for free when someone working right beside you and perhaps considerably younger than you is getting paid for his time. I think the feds got this one right, frankly.

Summary. Hiring good people to fill your lab and to whom to delegate responsibility is probably one of the more challenging aspects of running a lab, and it's a skill that no one can really teach you. Only experience can help you become expert at not only knowing whom you need to hire (i.e., what skill sets you are specifically looking for) but also candidates who will mostly likely succeed. Ultimately, with practice and after a few mishirings, you will eventually be able to find winners who will make coming to work every day a true pleasure.

Chapter 12
Strategy and Tactics: Running a Successful Laboratory

Sketching out a grand scheme for your research may sound utterly daunting, but having a broad sense of your long-term general direction of research is extremely important. I would call this theme the strategy of your research. It would be the kind of thing you could describe in a so-called *elevator pitch*. It's as if you walked into an elevator and someone you didn't know asked you what you were researching and why, and you had to answer before one of you had reached your floor and had to exit. What would you say? How would you crystalize multiple ongoing projects in multiple directions into just a few neat sentences? Now of course, as your laboratory matures and you develop new collaborations that have very different aims, your lab therefore may not have one clean common theme (and in fact it probably *should not*—see below on the Lean Laboratory). But to some extent those few major themes may all work off of one another in some complex and perhaps elegant way. If that is the case, so much the better. But understanding your general area of interest and focus is really critical, lest you lose sight of your long-term goals.

As I write this chapter, for example, my research continues to be focussed on novel biomarkers for assessing neuromuscular diseases in human diseases, but I also have a study focussing on novel electrode arrays for animal use, work focussing on assessing muscle injury due to overuse, and a new off-the-wall idea regarding treatment of amyotrophic lateral sclerosis. What would my elevator pitch be? Something along the lines of, "My laboratory is focussed on the investigation of neuromuscular disease. Our work is mainly focussed on the application of new therapies and improved ways of monitoring their impact on the health of the individual. We study both animals and humans in an attempt to ensure that the outcomes of our work have immediate pre-clinical and long-term value. This research will improve the lives of all people suffering with a variety of neuromuscular disorders, from muscle wasting in the older men and women to children with muscular dystrophy."

The Lean Laboratory. In 2011, Eric Reis authored *The Lean Startup*. The subtitle of the book was "How today's entrepreneurs use continuous innovation to create radically successful businesses." Obviously, this book was not about doing

© Springer Science+Business Media New York 2016
S.B. Rutkove, *Biomedical Research: An Insider's Guide*,
DOI 10.1007/978-1-4939-3655-7_12

research or about running lab—rather it was about trying to get a startup company off the ground on the way to stunning success. But the ideas that Mr. Ries espouses for use in the business world actually can be very effectively applied to the world of scientific research.

The basic premise of the book is that you should at all times remain continually lean and flexible and not mired in predetermined plans or ideas. He gives examples of startup companies that are initially focussed on one product or service and then morph, virtually overnight, into companies that are focussed on a completely alternative trajectory. For example, a company first works on creating a product that the directors believe will have a market in one group of people but then discovers, as they start actually trying to sell the product, that there is little interest from this group as a whole; but they learn that there is a subgroup of this population who are actually very interested in it. So they modify the product to appeal to this subgroup and another larger allied group.

One of the major premises of that book is the concept of the "Minimal Viable Product", or MVP. Basically, you shouldn't waste your time making a product that you perceive as perfect from the get-go. You want to create a product that will sell and introduce your concept to the world without breaking the bank. What you learn from that experience will help inform future decisions as you make second and third generation products. So I propose here the research parallel: the "Minimal Viable Study," MVS and suggest the concept of *Lean Laboratory*.

While you cannot expect to divert your lab from one effort to another, many many successful researchers have a number of projects going on in different areas—borrowing from another business concept of diversification—the same basic concept can hold. Do not devote excessive time and effort to any one project unless you are convinced that it is going to pay off in the long rung. In a Lean Laboratory, you always start small, with pilot projects and see if there are positive results before embarking on huge undertakings that eventually might fail—in other words, try performing an MVS. There is still the risk that when it is time to undertake the larger effort that it may still fail even after making those initial investments, but at least the likelihood will be lower.

Let's examine two starkly different examples of the Lean Laboratory at work to show how this basic concept can be employed—one at the bench and one in the clinic.

1. **Drug studies in mice**. Let's say you have been reading the literature and see that there are some nifty new approaches for treating a disease of interest to you. Researchers have been focussing on a set of drugs that seem promising and published *in vitro* studies seem promising. But you've realized that perhaps a related class of compounds is perhaps even more effective. It seems so good, that you suspect other people may have had this same idea, but after you've thoroughly reviewed the literature, you cannot find any evidence that is true. So one approach would be to make a major investment and study say a relatively large number of mice at different doses using say 1 or 2 of these new compounds and treat the animals for say 8–12 weeks at which point they would be sacrificed and a variety of analyses completed, including pathological analyses and running assays. Moreover, you will do

everything to the highest possible standard, including blinding of the researchers to drug versus vehicle and animal status, as discussed in the earlier chapter on animal studies. You know that if you do it all well that even if negative, you will at least get a paper out of it. So it seems like a worthwhile venture, but it is a pretty big commitment. In fact, as you actually start to write out the detailed plans you realize, it is actually going to be a huge effort. And if it turns out to be negative, you will be kicking yourself for wasting so much time and money on a dead end, even if you can manage to get something published. After all publication in itself should probably not be an end goal.

So instead of doing a huge study, you metaphorically just dip your toe in the water instead. You decide you will only test the most promising of these compounds at 1 dose for just a couple of weeks in just a few animals. Since you know that you may not be able to see a substantial effect of the drug in such a short period of time, you pick a couple of sensitive biomarkers a priori. You also toss out the blinding idea because it adds an extra layer of complexity. So now you run the study in a truly bare bones kind of fashion; just a handful (say 12 animals are used, 4 with higher dose, 4 with lower dose, and 4 with placebo). You treat them daily and then at the end of just a month, you do your assays to determine whether there is a noteworthy effect or not.

Now, no matter what happens, you will have learned something valuable in the process—perhaps just in terms of potential side effects of the drug or challenges with handling it or other entirely unforeseen issues, such as your assays not working properly. And if you are seeing evidence of the biomarkers at least trending in the right direction, you will have reassurance that perhaps this approach might work and feel prepared and committed to take on a larger more conclusive study. On the other hand, if the data are all going in the wrong direction, it may mean you should cut bait and move on to your next project; or if you feel very committed, reconsider dosing and your choice of biomarkers and try again.

Of course, there are some flaws in this logic. As discussed in the earlier chapter on doing top-notch research, a statistician will point out immediately that this approach is a recipe for Type 2 error and nothing more—namely rejecting a hypothesis prematurely because your sample size was too small. While there is truth to this of course—in other words had you studied 20 animals you might have seen that those first few were actually an aberration and everything trended in the opposite direction—it is also shortsighted. Every day we are forced to make hundreds of non-science-related decisions based on limited data sets—from choosing the best dinner at a restaurant to deciding whether the long line at Starbucks is going to make you late. You don't have the luxury of applying statistics to these analyses. So buried within the decision to run a Lean Laboratory is the recognition that you will make miscalls, but that overall the time and money lost on the effort will pale in comparison to the grandeur and scale of the miscalls you will make by taking the other approach. But even if you decide to proceed, the amount you have learned in the process will be huge and will help ensure a more definitive success or failure on the next go-round. By taking a Lean Laboratory approach, you embrace constant learning, continually modifying and improving your methods.

2. **Drug study in human subjects**. Employing a Lean Laboratory approach to the study of human subjects is considerably more challenging than doing so at the bench. Obviously, you cannot simply start doing studies without IRB approval (the case is also true in the world of animal research, but getting quick approval from the IACUC is a lot less painful). And IRB's don't always see kindly to doing studies that are only geared to collect pilot data (again, to be clear, all studies need IRB approval, including those collecting pilot data), where a simple calculation of the sample size will show definitively that you are wasting your time by just studying say six people, half placed on drug and half placed on placebo.

However, there is an alternative, more rational approach that is scientifically valid that I think many researchers overlook: N-of-1 studies. As applied to therapeutics, the concept of an N-of-1 study is to see whether the drug offers a therapeutic benefit in just a single person. Now depending on the medical condition you are studying, the type of drug, and the effect you are looking for, this can be more or less challenging. First, the drug has to be available. The easiest example would be using an FDA-approved medication in an off-label use. This is entirely legal (but again since you are actually doing research in this hypothetical situation you would still need IRB approval). Let's say the drug was approved for treating hypertension but you are interested in whether it works in treating headaches—a not uncommon situation since this is true with beta-blockers and calcium channel blockers. You identify a reliable patient with refractory headaches and begin treating them for 1 month on the drug while they maintain a headache log. Nothing is blinded. You then have them stop the drug and maintain the log. You then restart them and then maintain the log. After doing this for a couple of months, you will see whether this therapy is working any better than standard treatment. Ideally, you could even do this with 2 or 3 patients, and see what the results have to show. At that point, you will have a sense as to whether this is really a promising intervention or the improvement is going to pretty modest and probably not worth pursuing on a larger scale.

Of note, you can also take this approach using a placebo in addition or instead to the removal of the drug. This is obviously a bit more challenging, but on the other hand is likely to provide you with a stronger data set than an open-label approach.

Now that is an easy example. Other N-of-1 studies are considerably more challenging. For example, showing evidence of slowing in a gradually progressive disease is far more complicated. For example, studying Alzheimer's disease in a patient—a disease that progresses over years—would be very challenging and probably not amenable to this kind of approach. N-of-1 studies work well for symptomatic/short-term improvement not for slowing progression. However, if you do have a potential therapy that is going to change disease course for the better, than you might have a shot at success with an N-of-1 study.

Another approach to being a Lean Laboratory in human studies is to attempt a retrospective data analysis that may at least provide some clue as to whether the question you are thinking of asking is worthwhile. Such a retrospective analysis, of course, doesn't need to come from your own hard work, but could reside in the literature in already published materials, or it could be obtainable in a publically accessible database of de-identified patient data. For example in my field of neuromuscular disorders, including amyotrophic lateral sclerosis (ALS), the Pooled Resource Open-Access ALS Clinical Trials Database (PRO-ACT) is available freely online and contains patient data from 17 different clinical drug trials and a total of over eight million data points in ALS. Of course, such a resource can't tell you if gene therapy is going to work in ALS, but it could help in guiding decisions to more basic questions. Other areas of medicine have similarly available open resources, such as the Yale Open Data Access program. This repository contains data from over 80 clinical trials and is constantly being enlarged. This is a growing movement, and being able to access raw data from other people's work can serve as a great initial step to help ensuring Lean Laboratory concepts in human clinical research. And best of all, for analyses of these de-identified data, you don't even need IRB approval!

Summary. I have offered up two parallel examples of a similar kind of study in two very different environments, animal and human. But this approach can be used with so many other ideas that it should really be, in my view, a modus operandi for all science. Gather as much data as you can with the least effort to provide some evidence to test your hypothesis. And then make a decision based on that limited data set, *accepting the fact that your decision may be wrong*. All you can do is to hope to improve your chances of being successful when you really go for the bigger goals.

There are so many possible questions to ask and so many diseases, etc., I cannot possibly hope to even fully scrape the surface of the concept of the Lean Laboratory. But I put forward the basic mantra that any experienced consumer knows: "Look before you buy."

Chapter 13
Everything You Ever Wanted to Know About Collaboration

Collaboration is the cornerstone of successful science in medicine and beyond. The days of doing work in an isolated laboratory or basement and hoping to reach some startling revelation are long gone. Yes, deep in all our hearts, I believe, we would like to think that individual discoveries are still just waiting behind the next corner. But the truth is that even those discoveries were extremely challenging to bring to fruition and did not happen alone in most cases. They often did happen through collaborations of a sort, but collaborations that were spread over time rather than through space. In other words, work of individuals over decades gradually culminating in some great "eureka" moment, and the discovery being attributed to that one person. For example, Alexander Fleming's discovery of the penicillium mold in 1928 was based on his knowledge of the broad field bacteriology. Most great new discoveries do not occur de novo, but rather are built upon previous work. Yes—there are exceptions—with Einstein's theories of special and generalized relativity being the most obvious—where one person revolutionizes scientific thinking virtually out of the blue. But even Einstein relied on the work of Bernhard Riemann's mathematics from the 1860s in order to successfully formulate his theory of general relativity.

OK, so back to the modern day. What is collaboration? How does it happen? How does it flourish? How does it end? What are the rules?

For the purposes of this chapter, I am going to use the term collaboration to refer to working together amongst peers, not mentor–mentee relationships or the laboratory staff you may hire, including post-docs and research assistants, who help you in your day-to-day work. To be sure, these people are your collaborators too and should always be treated as such. As one of my own mentees likes to say, research is definitely a team sport and we each make contributions. And advanced post-docs in your lab certainly may serve the role of collaborator as they will have gained expertise that is somewhat different than your own in their previous graduate or post-doc work. But what I am talking about here is peer-to-peer collaboration with other researchers in your own department or at another institution in your town, across the country, or abroad.

© Springer Science+Business Media New York 2016
S.B. Rutkove, *Biomedical Research: An Insider's Guide*,
DOI 10.1007/978-1-4939-3655-7_13

Forging a collaboration. In your field of interest, at your own institution. How do most collaborations begin? I think most begin naturally amongst your closest work colleagues. If I look through the papers I have published, most also bear the names of my colleagues at the hospital in which I work—other physicians who worked with me on creating a research idea, collecting data, analyzing it, and finally writing a manuscript and seeing it through to publication. The colleagues at your job are people you know and work with on a regular basis and therefore form a nucleus of sorts from which all your research endeavors will grow. And if you are pursuing clinical work, they also may be critical in providing assistance in the recruitment of patients with a certain disease.

However, such close collaborations are often limited in a certain respect for several reasons. First, you are all in the same field. That means you are all thinking along similar lines and have similar, if not virtually identical, areas of expertise. This is not the way to come up with new great concepts that can lead to a sustained research endeavor, but it is an important way to start a career and learn about collaborating with other people effectively. Another issue is that since you are all in the same place you may share similar educational or training experiences—or perhaps you have even trained one or two people who are now your colleagues. So while extremely important, these kinds of collaborations have their functional limits. Thus, it is important to branch out.

In your field, but outside your own institution. The next tier of collaboration is between you and other people in your field but at different institutions. Such collaboration may yield greater rewards in the long term for a number of reasons. First, it is likely such people will add a much greater breadth of knowledge and experience, having been trained and researched/practiced in different places, coming from widely different regions, and perhaps, in the clinical realm, dealing with different populations of patients. And moreover, if you are considering running a multicenter study, where you are aiming to recruit a large number of patients, having multiple sites assisting with the data collection not only ensures that you will help reach your recruitment goals, but it also helps to solidify the robustness of whatever you are studying—whether it be a new drug, questionnaire, or biomarker. And if you are doing studies in a rare genetic disease, such collaborations are even more critical, since it may be impossible to identify a gene or gene product without all the centers contributing and sharing in the work. Moreover, some of these far-flung colleagues may have pet projects of their own that they are interested in working on and thus they may want to share the wealth in both directions, offering you something in addition to your giving something to them. And those smaller pet projects may in turn inform your own project. In other words, collaborations with individuals outside of your own institution but in your general area of expertise begin the all-important process of cross-fertilization.

How does one go about forging these types of collaborations? Well generally, this means attending meetings in your field and networking and being social and making new connections through your friends, mentors, and other far-flung colleagues. It is interesting to me how some of my closest collaborators are people who I have met through meetings because of areas of common interest and expertise. If you never attend meetings or conferences, it is very difficult to begin to develop these important kinds of networks that you can draw upon when you have a new idea. Equally important, these people may reach out to you as well when they have a new idea for a study and they are seeking input and potential collaboration. For more on developing this kind of symbiosis, see the chapter on successful networking.

Outside your field. The third and what I would call highest order of collaboration is one in which you begin working with people far outside your field of expertise. Now, I must say that these types of collaborations are really the most exciting and fruitful, because it is here where you begin to truly cross-fertilize and bring together very disparate sets of ideas to potentially create something much greater than the sum of the individual parts. Examples of these kinds of collaborations could be straightforward and common—for example, working with a biostatistician when planning a new clinical study or analyzing animal or other more basic data. Biostatistics, however, is a very special type of collaboration since biostatisticians are specifically focussed on collaboration; in fact, their actual existence as a practicing area of study is almost entirely predicated on working with other biomedical researchers.

Another more meaningful example would be reaching out to a PhD researcher who has expertise in a specific type of disease or disease mechanism. Perhaps you are studying a new drug therapy in a particular mouse model of disease when you realize that someone across town is studying the same animal model, but trying to understand the basic biology of disease pathogenesis. Or perhaps you are thinking about something even further far afield from your work. For example, perhaps you have an idea about a new type of pharmacological agent and wonder whether it might be effective in a specific disease but need the expertise of a medicinal chemist to answer that question. Or perhaps you are studying a microbe but are focussing on its impact on the gut whereas another individual is focussing on its impact in the lungs. Or maybe someone has a new assay or other technique that they have been applying to one area but not to another.

These types of collaborations generally emerge not because you started up a conversation at a meeting—in fact, most of these people would not attend the same meetings as you, so there would be very little opportunity to meet in the first place. Nor do these collaborations form out of mutual interest or for simple practical reasons. Rather, these develop from premeditated efforts on your part to reach out because you need help of some sort. For example, you may recognize a deficiency in your own research expertise or an unanswerable scientific question and recognize the imperative to extend your work in a new direction to make it more effective and successful; while you could learn some new skill or buy some new piece of equipment, it makes more sense to have someone who knows the landscape well help you out. Another possibility is that you have a brand new idea and realize that you simply can't do it on your own since it will entail incorporating an area of science with which you have no familiarity. And the third is because you come across someone else's work—perhaps through accident or because someone mentions it to you— and you realize that what she is working on could greatly impact your work in a positive way.

Forging these collaborations with people outside of your field is a special and complicated case and deserves some detailed discussion. The first thing to recognize and appreciate is that the "culture" of their field and work may be very different from your own. These cultural differences can be subtle or stark depending on the field. When I mean, culture, I am speaking broadly about the standard social and political order of a field. Some fields are more hierarchical than others or may be more experimental or theoretically based, whereas others may be more organic in their general approach to ideas and experimentation. And the individuals in these fields may be unfamiliar or only vaguely familiar with your field and likely quite unfamiliar with your small territory within that field. So those differences can be quite challenging to navigate. On the other hand, if they are in an allied field, the culture may be similar and the researcher may already be working with other biomedical researchers.

For example, I have had the good fortune to collaborate with several engineering professors at the Massachusetts Institute of Technology (MIT). As you probably know, MIT is one of the world's premier engineering institutions and the school can boast a bevy of Nobel laureates and other notables on their faculty and amongst their graduates at any time. But the culture of MIT is unique and very different than my own world of healthcare and biomedical research. For example, most professors at MIT have a group of graduate students and maybe a couple of post-doctoral students doing much of the research. The professors oversee the work and stay involved, but the graduate students themselves often drive many of the day-to-day research decisions. The professors have a variety of other obligations and overseeing the student's work is only one piece of a much bigger set of responsibilities and interests. This is very different than my situation where I am constantly in the trenches, guiding my team on a regular basis as we try to move our whole research effort forward.

Thus, when I first extended out my interest to a potential collaboration to an electrical engineer (whom I had actually met through my wife through a social context), I was a little surprised about the approach taken. Yes, the researcher had some broad ideas about the work and assisted in the grant application, but once we were funded, nearly all the day-to-day work fell into the hands of a group of graduate students. The professor would meet with the graduate students weekly to discuss progress for 1 hour or so, but that was, for the most part, the extent of the involvement. I ended up working directly with the graduate students involved in the project quite a bit. But the work progressed well and in the end we had a lot to show for it.

Another example of what could be considered a huge cultural difference is when you are collaborating with industry, such as a pharmaceutical company. Working with industry is sufficiently complex that I have devoted a separate chapter to that entirely (see Chap. 32). But I would just mention here that while industry may be used to working with physicians and outside biomedical researchers, depending on the type of company you are dealing with, the interactions could be quite strange for you since the cultures are so different. A company may be surprisingly cautious about what it reveals about its ongoing work and recent data or its long-term strategies and interest. Moreover, companies can be remarkably "stovepiped" in their strategies, with one group within the company working on one area of interest and another working on something quite unrelated, with very little interaction between the two. You may find yourself communicating with people who often don't have any idea what another person is doing. Also, the time scale can be remarkably slow. Pharmaceutical companies, for example, have a time line toward drug approval that can stretch out for a decade or two. Getting a drug to market is not a sprint but something more akin to an ultra-marathon. But as an individual academic researcher, you are not likely to be thinking 10 or 20 years ahead in terms of our own research or lab, but rather toward the next grant application. Finally, when working with companies, especially larger ones, you may feel like you never quite know who is making the decisions and that uncertainty as to who is in control can seem strange.

Other cultural differences may be more field-specific depending on what you are doing. For example, early in my work, I collaborated with physicists, who did both experimental and theoretical work. While they were interpersonally terrific people, seeing clearly across the aisle between our fields was something of a challenge. Physicists tend to view ideas as unalterable laws with rules that make sense in some deep, fundamental, and ultimately elegant way; most physicians and biomedical scientists, in contrast, see physiology and disease as an incredibly complex web of interacting parts that are often very hard to understand and not always very elegant. In the medical field or biology more broadly, as soon as you conceive of a rule or a relationship, you can usually find many exceptions to it. Moreover, it is often ridiculously challenging to even be sure what is cause versus effect or whether a potential mechanism is the critical link between disease and health or an unimportant sideshow that you shouldn't be wasting too much time on. These differences in culture were very challenging to navigate.

Another challenge is terminology and language. It is actually quite a strange experience to start working with someone in an entirely different field than your own. First, you feel like you have to explain some of the most basic concepts—concepts that you think everyone who finished grade school should know—recognizing that you have forgotten how much you have learned and incorporated into your own vocabulary without even being aware. Even the simplest of acronyms may require a detailed explanation. And, of course, the opposite is true for your potential new colleague, in that he may also find himself struggling to explain what may seem to him to be so "obvious" as to not even require a moment's consideration. For the most part, this simply requires a concerted effort on both of your parts to make sure that you understand each other's work to the best of your capability and to be empathetic toward the other person's relative ignorance with your own field.

Once you have committed to working together on a project, it would seem to make the most sense to start small. But, in fact, many collaborations emerge at the time of a grant application—perhaps because an investigator recognizes the need to have input from someone in a different field, far removed from his area of expertise. But before the application is submitted, some preliminary data may be needed, and thus the two begin collaborating often hoping to generate some data in short order. Regardless of the exact mechanism, working on a small project together is generally a good way to start rather than biting off too much at once. Perhaps focussing on a small study, which involves limited data collection and paper writing, is a good way to understand each others' idiosyncracies, general work practices, including email habits and work hours, and how many other projects they have going on.

Practical aspects of collaboration. Once you have established a working collaboration with another investigator or lab, things generally settle into some kind of rhythm, depending on the nature of the collaboration. Close collaborations could entail frequent emails, phone calls, teleconferences, and Skype meetings either on a weekly or even more regular basis. Other collaborations may require considerably less frequent interaction, perhaps just biweekly or monthly. Regardless of the nature of the relationship, however, it is important that communication always remain open and that everyone remains accessible to one another.

Moreover, the collaboration is likely to be much more than just your working with another investigator. More likely than not, your entire labs may be involved in the collaboration to a lesser or greater extent. This means that you will need to ensure that there are multiple levels of communication, which will hopefully prevent individual misunderstandings from interfering with the overall research effort. It usually works best if individual members of your team know whom to reach out to on the collaborative team rather than always working through you or the other PI. For example, a post-doc from lab may interact preferentially with a post-doc from the other lab or a graduate student in one lab may work with a research assistant in the other. Generally, whatever is set up should not be necessarily hierarchical (i.e., post-docs only conferring with other post-docs) but build organically from whatever the specific situation demands. For example, a research assistant in one lab may be supplying the data to the post-doc in another lab for analysis. The more closely you work together, the better considered the infrastructure needs to be. Leaving everything to chance or simple evolution may be risky, and thus some forethought to sort these things out may be useful.

Regular combined meetings, if you are working closely, are very important. But both PIs need to be involved in these to help ensure that everyone is moving together in thoughts and actions. These can be in-person, via teleconference call, or via the Web, but whatever means is taken, they should be on a standing schedule. This is especially important for collaborations that are somewhat less well integrated. If there are not regular opportunities for all the team members to interact with one another, the likelihood of miscommunication or weakening of the collaboration is quite possible. I cannot overstate this point: it is very critical to have regularly scheduled meetings at a minimum on a monthly basis to help ensure a fruitful team effort. Sometimes you may feel that a discussion is not really needed, and that the project is moving along smoothly and you are wondering why you are even bothering having the meeting. Yet, inevitably, you will find that issues will arise simply because you are all discussing the project that just were not voiced during regular day-to-day business. You may suddenly find that one minor issue brought up as an aside by one of the research assistants at the end of the meeting turns into an entirely new discussion with important implications for the whole effort. This underscores once again the critical need to have regular meetings, even when there don't really appear to be any agenda items to discuss beforehand.

Another important aspect when setting up a collaboration is to ensure that issues like authorship on publications is discussed and agreed upon ahead of time. In my personal experience, this has generally not been a major problem, since most papers resulting from the work generally have a clear hierarchy as to who did what work and who should have the highest ranking (i.e., being first author), with usually one PI serving as senior author and the other PI as second senior author. If there are issues concerning who should get top billing, one way of settling the matter is by giving both first authors (and/or both senior authors) that recognition by placing an asterisk by the name and noting that both contributed equally to the manuscript. This is not an ideal solution, but it is an effective way of helping to ensure that everyone gets their due. And, of course, you can switch order on the next publication just to keep everything even.

Similar decisions relating to grant applications and financial decisions should also be set up a priori. For example, if applying for NIH funding, do you want to apply as co-principal investigators or would it be better to go separately, perhaps with one serving as PI and the other as co-investigator? There are advantages and disadvantages to both decisions. Submitting an application as co-PIs means that you are both getting equal billing; on the other hand your project may be lopsided in responsibilities—i.e., one team doing a lot more work than the other—and in that case, it is probably better to go with the approach of having one person serving as PI. A thorough discussion of grant finances also goes along with this, and it is important that both groups request the money they need to actually do the planned work.

Disputes. No collaboration is generally entirely without some friction. Unlike your lab, perhaps, in which there may be a pretty definite hierarchy and no one is going to get into a major argument with you, the principal investigator, in collaborations, no one is clearly boss and it may be that there are times when some of the research staff are not getting along perfectly with one another. Generally, if communication is open, things work well, but at times an issue may get escalated to the point that you need to intervene to help ensure that everything keeps functioning smoothly. Better yet, however, is to check in regularly with your staff to ensure that things are working. And just asking "how is it all going" may not be sufficient. You may need to just sit down and talk for a while. It is always amazing to me how things generally start being brought up when people have been talking for a while that may not arise with a directed question. An ounce of prevention here can be worth a pound of cure, and your identifying an incipient problem could help head off a major problem down the road.

The problems are more substantial when the PIs start to have a dispute about some aspect of the research. Perhaps it is over the distribution of grant money, or authorship, or perhaps on the day-to-day running of operations, or perhaps simply on the philosophy of the enterprise. People do research for a variety of reasons, and you may discover that your goals may not be entirely aligned or that one individual's personality, which you were willing to accept as "difficult" at the start of the collaboration, has transformed into something more akin to "intolerable." Another area where there is cause for a potential problem is if there is friction between team members between your two groups that gradually escalates because neither of the principal investigators are willing to take responsibility or to try to help fix the situation.

Regardless of the specifics, I think significant disputes between PIs are actually fairly rare. Politeness and general goal-oriented behavior prevents two successful researchers from becoming too enraged with one another, and if there is a problem, these can generally be worked out. However, in the rare circumstance that a problem develops in which there is no resolution, sometimes it is necessary to appoint a third person to serve as a fair arbiter. In fact, NIH grant applications in which you are planning to have two or more co-PIs, require a brief section on dealing with potential conflicts. One way of achieving this is by naming a person to serve as adjudicator to deal with this challenge. This person would presumably be someone you would both trust and feel would not show favoritism to one side or the other and who could withstand the trial of being put in such a challenging position. Alternatively, you each could reach out colleagues to serve as your "seconds" (to borrow from the dueling vocabulary) and see if they can settle the dispute. It is important to recognize that such methods of problem solving still depends on both researchers generally respecting one another and being willing to accept the decision of an independent party. If the interactions have deteriorated to the point that there is actual acrimony, it maybe impossible to find an amicable resolution. But if there is a large ongoing funded grant application, it is better to work through these issues than simply telling the funding organization that you had to quit because you couldn't get along. While fortunately these situations are decidedly rare, it is good to be aware that they can occur so that you can try to avoid things escalating to the point of intolerability.

The life cycle of collaboration. As the previous section has pointed out, collaborations can and usually do come to an end, usually amicably. And thus to some extent, like any research effort, a multi-laboratory collaboration may at some point live out its useful life and it may be time to bring it to conclusion. Collaborations have beginnings—tentative steps toward working together, perhaps in the acquisition of pilot data together or the writing of a manuscript in which one group needs input from another group—to mature years—when the collaboration is going full-swing and data are being collected and analyzed and papers being written. Usually the mature years are associated with a significant amount of funding helping to ensure a successful effort and also to have a new goal established by the grant itself. And then after a period of time, the groups may start to diverge. Perhaps the question or research area that brought the groups together has been settled for the most part or perhaps the work can no longer be successfully funded. Or, less likely, perhaps friction has developed to the point that the group effort is no longer sustainable. Or perhaps one of the collaborators has retired, has taken a distant job and moved to a far away location, or has had unexpected health problems or has even passed away.

Whatever the case, it is important to recognize that most work, including even very successful collaborations will not last forever or even as long as you would like. Taking the long view toward collaborations, like all of research, is a healthy behavior, since it helps keep your eye on the big picture and less so on the moment-to-moment concerns of getting a paper published or a grant application submitted. But also remember, just because a collaboration comes to an end, does not mean it may not be reborn at some later date when a new interest or idea or perhaps a specific grant solicitation is announced.

Summary. Like so much of research, successful collaboration is a skill that is acquired gradually over time, not something that you've been specifically taught how to do well during your training. While collaboration can have its challenges, it can also have amazing rewards and if you want to achieve anything truly great in the realm of biomedical research in the early twenty-first century, it is almost a necessity. Just remember that it is not usually just you and the other PI collaborating, but your entire research teams, and making sure that things are running smoothly requires some degree of integration and constant attention to communication, aiming to head off problems at the pass. I think of all necessities in research, becoming a successful collaborator often requires the greatest skill and takes the longest time to learn, as you try to understand the specific knowledge and terminology of a different area of science, the personalities and work habits of your peers, and the very distinct culture in which they work.

Part III
Successful Paper and Grant Writing

Chapter 14
Writing a Successful Research Paper. I—Up to the Point of Submission

Entire books are devoted to the writing of research papers. And thus my effort here is not to emulate those efforts in exquisite detail, but rather to provide an overview to the creation of a successful paper and seeing it through to publication. Writing papers, like writing grants, is something that improves and speeds up with time. However, there remain several key elements to making the entire process less painful. I hope to share with readers some of my ideas here.

So where to start? Say, for example, that you are in the midst of collecting data for some grand study but realize that you already have something useful and important to put into print. And in fact, as a general rule, if you are involved in investigator-initiated research, you should be thinking about potential early papers supporting your hypothesis prior to any major publication that may come at the end of the entire effort. So as you start to think about writing a paper, there are some basic questions you should be considering:

Who is your audience? As you start to craft your manuscript, it is extremely helpful to decide on your audience before you do anything. Is this going to be a paper geared toward basic scientists working in a very specific area in your field? Or is it a paper that is going to be geared toward a subspecialized clinical audience, such as cardiac electrophysiologists or thyroid cancer specialists? Or is it a paper with broader research appeal—perhaps an epidemiological analysis of health care patterns?

What journal(s) should you consider? Once you have decided on your audience, I think it is very helpful to decide on a journal next. The advantage of selecting a journal early in your writing process is that it can help you gear your writing to the journal's audience. This is important because knowledge assumptions are always made when writing an article and even though you may provide background information in the introduction that may help even a reader inexperienced in the area access the information, it is unrealistic that you can provide all the background necessary regardless of a person's specialty. Thus, picking a journal makes your storytelling simpler from the beginning. On top of that, the article structure, as outlined by the journals, is often different with some imposing limitations to the word count in the introduction or in the methods sections or the number of tables or figures.

© Springer Science+Business Media New York 2016
S.B. Rutkove, *Biomedical Research: An Insider's Guide*,
DOI 10.1007/978-1-4939-3655-7_14

Also, you may find yourself wanting to write the article for a specific type of research article (such as a brief communication versus a full length research article). Knowing those options right at the beginning of the writing process can be extremely helpful. Moreover, abstracts often vary markedly in style between journals, some requiring subheadings and some a freely organized paragraph, usually with vastly different lengths. Titles also have different limitations in terms of length and use of abbreviations. In addition to all of those issues, it is also very helpful to know the citation formatting ahead of time since this may become time consuming. Although reference formatting programs such as Endnote® and Mendeley® are extremely useful (more on this later), there are still some issues with references that are good to know ahead of time, saving you effort down the road, the main one being the placement of the citations within a sentence. The bottom line is that choosing your target journal early will save you a great deal of time down the road.

But what journal should I choose? One of the biggest mistakes new investigators make is aiming to get their article into the highest-level journal conceivable. I recall I sent one of my early publications, which was evaluating a specific type of electromyographic test, to *The New England Journal of Medicine*. This may sound silly, but it was on a relatively broad topic and my co-authors and I convinced ourselves as to the article's broad reach and potential importance. Of course, it was swiftly rejected. So you should realize that there is no specific need to get all of your articles into *Science or Nature*. Sure, if you end up in the position of sending an article there, great. But generally, the breakthroughs most of us make in our work are fairly modest and of sub-sub-specialty interest. Therefore, don't fall victim to visions of grandeur and keep your goals modest. In less high-profile journals, you will find the reviewers much more accepting and the editors easier to work with. Aiming too high could also waste a lot of time. If you are repeatedly sending articles to high-level journals, the amount of effort in reformatting to a different journal is painful, plus you may be waiting weeks or months to hear back on each submission. It is much better to get an article moving through the review and revision process than repeatedly having to start over again.

How important is the impact factor? Many researchers focus on a journal's impact factor when deciding whether to submit an article to it. The impact factor refers to a number generated by the average citation rate for an article published in that journal in the 2 years after it is published. The higher the impact factor, the more the articles that are published by the journal that end up being referenced in future articles during those 2 years. A journal with an impact factor of 2.3 means that, on average, each article published gets cited in another article 2.3 times in the first 2 years after publication. Similarly, a journal with an impact factor of 20 means that on average an article that gets published in that journal gets cited 20 times. And to some extent impact factors are self-generating. The higher the impact factor a journal has, the more often those articles get cited, since people consider that journal high profile and would rather use an article published in that journal as a reference. So the process of "maturing" a journal from one with a relatively low impact factor to one with a high impact factor is actually a pretty long and arduous, and there is only so much the editors can do to achieve that, especially if it is in a pretty subspecialized area of work.

Impact factors are also problematical in that they are calculated from the arithmetic mean of citations to published articles; but in fact, publication citations, like wealth distribution, follow the power law. This means that just a handful of publications that are cited extremely frequently can raise the impact factor for the entire journal. Journals can also help manipulate their impact factors by publishing review articles which generally get cited more than articles describing original research; they may also "bury" some smaller articles and make them non-citable.

Another issue with impact factors is that they only count articles cited within 2 years of publication—a very arbitrary cutoff. In truth, much work builds gradually over time, and early work in a new area may not be noted or cited (except by the authors themselves on future articles) for years. For this reason, many individuals have been downplaying the value of the impact factor in recent years, although the journals that have high impact factors are always happy to tout them. I personally think the whole impact factor argument is a bit overstated. It helps to have high-profile publications when you are applying for jobs, submitting grant applications, and looking for a promotion. But honestly, having a number of strong articles with excellent science, in smaller subspecialty journals with relatively low impact factors, is far more valuable than having just one or two articles in very high-impact journals.

Should I publish in an open access journal? Everything today is about open access, and ensuring that your paper sees the light of day by having it freely available online is a superb idea. The problem is that the open access movement has also led to creation of many journals that are pretty much only out there to make a buck by publishing virtually anything and charging the authors several thousand dollars to have the imprimatur of its having been published in a peer-reviewed journal, and being available on the web as a free download. While I strongly suggest all authors consider publishing in open access journals, there are several pros and cons to consider.

First, and perhaps most importantly, if the National Institutes of Health or other US governmental organizations funded your work, it will automatically be made open access 1 year after the date of publication (that is, as long as the appropriate online forms have been completed) in PubMed Central (not to be confused with PubMed). Thus, there is really no value whatsoever in publishing such funded work in an open access journal for thousands of dollars, unless you need the article to appear in freely accessible print immediately after it is published. Now, if your work had no funding or was funded by a foundation, you will not be able to have it published in PubMed Central for free. Thus, if you feel that your work would benefit from open access publication, you should strongly consider this option. But remember, most researchers, if they are working at a university and the journal is not excessively obscure, will likely be able to access the journal and the article through their online resources as soon as it is available from the journal. Finally, there is no reason that you as an author cannot simply send an interested reader the article as a PDF (presumably even in non-open access journals the submitting author is provided a free electronic copy). There is nothing illegal in this and in fact author contact information (i.e., email address) is typically accessible on the Web exactly for this purpose.

Since publication costs for open access journals add up quite quickly, it makes sense to use this sparingly and hopefully achieve open access through free mechanisms, such as PubMed Central. And importantly, there are some journals that actually provide free open access. Also, if you are from an underprivileged country or have minimal funding, many open access journals will discount the cost to you, so it is always worth checking.

The bottom line is that the open access movement is very much in its infancy and I think we will continue to see substantial changes in this over the coming years. But the idea that all literature should be available to all people is definitely taking hold, and I strongly endorse it. Just don't be bamboozled into paying huge out of pocket costs when you don't need to.

Are there authorship issues of which I need to be aware? Usually, figuring out authorship is not a huge problem for papers. There is one primary person involved in the research—usually the more junior person doing the grunt work and generating the first draft of the article. This person may be a junior faculty member, a fellow, a resident, a post-doc, a graduate student, or perhaps even a very dedicated research student. Occasionally, there are two or even three people who contribute evenly to that effort. In that case, as noted earlier, you may want to make them all first authors, which can be done with the use of asterisk after the names of each and a clarification in the header beneath the title explaining that all contributed equally to the paper.

There are a few other worthwhile authorship issues to consider. First, it is usually a good idea to decide on authorship before the writing of the article ever commences, and perhaps more importantly, even before the project commences. That way expectations will be set accurately from the beginning. If each person understands his or her own role in the project, they will set their prospects accordingly and will dedicate time and effort commensurate with the amount of recognition they expect to deserve. Of course, this doesn't always work out neatly. Sometimes the person who takes primary responsibility in article loses interest or becomes distracted with other efforts and another team member, who was supposed to have only minor role in the project, ends up doing most of the work. So keeping the conversation dynamic as regards everyone's role in the project is important.

Another useful thing to remember is that there may be more than one paper coming out of any single project. "Slicing the salami too thinly" may not be great for the overall research effort and thus should be avoided. On the other hand, if the work does lend itself naturally to division in some fashion, this may be worth considering since it will allow multiple people to enjoy being first or last author on article.

People who have only contributed minimally really should not be included as authors, but all people who have been involved in data collection, analysis and writing, and reviewing of the paper can be included. (Some journals offer specific guidelines as to what they consider appropriate for people to be considered authors. The number of authors on scientific papers has increased substantially over the past few decades, for a variety of reasons, and I am not certain that this is all bad, as long as everyone has done their share.) For those people only peripherally involved in the project, a simple acknowledgement may be all that they expect and all that they should receive.

In short, determining authorship and author order on a paper is not usually a huge issue. And some simple preventive medicine can really help obviate any problems down the road.

Who should do the writing and how? Another obvious aspect to authorship is the actual writing of the paper. To be an author on the paper does not mean you actually have to write any part of it, though it should include at least a review and approval by each of the contributors. But the writing of the first draft of the paper itself is a task that is sometimes hardest. Clearly, if you are just starting out, writing that first draft of a paper should rightly fall in your hands—your mentor would probably strongly suggest this, so that you can get as much practice as possible in the art. In contrast, as you move up the ranks and gradually increase in seniority, it is important to give other people the opportunity to write various sections of the manuscript and possibly the whole thing, when you yourself someday become a mentor. So for a given article, it depends on how much of it should be a learning experience for the younger investigators versus its simply being the report of a scientific investigation and nothing more. Clearly, if you are working on a project and it is very time sensitive (e.g., a new gene discovery or important mechanistic insight) that really needs to get out immediately, it is probably better for the most experienced member of the group to take charge and write much of it, with contributions from the rest of the team as needed. If a more leisurely pace can be taken such that others can participate, it makes sense to give the entire initial manuscript development to the person or persons primarily responsible for the work.

When larger teams are involved in a project, I find sometimes it is more efficient, and everyone is happier, when we divide up the sections a bit, with the people who were doing the experiments writing the methods sections, the people more involved in the analysis helping with the results and drafting the figures, and the people who understand the big context of the work (usually senior members and I) taking the lead in the introduction and discussion sections. Without fully understanding the context and broader applicability of the work, those last sections can be really challenging to compose, and you'll find yourself rewriting them in their entirety. While this can be a useful exercise for a junior person, it can also be a huge waste of time. Again, much of this depends on the urgency of the getting the publication and the specific roles of the people involved in the study.

One final comment on writing: if there are people who are non-native English speakers, or you are not one yourself, they should be given the opportunity to compose a first draft. Although this can be very challenging, it is an incredible learning experience, and it is the only way they will start to learn fluency of the scientific language. As an aside, English has become almost international language of the biomedical sciences, so if you are thinking of submitting a paper to a foreign language medical journal, I would probably just forget about it.

Where do I begin? OK, you have decided on your audience, you have selected your journal, you have figured out who should be authors, and who should take on specific aspects of the writing, so what next? You will first need to know what you are going to say and, in my view, that generally means looking at your data and creating the figures and tables that really are the backbone of the results section and the research article as a whole. Why did you do the experiment in the first place and what are the results showing you? What are the most salient aspects of the results that have the biggest scientific meaning and overall impact? This is really the first effort that should be made since knowing the results you want to highlight (or perhaps need to highlight depending on your study design and pre-specified outcomes) is critical to getting the right message across. And then you can ask yourself, what other ideas do you want to get across in terms of outcomes?

Once you have sorted out the main figures and tables that you envision in the manuscript, it probably makes the most sense to write the results section. I think starting with the results section is often simplest since that information is ultimately the most important thing that you want to convey. Remember, the results section itself can be relatively low in word count if much of what you are trying to say can be conveyed in the figures or tables that are part of the results section. It sometimes amazes me how short result sections can end up being, especially considering the length of the methods section, the introduction, and the discussion sections. Yet this section is what the entire paper is built around. In one sense, you can think of the article as a bird's nest with a couple of eggs in it, the eggs being the results themselves. The rest of the article is just there to support the results.

The methods section. The methods section is usually relatively straightforward to write since you are just describing what you did. Breaking the tasks down sequentially or into smaller categories, such as "Subjects, Measurement Techniques, Genotyping, and Data Analysis" and such can greatly simplify the organization of a methods section and not force you to connect up often dissimilar areas. One point of caution especially with the writing of methods sections: don't plagiarize. If you are using well-established methods or those you or other have published elsewhere, try to ensure that you are using your own words to describe the technique and reference accordingly. Remember, you can greatly simplify your methods section by referencing liberally. To avoid inadvertently plagiarizing, even if it is just a very mundane section of the data collection process, just make sure you are altering the wording sufficiently to ensure it is truly different. Many journals now have automatic plagiarism detection software, so you need to be especially careful about this. It would be bad form to get accused of plagiarism even if you are doing it inadvertently or because you are rushing to get a paper submitted. And it is even more embarrassing to be found having plagiarized your own work. Remember that just because you wrote the earlier language, the moment it is published, the journal usually holds the copyright.

The introduction and discussion sections. I usually work on these together since to some extent some of their material may overlap. As the introduction implies, it introduces the topic and explains the rationale for studying a topic and the expected results. The discussion, in contrast, provides insights into the results in relationship to the wider body of literature that already exists and probes deeper into the meaning of the results and its limitations. One good way of thinking about what should be in the introduction and what you should hold for the discussion is to outline the points of interest, and then err on the side of making the introduction too short (in fact, some journals have word limitations to ensure that introductions don't drag on). Most readers generally want to get to the meat of the experimental work and results and a long, drawn out introduction section can just be distracting and boring.

The first paragraph in the introduction can begin with a simple few sentences discussing the current state of affairs on the topic you are introducing, and moving from general to specific—namely your study. Though, I would make an admonition against starting too broadly. For example, many papers in the field of amyotrophic lateral sclerosis begin with a very similar sentence, something along the lines of, "Amyotrophic lateral sclerosis remains a uniformly fatal disease without an effective therapy." Virtually any reader who is interested in your article knows this fact and to simply reiterate the concept in the introduction serves little value. So start broadly but not to the point of obviousness.

The next paragraph or two in the introduction should gradually hone in on the specific area of interest that you will be studying and set up the research question to be studied. And then I like to respond to that question with an answer of sorts—namely here is how we are going to do that and this is what we are going to talk about. In that way, the introduction will end by leading you directly into the methods section. And this approach of first introducing the section and then creating the problem to be solved provides a nice "arc" of sorts—building tension followed by resolution, even before you get into any of the experimental details. Just because you are writing a research paper does not mean it can't have some modest drama to it.

Introductions are generally devoid of figures, but sometimes a figure in an introduction can help effectively set the stage or help explain a more complex topic to assist a reader in more easily understanding the main thrust of the article. If such a figure can also save words and streamline the text, it is also worth considering.

Then you will get to the discussion section, which I personally find the most enjoyable to write, in part because you can take the most liberties in the structure of this section. The goal here is really to put the details of your results into context of the broader body of literature, discuss some of the unexpected aspects of your findings, some of the limitations of the work (and even the best work has a multitude of caveats and uncertainties), and then ideas for future studies that might build off of this one. Small bits of the discussion may overlap with the introduction section, and that is okay, as long as you find yourself not simply repeating things. Like the introduction, if it is possible to include some tension-release in the discussion section, you should try to do it, though the discussion tends to not lend itself to any real drama.

As a general rule, don't overstate the importance of your work. Reviewers and readers usually don't like it when the author sounds like he is boasting about the results of his study. Try to stay as dispassionate and self-critical and skeptical as possible, since in all likelihood this skeptical interpretation of the results is closer to the truth than a more unabashedly enthusiastic one. I also find a paragraph specifically delineating the limitations of the study as an effective method of capturing and solidifying that self-criticism. Really try to think through all the ideas you may have missed in designing the experiment or interpreting the results and try to include those concepts in this section.

Writing the abstract. Once you have written the article, go back and write the abstract. I generally hold off on this until last since it is only at that point that I have a good sense as to the entire thrust of the article and the ways in which it is most important. As mentioned earlier, journals have widely varying abstract formats, from single blocks of text to formatted sections that mimic a mini-paper of sorts. Make sure you know what format you need to use for the specific journal you are writing. Also, make sure to actually include some real data in the abstract and not just vague statements, since 90 % of your readers will only read the abstract. If at all possible, make sure this data will help convince a casual reader that your conclusions are based on facts.

Referencing. Frankly, it is never exactly clear to me when one should start adding in the references; I think this mostly depends on personal preference and one's familiarity with a specific topic on which she is writing. If you generally know the subject matter of your paper quite well and that all the information you will be including in the introduction and discussion is actually accurate, then it probably makes more sense to write up most of the article and then go back and start finding references to support the declarative sentences that would not be considered general knowledge. On the other hand, if the topic is relatively unfamiliar to you, it sometimes can be more effective to add in references as you write to help ensure you are not veering off into inaccuracies. Regardless, before you begin writing you should be sufficiently familiar with what you are going to say such that you do not need to read up on everything that you are putting down in words. In practice, I tend to write a rough first draft without references, adding in a simple notation (e.g., an asterisk) to point out where I should add in a reference later; that approach helps speed things along nicely when I come back to the paper later.

Using a referencing program is critical, of course. Not only will it speed your referencing for future papers, but also if you need to revise the paper later, it will allow you to add in new references easily and automatically renumber them all. Another advantage is that if you end up needing to submit the paper to a different journal, it will save you considerable time in changing the references since it often seems that no two journals have identical citation or bibliographic formats. One note of caution: if you are working with collaborators, it is important to make sure you are all using the same referencing program and that you've created a shared library.

Finish off your tables, figures, and figure legends. Once you have the bulk of the article written, make sure you go back and clean up your tables, figures, and figure legends to ensure they are clear and easy to interpret and that the figure legends provide the needed information. I find that figure legends often get the "short-end of the stick" in terms of attention, since we end up spending so much time on other aspects of the paper. But these are really important since the reviewers and future readers may only focus on the figures and their legends and only skim much of the rest of the paper.

Avoiding excessive complexity in tables is also a good rule. Huge tables are a complete turn-off to most reviewers and most readers, so keep these as simple as possible. Most people will never even look at the detailed information in a table, even if this is the simplest and most efficient way to present the data. There are also a number of tricks to shrinking tables down by not making individual columns for every parameter. Many journals also allow supplementary data to be uploaded at the journal's website or to refer to the data at an independent website. Such approaches can be helpful when you find the tables growing too large.

Now take a break for at least a week. Eventually, you will have finished your complete first draft of the manuscript. At this point, the best thing you can possibly do to improve it is to go away from it for a week or longer. After poring over the details for many hours, you will have entirely lost perspective on what is important and what is not, what is well written, what is awkward, and what makes absolutely no sense. So the best thing you can do to get away from it is to simply not look at it for a self-imposed editing hiatus, no matter how badly you want to submit it.

When you do come back to it, it will seem like someone else's work, which is exactly what you want. You may be patting yourself on the back for some of what your earlier-self put into words, but you also may read sections that make absolutely no sense to you. But this is why it is so important to wait. To be able to come back to it with clear eyes and head will make the paper much stronger. You may even identify complete flaws in your logic or omissions that seem to be so obvious that you'll wonder if you were drugged when you had written the first draft. So be aggressive with the editing at this stage and make sure it all makes sense.

Once you have done this, it is probably a good time to give it to a friend, colleague or one of the other co-authors to read and provide feedback. They will likely uncover a number of mistakes and typos that you have completely overlooked and point out areas that make no sense to them. You will be amazed to see how many things you have entirely missed even though you have read the manuscript a number of times. After you have accomplished this set of edits, I will usually put it aside for another week or two and let it age before I take it out and reread it. At this point, you should be coming close to a final version for submission. Reading it aloud at this point can be helpful to catch any remaining typos or small glitches, including sentences that are too long or clumsy.

Writing a cover letter. Most journals require that you include at least a brief cover letter. Nearly all journals also specify other things you need to include in the letter such as how each of the authors contributed to the article, whether there are any conflicts of interest, or whether certain reviewers should be excluded. But in addition to these issues, you also have the opportunity here to make an argument as to why your work is significant. I used to not pay much attention to cover letters and pretty much let the chips fall where they would with the submission of the manuscript itself. However, after serving as an associate editor for a major neurology journal, I have come to realize that the cover letter is a good opportunity to put your best case forward with the editors as to why the work should be published. Often the cover letter is not provided to the reviewers, but in cases where the reviewers are perhaps sitting the fence on the reviews, a strong cover letter providing context for the article may persuade an editorial team to allow the paper to proceed to revision rather than outright rejection. So spend some time on the cover letter and make sure it gets the most salient and important aspects of the article across.

Submission. Submitting a manuscript online is usually a pretty straightforward process, although every website is somewhat different. Some of the larger publishing companies such as Elsevier, Springer, and Thomson Reuters have standard menus to wend your way through. You'll need to list all the authors, titles, submit an abstract, and a cover letter. There are also opportunities to provide any conflicts of interest for any authors. You may also have to state that you are only submitting the article to this one journal (note: while you can and probably should submit grants to multiple funders at the same time, that is not the case with research articles, in which you must submit to only a single entity; if you do more and are found out, sanctions and other issues may apply). You may also have to upload some additional forms such as copyright forms or authorship forms; however, most journals do not require that you do this until the paper is reaching a point closer to acceptance, since it may create unnecessary nuisance work for both, you and for the journal personnel.

Reviewer suggestions. Most journals will give you the opportunity to suggest reviewers and also to request those to whom you would not like the manuscript forwarded (sometimes called "preferred" and "non-preferred" reviewers, respectively). The editors are under no obligation to use or not to use either group. The group of preferred reviewers strictly speaking should really not be friends or collaborators but rather people who are familiar with the topic and can judge the paper in a fair and knowledgeable fashion. Most journals don't make any distinction between friends/collaborators and impartial reviewers, but some do. Journal editors, seeking people who may be able to review a topic effectively, will reach out to them, especially if they are having a difficult time identifying other reviewers.

Non-preferred reviewers—i.e., those people to whom you don't want the manuscript sent—are usually honored, since journal editors realize that there may be a variety of conflicts that could arise, from interpersonal disagreements to different philosophies about a subject to competition in a research area for funding. The only time the non-preferred request is not followed is when the authors submitting a manuscript offer a long list of non-preferred reviewers (which I have seen more than once as a journal editor). If the authors need to exclude such a wide range of people from reviewing their manuscript, there is obviously something amiss. Non-preferred reviewers may also be asked to review a manuscript if no other reviewers can be identified. But if the reviewers are excessively critical a thoughtful editorial team will take these reviewers' non-preferred status into consideration and try not to unfairly penalize the author for having mentioned them.

In many journals you will be asked to include at least one or two suggested reviewers; but in most none will be required. I have suggested reviewers and have papers rejected and not suggested anyone and found the papers readily accepted, so it is all a bit of crapshoot in my mind. And from the other side, I have seen preferred reviewers to whom the article was sent to review come back with scathing commentary and very low priority scores, whereas a reviewer identified by the editors alone came back with glowing comments. The bottom line is that you really don't know what anyone is thinking. The anonymity of the review process may allow people to speak their minds in ways that they would not otherwise do.

Waiting. Once you've had a chance to review the entire document (usually downloadable as a PDF that the reviewers will actually see) and you press the submit button, the work is done, and you can at last relax. The waiting process can be short or long depending on the journal; most journals will take a minimum of 4–5 weeks to get back to you with a decision. Others will take several months. The wait is not usually a result of slow processes at the journal's editorial office. Rather, it is usually dependent on the speed of the reviewers. Reviewers are generally given 2–3 weeks to finish a review after accepting it, and if they are speedy about getting it completed, a decision about the article can be made and relayed to the authors in relatively short order. On the other hand, for most reviewers, reviewing someone else's work falls to the bottom of the priority list and only gets completed after it reaches the top of their queue, which could be weeks, or they are guilted into completing it after receiving nasty notes from the editorial office about not having completed their review. As an ad hoc reviewer for a number of journals, I admit that I generally fall into the middle ground—not taking care of the review immediately, but getting it completed just short of the deadline. That of course would be dependent on my other activities and the personal interest level of the paper for me. However, I always get them completed and almost always on time. Sitting on the other side of the table as an editor has given me a new appreciation for people's review habits. Some reviewers are fast and thorough. Others are slow and superficial. There are certainly those who are fast and superficial and those who are slow and thorough as well. Some are generous with their scores, others are miserly, being critical of everything that crosses their path. I would say, however, most tend to be fairly generous, with few people clamoring for rejection of an article. But there are some reviewers who will agree to review a paper, and then never submit their review, despite repeat personal requests not only from the editorial board staff but also from the journal editors themselves. They'll answer emails saying that they will take care of it in the next few days and then completely fail to do so. Journals make a note of these types and generally will not send papers to them again. And I think the editors will find it hard to look favorably upon articles that they later send to the journal for review.

At any rate, all this is to say that the review process can be extremely variable both in terms of time and the quality of the reviews that are done. But at some point, several weeks or months later, you will receive an email letting you know results of the review for better or worse.

Summary. The development of a research article is a slow process and rushing it is generally not a good thing. However, thinking through each of the multitude of steps from piecing together that initial outline to doing the final submission can actually follow a reasonably logical progression. The major points to remember are: (1) settle author order early in the process; (2) know your audience and preferred journal early on; (3) focus on creating the results section first since those are the jewels that you are going to present and the rest of the article is going to support, and make sure those figures and figure legends are really, really strong; (4) put the article aside at least twice to get fresh perspectives on it as you and your colleagues edit; (5) try to write a strong cover letter since it will help act as insurance if your paper ends up sitting the fence and the editorial team is wondering whether to proceed with it or reject it outright; (6) do not overthink your preferred and non-preferred reviewer lists since in the end it may not make a huge difference one way or the other; (7) enjoy the good feeling that comes with pressing the "submit" button; at least the challenge of putting together the paper will be over until hear you back … usually in several weeks or to 2 or 3 months.

Chapter 15
Writing a Successful Research Paper. II—Revising, Resubmitting, and Post-Acceptance Tasks

Ok. You have submitted your article and you have patiently been waiting for 6 or 7 or 8 weeks. Then as you working through your emails you suddenly see one pop up from the journal to which you submitted the article. You open the email with under-standable tentativeness. As you start to read the response from the journal, you may be surprised to find that the wording is not entirely comprehensible. You were expecting a simple yes or no. But, in fact, there are rarely clear yeses and even a "no" may not mean it is rejected. Thus, one often needs some assistance in interpret-ing the journal's decision letter. So that is what we will approach first.

Interpreting the journal decision letter. Journal decisions generally come in three basic flavors: reject, revise and resubmit, and accept. Let me discuss each of these in detail.

1. *Reject*. If your article is rejected, then it means that the journal is not interested in publishing your article, even if you were to extensively revise it. My recommen-dation on this is simple: read the reviewers' comments, take heed, and revise what you think is reasonable and ignore what you don't think is unreasonable, and send it to another journal. There are many journals out there, and even if you didn't get into your top choice, you will certainly find another. Move on with it. Some authors feel compelled to rebut the rejection, especially if the reviewers seemed to have missed the point or if the reviewers' comments don't seem that damning. But rebut-ting a rejection is almost always a complete waste of time. Even if the reviewers were substantially off the mark in several of their concerns, most editors will not allow for a resubmission of the article. It destroys the peer-review process if they allow themselves to cow under pressure from the authors. They would rather be wrong in rejecting an article than wrong in accepting it.

Some journals, however, do have strange rejection policies. They may say that your article is rejected but then say that if you substantially revise it, you may be able to resubmit it as a new article. Basically, what they are telling you is that the article in its current form will not survive the review process, but if you take heed of the reviewers' comments and completely redo the thing, you can send it in as a

© Springer Science+Business Media New York 2016
S.B. Rutkove, *Biomedical Research: An Insider's Guide*,
DOI 10.1007/978-1-4939-3655-7_15

new article and it may succeed on the second go-round. Generally, smaller, low-impact journals will take this approach. High profile, high-impact journals will generally not waste a great deal of time on an article that was rejected outright though even those may give you an opportunity to resubmit if the editors feel there is something really worthwhile in there.

2. *Revise and resubmit.* A revise and submit decision is usually the best you can hope for on an initial submission. This means that you need to rewrite the paper taking into consideration the comments of the reviewers and the editorial staff. If you are able to do so, the journal will eventually accept your manuscript possibly after one or more additional revisions. So when you get a revise and resubmit decision, you can usually take it that you have crossed the threshold and you probably have a considerably greater than 50 % chance of getting the paper accepted. Though this is not always the case, as I describe next.

In reality, revise and resubmit decisions can often be categorized into two basic types. The first are those articles that are real fence sitters. The editors/reviewers are not wholly convinced that it is worth publishing but it may be. In this situation, if you are able to revise and really deal with the concerns of the reviewers it will ultimately be accepted, but if you do not, it may still be rejected. The second are those that are clearly going to fly with an acceptance, but need some improvement. Unfortunately, the wording of the letter can sometimes make it pretty tough to discern between these two types, since the letter is usually written in a pretty firm style, so as to make sure you take the concerns raised seriously and that you will do your best to fully address them. Here are a few examples of letters from journals (unnamed) that I have received over the years to give you a flavor of the variety of comments and the severity of the language as to the extent of the revisions. I start with the most benign/gentle comments and progress, as best as I can tell, to responses that are more tentative.

1. "The reviewers have now commented on your submitted article, _____, and suggest minor revisions prior to its publication." This is as good as you can usually hope for on an initial submission. It will happen only rarely.
2. "If you can address the points raised by the reviewers, we will be happy to receive a revised version of the paper, but it may be subject to re-review." This too, is unusually positive language on an initial submission of an article.
3. "A number of concerns were raised by the reviewers. If you can address the points raised by the reviewers we will be happy to receive a revised version of the paper, but it will be subject to re-review." This is more typical. You will need to address a number of concerns raised by both reviewers and the editors may send it back the reviewers for their comments (they are keeping their options open).
4. "No guarantee on acceptance can be given at this stage. That will depend not only on your addressing the issues raised by the current Reviewers, but also their numerical ratings of the revised manuscript and the reports of any additional Reviewers that the Associate Editor may need to consult." This too is a pretty typical response in the "revise and resubmit" category.

5. "Although our reviewers found your manuscript to be of interest, they also raised substantive issues about your study. Major revisions would be needed to consider it further. Please weigh carefully the reviewer and editor comments below, and with your co-authors make a determination as to whether you can address the criticisms. If you prepare an appropriate revision, your manuscript will be reviewed again. Please understand that an invitation to revise is not a guarantee of eventual acceptance." This one also is pretty typical, but is starting to increase the uncertainty that it might not make it in, even if you do fully revise it.

6. "Thank you for submitting your manuscript to _____. After careful consideration, we feel that it has merit, but is not suitable for publication as it currently stands. Therefore, my decision is "Major Revision." We invite you to submit a revised version of the manuscript that addresses the points raised by the three expert referees (reports are copied in full below). All three referees raised concerns regarding your study design, interpretation, and conclusions that would need to be addressed for the manuscript to be considered technically sound and therefore suitable for publication. In particular, Referee 1 and Referee 3 remain unconvinced that your conclusions are robust and fully supported by the data presented." This one is getting pretty serious and it sounds like there is the possibility that you may not be able to succeed.

It might of interest to learn that the second to last example (#5) had quite positive reviews, whereas some of the earlier letters were from papers that had decidedly less positive commentary. So if there is anything to be learned from these examples, it is that the language of the "revise and resubmit" decision may or may not say much as to the actual likelihood of paper acceptance. I think the bottom line is that the editors want to reserve the option of rejecting a manuscript for which the authors respond inadequately to the concerns raised regardless of the actual likelihood of acceptance. Some journals use stricter language than others and so what ends up getting written is somewhat arbitrary and hard to compare across journals.

From my own personal experience, only on two occasions have I had an article rejected after receiving a "revise and resubmit" request, and in both cases it happened only after I had redoubled my efforts to address all the reviewers' concerns adequately. These tend to be very frustrating situations because you already feel like you have expended a huge effort and resubmitting a paper not to mention all the weeks or months that have passed as you waited for the reviews to come back. Thus, perhaps the teaching point here is that if you have a paper that sounds like it is going to have a tough time during the resubmission process, it might make sense to send the paper to another journal for review rather than spending a great deal of time and effort revising it for the original journal that may ultimately end up rejecting it after a great deal of time has passed.

Accept (or Accept with minor revision). Usually, you will not receive an acceptance letter until you have revised the paper at least once or possibly twice or thrice. If there are any hesitations about providing a full acceptance, it is usually because there are a few typos or sentences that have been poorly phrased that the editor or one remaining reviewer feels need to be corrected. But, of course, an acceptance is something to feel good about—your paper is going to see the light of a day in a peer-reviewed journal. That is no small feat.

Revising your paper. The process of revising a paper at first can seem a bit daunting. You may have a litany of critiques from two, three, or even four reviewers. Most of the time, reviewers won't write long dense paragraphs of criticisms, but will itemize their concerns. Though some reviewers can go on and on in large, solid blocks of painfully inscrutable text. In such cases, you should go back to that long dense paragraph and start breaking it down into individual digestible points that you can address, one by one.

Once you have itemized the list of concerns, work through them to see which are the most damning—those are usually the ones that require a reanalysis of the data, or worse yet, additional experimental data that you may not have. Addressing the latter type can be very time-consuming and you might need to first consider whether you really want to go through this since it could add many weeks or even several months to the entire submission process. And with additional experiments and analyses, it also possible that the results obtained will be unexpected and potentially in conflict with your earlier results, so you may find yourself rewriting much of the paper or even potentially withdrawing it altogether. Of course, that last possibility would really be a good thing—it is better to forgo a publication than to have poor or inaccurate data out there in the literature. There is plenty of that already.

Importantly, you do not need to do everything the reviewers suggest, as some of their comments may actually be wrong or misguided. Naturally, it is better to generally assume, initially at least, that the reviewers are correct and the paper, as written, is at fault. But at some point you might identify critiques that in your view are just plainly off base, perhaps due to an obvious bias of the reviewer or a misunderstanding of the language used. But be careful: make sure you fully understand what the reviewer is trying to say. It is easy to blow off a concern only to later realize what that the concern was actually quite legitimate, but was phrased in an odd or incomprehensible way. Often reviewers are not spending an inordinate amount of time on crafting their commentaries into beautiful, clear language so, deciphering what they are getting at can be trickier than you might think. And for many, English may not be their first language, so it is important to be forgiving about clumsily written commentary.

As an editor, I have seen a variety of styles that people utilize in responding to the reviewers. Some are sharp and succinct, e.g., "We have rewritten this paragraph for improved clarity" or "Figure 2 has been omitted," and also those that attempt to be more placating, e.g., "We agree with the reviewer that the word choice was unclear. We have rephrased this for clarity." I don't think which approach you take makes much difference. Do whichever feels most comfortable and natural to you.

The greater concern really is when you disagree with the reviewer. If you flat out think a comment is wrong, you should say so and explain politely why the reviewer misinterpreted your meaning. And if at all possible, toss the reviewer a bone. It will help placate the reviewer since they may see the paper again and not take lightly to your summarily ignoring one of their criticisms with a curt, "The reviewer is incorrect." If you simply dismiss their concern out of hand, she will feel that you have not taken it seriously and will be highly critical of the paper on second review, possibly recommending rejection. On the other hand, if you have been careful and polite, at the very worst, she will give you another chance to get it right. So a bad terse response would be "The reviewer is incorrect in the interpretation that the data represents a mere medication side effect. No change has been made." A much better approach would be, "We agree with the reviewer's concern that the findings could represent a medication side effect. Yet, there are several factors that we have identified, that we believe make this unlikely. These include: X, Y, and Z. We have reworded the paragraph in the discussion delineating these for clarity and have also added in two additional points supporting our view. While it remains impossible to exclude this interpretation, we believe the preponderance of the evidence argues strongly against it."

As you start drafting responses to the reviewers, start editing your original paper using "track changes" mode, assuming you are working in Word or another standard program, so that you can keep an accurate measure of what you have changed. I usually go back and forth between a written response to reviewers and the change in the manuscript so that I am not forgetting or skipping over changes. You will need to provide both a written letter of response addressing each concern raised as well as the fully revised paper.

Eventually you will have worked through the litany of criticisms, having addressed each response in a separate document that you will upload along with the manuscript in track changes in mode as well as a manuscript with all the changes accepted. Do make sure you read through the version with all the changes accepted since you will undoubtedly capture some typos along the way and it may be hard to see them when it is all marked up. Then go ahead and resubmit.

The review of a revised paper is much different than the review of original version, unless the paper is real fence sitter in which case the reviews will either make or break the decision for acceptance. If that is the case, and hopefully that status was made abundantly clear in the initial decision, all bets are off. If you have not adequately addressed the concerns you might find yourself rejected. However, in most situations, the reviewers and to some extent the editors feel that they have already done the serious effort of reviewing the paper on the first go-round and will simply look through your responses and edits to make sure they pass muster. It is pretty rare for reviewers to start disagreeing with your individual responses, though it does happen. Most reviewers and editors have too much on their plates to be dealing with such minutiae. If the overall gist of the responses looks reasonable, then the paper will move forward through the review process pretty smoothly. You may still be requested to address several more minor lingering concerns, but once you have been asked to revise a paper a second time, it is pretty rare that your third decision will be a rejection. Most editors realize that is not fair at that point and will try to see your paper through to acceptance. After all, it is not the reviewers' or the editors' job to write the article for you—it is your work that should stand or fall on its own merits. If other people down the road read your paper and disagree with your data, your logic or your discussion or conclusion, they can always send a letter to the editor or email you personally. There is no such thing as perfection. The best you can do is honest, high-quality work. Only time will tell whether the paper is considered valuable.

Post-acceptance tasks. Even after you receive that happy email saying that your paper was accepted, you need to temper your enthusiasm, at least slightly. There is still more work to be done. First you will probably have some online forms to complete—such as the copyright transfer and authorship forms. This is not a huge deal, but does require a little time to complete. Then, usually within several weeks, you will receive the proofs of your paper. Although authors (including me) have a tendency to want to just say everything is OK without giving them a thorough once over, this is a huge mistake. You should definitely slow down and spend a good amount of time working through the proof to make sure that there are no typos or other errors, such as the wrong figure legend being applied to a figure or authors names being misspelled. Today, most proof corrections are done in Adobe Acrobat® or with other online, web-based programs provided by the publisher and it is pretty straightforward to make the changes. But do expect to spend a couple of hours ensuring that everything is as close to perfect as it can be. On the other hand, it is also important to note that you cannot make endless edits to a proof. You need to keep your changes limited to errors and occasional language improvements. If you start making major changes to the manuscript the publisher may contact the editor of the journal to get their approval, which will slow down the process.

Even after submitting the proof, you are still may not be quite done with the article. If your paper was based on funding from any United States governmental agency, such as NIH, NSF, the CDC, NASA, or the Department of Defense, you may now have to upload the manuscript into PubMed Central. This is a good thing, since it means that even if you did not choose an Open Access version for publishing, as noted in the preivous chapter, it will eventually be open access (1-year after the article is officially published). However, this too requires work since you need to ensure that whatever was uploaded into PubMed Central is correct and that there were no mistakes made in the process. Usually, this is not an issue, but the PubMed Central paper, if based on your final submitted and accepted documents and not the final corrected proof, may contain errors that you caught in reviewing the proof. So you'll need to go back and correct those in PubMed Central based on your earlier proof corrections. If the version uploaded into PubMed Central was based on the final published article (usually because you had to do the upload manually rather than its going from the publisher directly, which is becoming more typically the case), you are probably OK, but you should still give it a quick once-over since it is this version that people are probably going to see more than any other over the long haul.

Once the proofs are submitted and the PubMed Central tasks completed, you can now actually feel that the paper has been published and you are done with it. What I find strange is that by the time this happens, the paper feels like stale news. It is usually research that you completed months if not years earlier and may seem virtually irrelevant to anything you are working on currently. So, unfortunately, that sense of real satisfaction is usually not there—the publication of the article almost seems like an aside compared to what is going on in your life at the time. But you should take a moment to take pleasure in your accomplishment—take your colleagues/co-authors out for a cup of coffee or lunch to recognize the success achieved.

As an aside, I will also use this moment to point out an emotional truism about acceptance and rejections. Rejections hurt a lot more than acceptances feel good. In many respects, I think this is analogous to people feeling more upset about losing money in an investment than feel happy when an investment does well. Human beings seem to have a lopsided response to good and bad new, and perhaps there is an evolutionary basis for this. But, regardless, if you get a paper accepted, you may feel "up" for a little while, but that sense of success is remarkably fleeting. There is other work to be done and as just stated, this is often fairly old news—at least to you. So it is hard to feel excessively positive about the whole experience, especially since it may have required a great deal of revision, etc. A rejection, on the other hand, can really sting. It may cast you into a negative state of mind for some time since you may take it as a direct criticism of your research abilities, your writing skills, and your sense of self. You may feel hurt and misunderstood and that the reviewers and editors were just a bunch of idiots. The thought of resubmitting the paper to another journal may seem beyond odious and so distasteful that you want to drop the entire thing. The best thing to do at this point, rather than despairing, is simply walk away from the paper for a week or two. When you come back to it, you will be in a much better frame of mind and will be prepared to do the work necessary to ensure that this work eventually sees the light of day.

Summary. The most challenging process of revision is trying to understand what the reviewers and editors are looking for to make the paper acceptable. It often takes reading between the lines and struggling with changes until you seem to have effectively addressed all the points raised. But with careful work and thought, you can usually bring a "revise and resubmit" decision to successful closure. For outright rejections, it is almost always best to give up and move on to another journal than wasting your time arguing with the editors that they made a mistake. But even after a paper is accepted some last remaining tasks remain, including editing the proof and, if needed, uploading it to a public database, such as PubMed Central.

The process of dealing with revisions on a paper can often be remarkably long and tedious, and at times you may wonder if it is all worth it. But, for better or worse, the basic currency of academic research is the peer-reviewed paper. You simply must consistently and determinedly work through the seemingly endless process of writing, editing, review, re-editing, and re-review until its final acceptance. After all, it is always surprisingly uplifting to have a colleague come up to you at a conference and say, "Hey, I saw your paper in *Journal X*. That was really nice work."

Chapter 16
Funding: An Overview

As a medical student, resident, and even as a junior attending, I spent little time thinking about money and where it came from. Sure, I filled out billing sheets for my clinical time seeing patients and doing procedures, and every month when my department administrator handed me my P&L statement, I glanced at it, not really paying much attention to the details, unable to interpret it. Frankly, at that time, I considered the economics of medicine and medical research somewhat distasteful and undignified. After all, I was an academic physician and my goal was to pursue medical science in its purest form, unsullied by things like money. Money would surely always flow freely because any worthwhile effort would be supported. Right? But exactly how that worked—i.e., the who, what, where, when, and how—I gave only glancing consideration.

But gradually it became clear to me that ignoring the financial aspects of the biomedical field or pretending it didn't matter was flat out right unrealistic. You couldn't expect people to volunteer hundreds of hours to pursue a research project of significance for no recompense. And anyway, the little start-up research package given to me by my department when I first took my job was already starting to dwindle. So I started to look toward foundations and the federal government to help out.

All meaningful biomedical research has had financial backers, and it is inevitable that if your goal is to achieve something truly worthwhile, you will need some kind of funding to start up that investigative engine and keep it running smoothly.

Funding sources. There are several major sources of funding that I will review. These include non-profit foundations, the government, including the National Institutes of Health (NIH), the Department of Defense (DoD), and the National Science Foundation (NSF), smaller intra-institutional grants, benefactors, and industry. In general, obtaining government funding is probably the most challenging and often requires your having some non-profit foundation or intra-institutional funding before you can successfully successfully obtain funding, unless you are

© Springer Science+Business Media New York 2016
S.B. Rutkove, *Biomedical Research: An Insider's Guide*,
DOI 10.1007/978-1-4939-3655-7_16

applying as a trainee—in which there are a number of programs available (see Chap. 21). Philanthropy will also be discussed, as it has its own special complexities, quite distinct from standard grants.

Intra-institutional funding. Generally, funding that is provided by an institution, department, or division is the simplest and most easily obtainable, especially when it comes to new projects being pursued by a junior investigator. Many larger academic research institutions often maintain some kind of internal funding program, but not surprisingly, these are fairly small. People often consider these types of funds as "seed" money since the goal is to provide a small starting point for a new long-term research endeavor. With this kind of money you may not be able to do all that much—perhaps hire a half-time research assistant or buy yourself a little free time to do more of the actual data collection, be it with animals, human subjects, or molecules. Or perhaps you just need one small piece of equipment to start collecting a new set of data that may lead to bigger work. In my view, these kinds of grants are pretty much "no-brainers" for junior investigators. In other words, they should be sought out and applied for. And that is not just because the people reviewing these are your colleagues and will be easy on you. On the contrary, dotting every "i" and crossing every "t" on these is just as important as on the big ones. In a certain respect, doing a top notch job on one of these will not only help to ensure you of successful funding, but will automatically raise your stature. A professional looking grant application means people will take you seriously. Plus it will help you hone your skill set so that you can write better and more compelling larger grants down the road.

The bottom line on these types of grants is to seek them out and apply for them whenever possible, especially when you are just starting out. And if there is no formal mechanism at your institution of which you are aware, make sure you check in with your superiors to make sure that one doesn't exist or if there is the possibility of creating such a mechanism for funding.

Foundations and other non-profits. I am always amazed at the number of organizations out there helping to fund research and support patients with a specific disease. For example, in one of my areas of research interest, spinal muscular atrophy, there are three major foundations: the Spinal Muscular Atrophy Foundation, Cure SMA, and Fight SMA. In ALS, or Lou Gehrig's disease, there are at least a dozen, including ALS Association, Prize4Life, ProjectALS, ALSHope, NEALS, ALS Foundation for Life, Les Turner ALS Foundation, Packard Center ALS Foundation, and the Muscular Dystrophy Association, just to name a few (there are in fact many others). Foundations vary wildly in their approaches to funding and often have a specific "sweet spot" of interests. Some may be more focussed on improving patient care than on actually supporting basic science research, but many are specifically seeking to fund researchers. The most thoughtful and effective associations try to have a 360° view of the disease, aiming to help people with the condition as well as trying to advance research in directed ways.

Depending on the size of the association, it may be more or less regimented in its approach to funding. Some foundations will have yearly or semiannual grant submission periods with a formal review process and pre-published times of announcement and funding initiation. Others may be more free-flowing, funding projects as they arise with a rolling funding process. So once you have found a foundation with which your research interests align, it is worth talking to the scientific director to get a better sense of the possibilities for future collaboration and potential funding.

Unlike government funding or institutional funding, working with an association often means becoming friends with the team and getting to know them at least a little bit, whether it is just at meetings or informally. Foundations also have a specific focus—usually a single disease—or perhaps a few diseases that are tightly associated. When you work with them, you are pretty much only speaking their disease language, since that is all they may care about. While you may be interested in diseases X, Y, and Z, but if you are dealing with a foundation that is focussed on disease Z, disease Z should really be your focus when speaking with them. You may be able to bring in your experience or research ideas as it relates to other conditions, but it is generally only in how it relates to disease Z. You may find yourself needing to become a little bit fanatical about the disease—not because you are putting on an act, but rather because you find yourself being increasingly brought into the field and how it genuinely impacts the lives of the people who suffer from it. Generally, foundations understand the fact that you are being pulled in many directions, but being able to really focus on their one area of concern can really mean a great deal to them and makes you part of the team. There is nothing better than when one of the leaders of the foundation thanks you for all the hard work you have done and continue to do on their disease focus.

Foundations can also be fickle. People change, funding situations vary, and while you may be working in their sweet spot 1 year, you may feel like you are now no longer quite in the fold the next. This is natural and is not to be taken personally. But as you think through your research and you think through who might be willing to fund it, always consider foundations. They are eager to help support a young and inventive investigator if they think this person will help come up with new insights into the disease that may someday lead to a treatment. And like many other sources of funding, they have special grant programs available for young or junior investigators, including fellowship programs.

Governmental sources. This section is meant to offer only a limited overview to the detailed complexities of grants from federal sources. I will provide a detailed analysis of my personal take on how to apply for these grants in the chapters that follow. But there are some general considerations:

The grants can be very large. While most foundational grants have limits of no more than a few hundred thousand dollars over a 2–3 year period, federal grants can easily exceed $1,000,000. The size of the grants allows for major efforts to be funded and sustained. These grants allow you to think big (see Chap. 6 on choosing a research niche) and try to bring a complex or challenging idea to fruition. And a big, expensive project may actually have a shot at getting funded since the vetting process considers the cost last, after the scientific merit of the project has been agreed upon. This is discussed in further detail in later chapters.

Federal grants provide indirect as well as direct funding. This is a concept that is pretty much unappreciated until you are actually in the world of regular grant writing. Direct funding refers to the money that is used to actually fund the research itself. It can be used for: buying reagents, paying staff member salaries, paying your own salary, purchasing animals, or paying healthy volunteers or patients with a disease for their participation. Indirect costs (also called facilities and administration costs or F&A) refer to money that goes to the institution supporting your work (i.e., the hospital or university you work for). These costs help pay for the actual space being used, maintenance for that space, for administrator salaries, utilities, and the like. They are the costs that you pretty much take for granted when you are running a lab but must be paid by someone. The percentage of indirect costs is directly negotiated between your institution and the federal government and will vary depending on the size of the institution for which you work and its location. For example, institutions in large cities will have higher costs than those in rural areas. The amount is negotiated as a percentage of the total direct costs that you bring in minus equipment costs; at my institution it is currently 73 %. This means that for every $100,000 dollars that I bring in to my institution in direct costs, the hospital gets an *additional* $73,000, making the total $173,000. I will pretty much never get to see that $73K, but without it, I wouldn't have a place to do my research.

Unlike the federal government, foundations will often simply not allow any of the money to be used for indirect costs or they will cap it at some low value, such as 10 % of the total direct costs. The foundations don't feel compelled to be paying for heating costs of your building, and it is hard to blame them. They have worked hard to raise their money. So to some extent, the foundations' research interests are being underwritten by the federal government which is helping to sustain the research operation as a whole.

You may ask why institutions even allow you to obtain foundation grants if all they pay is direct costs and your hospital/university is doing it pretty much at a loss. The reason is simple of course: they know that foundation grants may lead to government grants. By not encouraging and supporting foundation grants, you are pretty much cutting your long-term supply-chain.

The different agencies have very different cultures. Most people in medical research receive most of their federal funding from the National Institutes of Health (NIH). This is probably the case since NIH is very large and the work to be funded is directly in their mission—i.e., health. However, the Department of Defense (DoD) and the National Science Foundation (NSF) can be excellent sources of funding. The Food and Drug Administration, the Centers for Disease Control, the US Department of Agriculture, and the National Aeronautics and Space Agency (NASA), also have grant mechanisms that may be applicable to medical-related research, so it is always worth looking outside of NIH. You never know what kind of solicitations are out there or how they might apply to your work. But what one recognizes very clearly when dealing with all of these agencies is that each has its own unique culture and perspective. The DoD tends to be very detailed about its oversight of how you are spending its money, the papers you are writing, and all approvals. NIH tends to be fairly liberal, giving the principal investigator considerable berth to do as he pleases with the grant, as long as he is staying true to what was described in their application. NSF is probably somewhere in the middle. Even within an agency you'll find differences depending on with whom you are specifically dealing. For example, one institute of NIH will be differently than another (e.g., National Institute of Aging versus National Cancer Institute). Part of this may be related to specific individuals with whom you may deal, but it is also broader than just that. Regardless, it is good to try to understand the culture of the people you are going to be dealing with, by talking with colleagues who have had grants from them before, and just interacting with representatives either by phone, email, or at conferences.

Philanthropy. Another important source of research funding is philanthropy. The challenge with philanthropy is that it is highly unpredictable and there is no way to apply for it. One certainly cannot expect large sums of money to just drop from the sky from a wealthy donor interested in your work or from a grateful patient. Moreover, no matter how desperate you are, you do not want to be going out soliciting wealthy friends or colleagues to help fund your research. The impetus to contribute really has to come from them. And if a patient, for example, expresses an interest in supporting your work that is a wonderful thing, but that may not quickly translate into anything tangible. On top of that, you may find yourself feeling that it is inappropriate for you to be asking them to write a huge check to support your nascent research idea or even for your well-established lab, since you should not be mingling your care of them with your desire to be a successful researcher. Even if you don't have those inhibitions or concerns, there is often still no free lunch. You likely will need to court a potential donor for months or even years before you actually see your efforts bear any fruit. In many respects, in fact, I find that applying for funding from foundations and the federal government is far more predictable. At least there are rules that are published and fair. When it comes to philanthropy, there really are no rules. But there are occasional free lunches. Somebody dies and has left a bequest to fund your work and never mentioned it to you. I've known a couple of people who have had the good fortune of obtaining such support. But it is relatively uncommon.

Now I don't mean to sound crass as I discuss this. Asking people for money to fund your research may sound self-serving and greedy. But one needs to remember that these individuals are looking to give away some of their money—they are just figuring out the best way to do it and to whom. If you end up being on the receiving end, it will be a way of their thanking you for pursuing research in something important to them. So don't think of it is as a one-way street. Many people in a position to offer large sums of philanthropy are fairly financially sophisticated and they know what they are doing. So don't feel that you are somehow stealing from them or doing something inappropriate.

Most institutions have development offices that try to help ensure there is a steady stream of philanthropic money. Generally, these offices are filled with intelligent and well-spoken people who can offer useful advice and, more importantly, can help get you out from being stuck in the middle of the process of obtaining money. They can also do a "wallet biopsy" to determine an individual donor's potential for giving. Unfortunately, these offices, while helpful, can't really do the heavy lifting and in the end, it is very much luck and your own efforts that will be needed to bring in successful philanthropic funding. There is no question, however, that these offices can definitely help initiate the conversations and move things along as the deal is getting close to completion.

Industry. Industry money can take many different forms. You can be a site of a large drug study, where you will be recruiting patients and in which you and your institution will get paid for your efforts. Or you may develop a contract with a company whereby you are testing a new drug in your lab using your special mouse model of a rare disease. Or perhaps you will create a new model or cell line that you will provide to industry (under a series of contracts, etc.). Or perhaps a pharmaceutical company will simply give you some new drug to study on your own without any cost but with the promise that they will be acknowledged in all publications. It is always worth keeping a close eye out for potential industry collaborations, because they can help bring an idea to practice very quickly—for example, a new assay that you developed being utilized in their research. Nothing feels better than when a behemoth of a company starts incorporating your new device or drug in their day-to-day research operations.

However, industry can also be remarkably fickle, especially if you are dealing with larger companies. If the vice presidents or Chief Operating Officers suddenly change or if the company is bought up by an even larger company, the focus may abruptly shift and you may find they are no longer interested in supporting you. And in all companies, nearly everyone needs to get approval from someone higher up. And if you are dealing with the pharmaceutical industry, the timeline may be unbelievably long. This makes since you need to consider it takes most new drugs 10 or more years to reach the marketplace—they are simply in no rush, even though you may be. There will also be limitations on publications and you may be forced to sign agreements, along with your institution, that may seem unacceptable, like not publishing on a topic for some preordained period of time or without their express permission. Outside of a large clinical trial where you know that you will be obtaining a set sum of money for your work, many industry relationships are unpredictable. But since the payoff may be large and multifaceted, it is definitely worth interacting with industry at many levels. I will discuss industry relationships in more detail in Chap. 32.

Summary. If you are hoping to be a serious and successful researcher, you are going to need funding. You may be able to complete some simple retrospective chart reviews or even basic clinical studies without any funding or with limited support from your institution. But for your research to survive and flourish, and for your institution to continue to support your work, you will absolutely need a steady flow of cash, and preferably with considerable indirect costs associated with it. Most researchers manage with a combination of sources: federal grants, foundation grants, a little philanthropy, and some industry contracts. But depending on your work and interests (and luck) you may end up finding yourself utilizing only one or two of these resources. No matter what though, grants specifically geared to support your research will likely be the single largest source of money that you will have over the years. So in the next few chapters, I will provide some basic insights into the do's and don'ts of the entire grant application process.

Chapter 17
Where to Apply for Funding: Making the Right Choices

The completion of a grant application is an immensely time-consuming and intensive process. It is therefore critical that you decide to apply for grants that you are most likely actually going to receive. But identifying those potential funding sources can often be truly daunting and a great deal more vexing. With an ever-growing number of foundations and other not-for-profits looking to spearhead research into a specific disease, a large and vast array of federal opportunities, and still other opportunities through universities and research institutions, deciding where to spend your effort in applying for funding is usually not simple. However, it is worth a great deal of time and effort to make the right decision about what to apply for. Submitting a grant application to an organization that is simply not interested in what you are doing is a tremendous waste of time and effort. Similarly, submitting a grant to the right organization but with the wrong funding mechanism is equally self-destructive. And finally, not only do you need to think through whether the funders are on the same page, but you also have to consider whether the people reviewing the grants are also in sync with the goal of the funder. The truth is that before submitting any grant application, you should learn as much as you possibly can. If, after extended review, you have decided that this is indeed a real possibility, only then should you start piecing together the complexities of the application. Bottom line: don't just start applying for the first grant that you come across or because you learn of a single promising solicitation.

Here is a basic approach to finding the best grant opportunities:

Go surfing. It may seem obvious, but the best place to start when searching for an appropriate funding mechanism is the Internet. Searching for the disease you are studying will likely reveal at least a couple, if not several, organizations that are devoted to funding research. Some organizations may be quite large and will fund research in a range of disciplines including the disease that you are studying. Others may be exquisitely focussed, perhaps just on a single disease, or a single type of genetic mutation in a single disease. Most larger foundations have specific descriptions of grant types available to help you hone your efforts more closely.

© Springer Science+Business Media New York 2016
S.B. Rutkove, *Biomedical Research: An Insider's Guide*,
DOI 10.1007/978-1-4939-3655-7_17

In addition to general searches, make sure you spend sufficient effort on the various federal funding sites, especially those of NIH. There is a wealth of information that is available there and you should exploit this to your advantage as much as possible. First, you may want to look at each institute's individual home pages and recent grant solicitations. The NIH websites and the individual institute's pages are very complex, so it is worth spending a great deal of time navigating through their information.

Through extended web searches, you may also be surprised to learn that some agencies fund projects that seem entirely in left field relative to their mission. For example, did you know that the Department of Defense has a grant solicitation specifically geared to muscular dystrophy in children? Or NASA has had grant solicitations evaluating the effects of bed rest on human physiology? So don't discount any one agency prematurely. There may be a lot more out there than you realize.

Actual phone or personal contact is the best way to learn of opportunities and make them realized. It is critical to actually interact with people at government agencies and foundations. At NIH, the people you will want to speak with include program officers at a given institute and also the senior research administrators, or SRAs who oversee the review process. You can usually identify these people through the NIH website and a couple of follow-up emails. Program officers work in a specific institute and are the ones who oversee the grant after it has been funded. They can also assist in helping see a grant through to funding if it is sitting on the edge of fundability—they will fight to have your grant funded, especially if they believe in it and your work. You may also see program officers at meetings as they are expected to interact with the broader research community; this is another good opportunity to meet them and let them get to know you and your work. I often find it extremely helpful just to listen to them—they have a wealth of information and you can learn a great deal about the application process, new initiatives, and new scoring criteria that might make or break a future application. While you can let them do much of the talking, there is also no harm in introducing your own agenda as well. They are used to it.

Similarly, and perhaps even more importantly, really get to know the people in the foundations. Most foundations will find a group of ad hoc scientists to review an application, and while the leaders of a foundation tend to abide by their decisions, they can certainly push things in one direction or another. By contacting people at the foundation, you will likely be able to make yourself and ideas a little better known to them. And even if you don't think they are a good fit, your simply connecting with them may bear fruit in the long term. Foundations really are looking for people to spearhead new research efforts and become part of their extended team. So don't be shy about reaching out more than once.

Who are the reviewers? Knowing who will actually be reviewing your grant is helpful, but not always possible. For example, in some foundations, this may be very difficult. But for NIH and NSF, if you can nail down which study section will review your grant (usually because you have been online looking at their list of standing study sections) you can find a web page that lists the members of the standing study section. Specifically, it will include the names of all the people who were involved in the last review session and the upcoming review session. Of course, you are not actually going to contact these people—in fact, *this is a complete no-no*. Under no circumstance should you actually try to influence a study section's decision by reaching out to the individual reviewers—and if you do, you will find yourself in hot water. However, if you recognize a couple of names on the study section as in your area of interest, and better yet, sympathetic to your ideas, it could certainly mean that this study section would be a good fit. If all the names are unfamiliar and they are in completely unrelated fields, this may suggest that this study section is not a good fit. Of course, if you submit an application that you think belongs in a specific study section and the SRA has agreed, they will likely bring in one or two ad hoc reviewers to help with the specifics of your application. So the people reviewing your grant may still be different than ones you read about on the web.

However, this can also play in reverse. Sometimes having people exactly in your area of interest serving on the study section can be detrimental. First, they may be in competition with you and although they may attempt to be fair-handed in their review, their take on something may not be quite the same as yours and thus their expertise actually gets in the way. Second, perhaps they simply have irreconcilable scientific differences—and no matter how well written or convincing your application and preliminary data, they just will not buy it. Obviously, you can't control for all potential outcomes, but knowing some of these potential issues upfront may help push you toward applying for one grant and not another.

Ideally, you would like a group of people reviewing your application who understand the significance of what you are doing—i.e., why it is important and critical to move the field forward—yet not so knowledgeable about every detail of what you plan that they can be endlessly critical. Obviously, you cannot tailor a group of reviewers to your liking, and thus it really becomes very much luck of the draw.

Follow the leader. If you are working with a mentor, he or she may be able to provide you with some valuable insights. Also, it is not unusual to have a foundation supporting several projects in a laboratory and perhaps seeking support for your work from the same organization as that which supports hers may make considerable sense. Similarly with federal funding, following your mentor's lead, and applying through a grant mechanism aligned with hers, is another good way to go, especially if considering applying for other research awards, such as fellowships and K08s or K23s and other career grants (for more on career grants, see Chap. 21).

Talk to colleagues. Talking to friends, colleagues and other people, not just your mentor, is another great way to learn about grant opportunities. You may learn of a new foundation. You may learn of another funding mechanism that you just overlooked. Or perhaps you will get connected up with someone else who is applying for a grant and would like to include some of your research efforts/expertise on the application to enhance it. The only way to make this happen is to keep an open mind and go along with new ideas even if you don't fully understand them or they seem way outside your wheelhouse.

Apply to more than one place. When submitting a manuscript of a new research article for consideration for publication, you are obliged to only submit to a single journal. You can't send out the article to five journals simultaneously and then choose the one with the highest impact factor that is willing to accept it. That is against the rules. However, when it comes to applying for grants, the opposite is true. You should apply to as many places as possible and as frequently as possible. Submitting grant applications is a little like buying lottery tickets. The more you submit, the more likely that one will actually end up paying off. However, you don't want to submit half-baked ideas to ten different places. A fully baked, well-constructed, and written grant will fare better than a poor one and so you have to balance time and effort with each of the applications you submit. And with NIH, you cannot submit the same application to different study sections simultaneously. Moreover, most organizations have different grant requirements and the specifics of what they are looking for may also vary. But the critical thing to remember is that you are not limited to submitting to one place. Generally, grant deadlines vary with the organization (NIH is three times per year, many foundations are only yearly or semiannually) and thus you should always be strategic with your applications and plan many months in advance. Also, with each submission, you may want to emphasize certain aspects and deemphasize other aspects to make sure your grant fits well with the planned mission of the organization or the institute.

What if you are unexpectedly lucky and you end up receiving multiple grants? Well, if you are in such a fortunate situation, the worst-case scenario is that you have to simply give one up since you can't ask for separate organizations to pay for the same work. In fact, this is a criminal offense as it is viewed as fraud, and you must be careful to avoid this. On the other hand, there are ways of planning your grant applications so that they are subtly different and you will be able to receive funding from more than one organization since the actual planned work does not overlap.

RFAs versus standard grant mechanisms. Requests for applications (RFAs) are a special type of grant mechanism offered by many institutions, including both federal bodies and non-profit foundations. These are usually focussed on a specific area of research. If one happens to fall right in the middle of your sweet spot, this may be a great opportunity. For example, if you are studying novel therapies in animal models of primary biliary cirrhosis and you happen to find a special RFA in this area one day while perusing the Internet, you should certainly consider applying. However, you should be wary, since RFAs are usually created with the intent of funding several projects by well-known investigators that fit neatly into a portfolio of research. This means that while there is definitely funding available for a project, it is going to be very competitive since only a couple of additional funding lines are likely to be given to be people outside this elite club. And since these RFAs garner a great deal of attention, they end up attracting many applications. In my experience, unless you are one of the lucky ones for whom this type of grant application is being tailored, it is not necessarily an easy road. Of course, if you get an unexpected email from a foundation or a program officer informing you of this new RFA in your field, you should take it seriously, and consider submitting an application, even if you are not sure you are a perfect fit.

Plan. One needs to be very strategic about applying for grants. Once you have identified a potential mechanism, be very careful not to submit a half-baked application. As I've said, this means planning out months and months ahead. I am often thinking about 6 months to 1 year ahead in terms of what grants I will be submitting. You don't want to submit to grants to the same study section at the same time, even if they are on vastly different topics.

And, going back to the idea of having two grants get funded on the exact same topic, if you carefully structure your grants so that they are overlapping but still very different, you may be actually able to have more than one grant funded and not have to give up any of it. Or perhaps, only certain aspects of it will be duplicated and you will only need to return a small portion of the money to one of the funders.

Look for grant opportunities geared for junior investigators. Finally, since this book is focussed on people just starting out on a career in research, it is important to recall that many organizations, from foundations to government agencies, offer grant mechanisms that are geared to new investigators. Many foundations desperately want to get new talented people into their fields and having special mechanisms for junior investigators is definitely one way of achieving this. These generally are somewhat easier to obtain, with higher pay lines, since you are not competing against big players with huge labs and a long track record of successful funding. If a foundation does not seem to make these opportunities clear on their website, you should definitely call and see if they have such tools available. Again, this is discussed further in Chap. 21.

Summary. Spending considerable effort figuring out where to apply is far more important than most people appreciate. There are, in fact, a multitude of opportunities and trying to ensure that you are applying your efforts most effectively so that you will have success is absolutely critical. The opportunity cost of applying for a specific solicitation or agency when another opportunity may offer you a much better chance of being funded cannot be overstated. Putting in intense effort *before* starting to work on an application is never a waste. Create a detailed list of all possible places to apply, their pros and cons, and then make a thoughtful decision. And if you end up still being unsuccessful, at least you will not be kicking yourself that you hadn't done your due diligence up front.

Chapter 18
Writing a Winning Grant Application

There are entire books devoted to the process and art of writing strong grant applications. My goal here is not to give you endlessly nuanced advice or specific details on different application types, but rather to share with you my personal insights and broad ideas and opinions as to what will help make the best grant application. But, not matter how much advice I give, I firmly believe that the only way to write a really strong grant application is practice. And even after you have your first successes, you will undoubtedly have some huge failures. It is inevitable. About all we can manage to do with practice is to improve our odds. Grant writing is definitely a very tough medium to master, and there is no definite recipe for success, except repetition and perseverance.

Before you begin. Before getting too deeply ensconced in your grant application, there are a few things you should consider doing. First, you should make sure you have a pretty good sense as to who is going to be on your research team, as you will likely need input from them as you work through the grant. This may include your mentor, colleagues in your department, perhaps a colleague or two in another institution, and perhaps a couple of experts in other fields. As already discussed, cross-fertilization is key. Coming up with new exciting directions of research de novo is not easy to do without outside influences and opinion. Often as you write the application, you may start to realize a glaring omission—perhaps an expert in another field who can really help you nail down one of the techniques you will be using or perhaps a biostatistician with expertise in your specific area. On the other hand, it may not be helpful to add in supernumeraries who really add little to the project except offering you their name recognition. (As an aside, I have found that having a big league, heavy hitter on your grant application generally helps minimally unless they are intimately involved in the work.) You also need to be wary to not bring on "hangers on" who really don't have much to offer but that you simply like or feel guilty about not including. All of your participants really need to bring something unique and critical to the table. Whatever the case, developing a pretty

© Springer Science+Business Media New York 2016
S.B. Rutkove, *Biomedical Research: An Insider's Guide*,
DOI 10.1007/978-1-4939-3655-7_18

good sense of who is going to be on our team and their willingness/enthusiasm to be involved should be one of the first things to sort out as you begin to put your application together.

Second, make sure you are thinking through your time line. Don't rush a grant application. Obviously, one shouldn't put off applying if it can be avoided (you have to be in it to win it), but sometimes it is better to wait an additional 6 months, as painful as it may be, in order to collect sufficient preliminary data and perhaps a publication or two to really strengthen your story. You have already figured out the best grant mechanisms to apply for (as described in the last chapter), so make sure you are set to tell the best story that you can.

Third, make sure to let your research administrators and anyone on the business side of the grant procedure know far in advance of your plans. They always appreciate having advance notice, and if there are snafus down the road during the application process, they will less likely drag their feet in helping correct them if they know you are a trustworthy and organized researcher.

How much preliminary data do you need? This question comes up all the time and is really a tough one to answer. Generally the more preliminary data you have, the better. In fact, one may sometimes feel that you actually need to do all the experiments that you describe in the grant application before applying for the grant to simply have sufficient data to convince the reviewers that you know what you are doing. That may seem ridiculous, but there is more truth in it than most of us would like to admit. You need to whet the reviewer's appetites by proving to them that you can do all the experiments and that the data really do look supportive of what you are trying to prove out. But you do want to stop short of actually doing the research you say you are going to do—the reviewers will complain that you have done it already, so why do you need the funding in the first place? Ideally, you'll have some data to support each specific aim of a proposal, but not too much. It is a tricky balance and one that requires practice to identify. But in general, I would say err on the side of too much preliminary data rather than too little. Some aims can have more data supporting it and some can have less. And hopefully you'll be able to build enough flexibility in your grant to show that if you achieve more than you expect, you have additional goals that you can pursue.

Outlining and not outlining. I recall as a high-school student reading a book on how to write better essays. One of things the author strongly recommended was, that before putting a single word down in your essay, you need to have a really detailed complete outline. The author gave some example (Dostoyesky, I believe) who took months to complete an extremely detailed outline of a novel before actually putting pen to paper and writing the thing. And then he would write the entire book in just a matter of a few weeks, his outline essentially paving the way to quick execution.

While creating a basic outline of what you want to do is reasonable—and you most certainly need to come up with a clear set of specific aims and experiments to test them—I have never found the excessively detailed outline very helpful. This is not only true for grants but also research papers. I find that when I start to write, new ideas naturally come to me, and it is only through the process of writing complete paragraphs and not merely telegraphic thoughts that I can really delve into something deeply and become excited about it. And in point of fact, excitement is very much what you want to get across in a grant application. Without excitement or enthusiasm, your application is dead in the water. By writing paragraphs you can allow yourself to go places you would not ordinarily travel. Sure, you can delete things that are ridiculous down the road, but let your mind wander. The process of creating a detailed outline I believe has a way of straitjacketing your thought process and turning your application into a dull, unimaginative work.

Writing the introduction and specific aims pages. The most important and challenging part of the entire proposal is your introduction and specific aims pages. It is here where you are going to set the tone for the entire proposal and positively or negatively bias your reviewers for the rest of the proposal. When a reviewer finishes reading the preliminary aims page she should be excited enough to start hoping that the rest of the application will be as good as the beginning. If it lives up to their expectations or exceeds them, then you are set. On the other hand, if the specific aims page is weak and leaves the reviewer questioning why or how you are doing this, you will be fighting an uphill battle that will be exceedingly tough to win. You need to come strong out of the gate, and the introduction and specific aims page is the place to do it.

I generally proceed here with a paragraph or two that introduces the reader to the area of research to be discussed and setting up the problem, going from general to specific. Each sentence needs to be very clearly written and a true guide to the readers bringing them directly where you want them to be for the hypothesis to be stated, assuming only limited knowledge. These sentences should be edited and re-edited until the story is as crisp and clean as possible and has a real driving force forward. One idea should clearly lead into the next. Some investigators will not place references in this part of the grant, since they will end up being included later in the introduction/significance sections anyway. The references also perhaps can be a little distracting. However, I strongly recommend referencing your specific aims. You can never be too compulsive or complete with references. Adding references to you specific aims pages will give it a sense of gravitas that will empower your entire application. Regardless of your approach, this introduction to the specific aims should be no longer than a few hundred words for most applications (and for some you won't even have an opportunity to include such an introduction). For an NIH grant application, it is generally half of the page or less.

Although not "standard practice," if you do have a particularly powerful image or diagram that is easily understandable at a quick glance that you believe has the potential of drawing the reader in, then it may be worth including. This has to be done judiciously since you also don't want to make the grant appear to be showy or as if you are trying to sell something (though in a very true sense you are). However, creating an emotional context to the grant can be very powerful, as long as it is done carefully.

The introduction should lead you straight into the hypothesis underlying the entire proposal. What is it that you are going to test here? The hypothesis doesn't have to be earth-shattering or of great complexity. It just has to support the underlying research effort that you will be explaining throughout. Frankly, I used to be freaked out by the concept of a hypothesis. I felt like I needed to be coming up with something like the principle of General Relativity or the Koch hypothesis of infectious disease. But they can be much more mundane than that. Here are a couple of simple examples:

"We hypothesize that diurnal fluctuations in C-reactive protein predict longevity and that inhibition of inflammatory pathways are effective at impacting this relationship."

"We hypothesize that test A will be more sensitive than test B for the diagnosis of condition X."

"We hypothesize that drug A will show greater efficacy than standard-of-care in disease Y."

Basically, your hypothesis is just your stating what you want to prove out in your work. It is the question that you want to test.

Once you have stated your hypothesis, you can then state that you are going to test it through a series of specific aims. The specific aims should number usually between 2 and 5 depending on the length and complexity of the application. Sometimes it is helpful to have, say, just 2 major aims and then each with 2 additional sub-aims. I generally find that 3 is a pretty good number that works well if it fits with your plans. Anything above 5 starts getting too complicated, and you will lose most reviewers. For each aim, it is generally a good idea to state the specific question of what you are going to study, what basic techniques you are going to perform, and the expected results of the study. The goal here is to provide a snapshot of one whole part of the grant. It is sometimes helpful to include simple sub-hypotheses here as well to support each part, but in my experience this is not always necessary. However, it is absolutely important to include expected results or at least hoped-for results. By talking about what you expect to find, it will make it considerably easier for the reviewer to understand what you are doing and why.

Once you have stated your aims, a very short concluding paragraph—perhaps no more than 1–3 sentences–is useful to tie up the story and provide some forward-looking information and long-term hoped-for outcomes of this work. While it is not advisable to be fantastical in this part and think extreme, it is not unreasonable to stretch the bounds a little. It will interest the reviewers and make them, perhaps, feel a bit more positive about reviewing your grant application.

Ultimately, the introduction and specific aims should be a tight package offering up a clear introduction into the area of research, the specific problem, the hypothesis you plan to test that in some way addresses that problem, the specific methods you will use to do so, the expected results, and how this ultimately will lead to important advances in medical science. Achieving this in a short amount of space and to make it clear and engaging to people who may not be exactly in your area, is no small challenge. It is for this reason, that it makes the most sense to begin working on the specific aims very early on as they will require constant and repeated refinement, usually right up until the moment of submission.

Writing a compelling and interesting introduction/significance section. The goal of this part of the grant is really to try to introduce the reader who may not be that familiar with what you are going to be talking about. But it also not to insult the reader who is quite familiar with the area, but to actually demonstrate your knowledge, familiarity, and comfort with the area. And, like the specific aims page, it needs to drive toward the logical effort of the research that you are planning to pursue. This section should be very well referenced and thorough but *not* exhaustive in its overview. You are not trying to provide a detailed review of the entire body of literature on a subject. You are merely trying to educate readers on those areas that are specifically relevant to your area of proposed research. Each paragraph should draw the reader in further, moving from the general to the specific, with the goal of leading her directly to "your doorstep" of the research you are going to propose.

It is usually a good idea to include a couple of figures or tables here that capture some of the basic information that you are trying to convey so a reader who does not want to read all the details can quickly scan the table or figure to get the gist of it all. The sections and paragraph breaks should be plentiful and should make logical sense.

Once you have introduced the basic ideas of your area of research, you can then introduce the specific topic or problem that you will be studying. Perhaps it is a new technique or pathway that might have important therapeutic implications. Or perhaps, it is an epidemiological question that will address an important but unanswered issue. Regardless of the topic, the basic idea behind this section is to underscore the significance of the study. It may not necessarily change the world but you should give the sense that, if successful, it will make the world a slightly better place. If the significance of the grant does not come through, then no matter how good the other sections, reviewers will not be enthusiastic.

One challenge that many grant applicants face is trying to make their little corner of the research world important. This can be challenging, especially if you are working on a very rare disease that only affects a handful of people or a complex disease mechanism or a technology that seems more like an aside than actually something relevant and mainstream. Why should you be spending so many taxpayers' dollars on something that will help so few or is so off the beaten-path? Well, one approach for dealing with this is to try to generalize the value of the work to be done. For example, perhaps the pathway being researched has a more general value and can be applied to other, much more common diseases. Or maybe the technique will have application ultimately to healthy individuals. Regardless, it is important to try to see the longer-term ramifications of the research and not just the narrow importance of the work being completed as part of this grant application.

Innovation. If you are applying to NIH for funding, you will have to complete a specific section on innovation. If you are not, the granting organization may not have a specific section asking for this. However, it probably will behoove you, regardless of who your potential funding body may be, to include at least a paragraph or two on innovation. Research does not necessarily need to be really innovative to be valuable, but highlighting innovative aspects of your work can definitely make a small but important difference when the grant is scored. And certainly there can be little harm to emphasize that your work is not just a reiteration of what has been done before. In fact, the innovations you are going to be pursuing don't have to be earth-shattering stuff. It can be a straightforward extension of previous work. If you have some innovative aspects buried in perhaps more mundane work, make sure you highlight those points. The whole project does not need to be pioneering.

Of course, if you do have a very innovative proposal you should definitely highlight this in every possible way. It will buy you some good will. But be careful. Excessive innovation is not always viewed in a positive light. It can be considered "risky" or perhaps not fully considered. Are you pursuing innovation in lieu of a step-by-step pursuit of an important answer to a big problem? This can be difficult to sort out, but if you are going to highlight something very innovative, make sure you build up to it carefully so that the reviewers understand that the underpinnings of the project are in fact really strong and the work is not so out-of-the-box as to be years ahead of its time and likely to find no practical application in our lifetimes.

Preliminary data. It is important to recognize that the presentation of preliminary data is key to obtaining successful funding. Exciting preliminary data can entice a reviewer's imagination while poorly presented or complex preliminary data can make a reviewer just get bored or make him/her feel like they are just not perspicacious enough to understand what you are getting at. Here are some specific recommendations to make your preliminary data section shine:

1. *State the individual pieces of preliminary evidence for your study in simple, comprehensible declarative sentences.* Examples of simple but strong declarative statements that summarize your pieces of data include "Cardiolipin antibodies levels correlate with the probability of peripheral thrombosis" or "X blood cell gene protects against HIV infection" as compared to titles such as "Correlation of cariolipin antibodies to thrombosis risk" or "Genetic determinants against HIV transmission." If you are going to give a title to section, you might as well make sure it actually transfers a piece of knowledge at the same time.

2. *Make your figures simple and straightforward.* Reviewers have limited patience. If you offer them complex figures that require prolonged and dedicated scrutiny to understand, you are asking for trouble. In fact, you should always try to make the figures comprehensible without the reviewer actually reading the figure legend or caption. What you are trying to demonstrate should be self-evident and virtually self-explanatory. Ensure that the figures are sufficiently large such that you are able to make them simple to read. While it is true that readers can readily zoom in on their computers or iPads, many still print out their applications or will simply be too lazy to change the zoom level; at any rate, you shouldn't ever make the reviewer have to do additional work when reviewing your application. They will either not do it or get annoyed: a definite recipe for receiving a low score regardless of what happens.

3. *Use color judiciously.* Once upon a time, all grants were printed in black and white. Since the virtual universal computerization of grant applications, color is being used more freely, sometimes to its detriment since color is not really required and people have varying abilities to discriminate colors (also remember that about 6 % of American men are red-green color blind)! So a reviewer that has color vision issues may not only be unable to evaluate your beautiful color figures, but may also be mildly annoyed that you didn't take his/her limitations into consideration. Plus if the grant is printed out, it may be printed out in grayscale.

4. *Make sure the order of the data you present is logical and follows the aims you have introduced earlier on.* Like the significance section, it should lead the reader forward, each set of data building upon an earlier set, if possible. I'll say it again:

make the reviewer's job as painless as possible. If they like you, they will like your grant a lot more.

5. *Put your best foot forward.* Grant applications are not manuscripts. While all the data you present must be absolutely real (more on ethics and falsification of data in Chap. 29), you don't necessarily have to torture yourself by showing all your bad data. Remember you are trying to convince reviewers that you have something worthwhile to pursue here. If you have strong data supporting one idea but other data that are not very strong supporting another, don't weaken your application by including weak data. You should be using only the data that are going to inform your research choices.

However, the inclusion of "weak" data can be helpful if it doesn't support something you don't want it to support. For example, if the data do not support one concept, you can use it to help show the reviewers why you are pursuing a different direction.

6. *Accepted or published manuscripts make the best preliminary data.* Generally, if you have work that has already been accepted, this is the best kind of preliminary data. However, sometimes it gets difficult to know whether to include this kind of data in the preliminary data section or include it earlier in the significance or in the innovation section. This decision very much depends on the nature of the data and its relationship to the research. However, the inclusion of such data is good since it already has gone through the trial-by-fire of peer review once. Where you place it in the application really depends on what you are trying to do with it. If you feel the data are relatively fundamental to the research, definitely put it in the background/ significance or possibly the innovation section. But if not, then it probably belongs in the preliminary data section.

7. *If possible, end with data that seem to imply future directions.* While a grant may fund just a single research project, remember that you are doing this for grander reasons than to just move your one project forward. You can really whet reviewers' appetites by providing easy-to-understand forward-looking data. For example, you could show just one example supporting some future application of the idea that you are envisioning in the long term. If it has big implications, this can really help increase enthusiasm for your application.

Approach and Methods

The experimental plan section of the application is in some respects the most important, since it is going to outline exactly why you are asking for the money and how you plan to utilize it. Moreover, a compelling experimental plan will convince the readers that you know what you are doing. The real challenge in writing up an experimental plan is that with your specific set of goals in mind, introduced during the earlier sections, a variety of approaches can be taken that all may work. As you'll see below, reviewers are not supposed to rewrite the grant for you or come up with a better research plan. They are simply supposed to evaluate the one you propose. Nevertheless, there is a very fine distinction between grading your ideas without thinking that there is a different and better way of doing something. It is difficult for the reviewers not to all become "cooks" of a sort and see better ways of doing something than you have put forward. In short, if there is one section of the grant application that is most open to potential criticism, it is the experimental plan. So writing up something tight, thoughtful, and at the same time planning for anticipated criticisms and concerns is essential and, obviously, very challenging.

The general structure of the experimental plan should follow along the lines of the specific aims, and actually repeating those aims at the beginning of the experimental plan is not a bad idea. Repetition is good, since by this point in the application, the reviewers may have already forgotten what you are planning to do in the research, having been mired in preliminary data and significance/innovation sections for some time. So a quick restatement of the goals is a great way to refresh their memories and begin a detailed discussion of the experimental plan.

This is also a good place for a broad figure that sketches the outline of the experimental plan and helps tie everything together. A cartoon or flow chart explaining how the experimental plan for each of the aims feeds back on the overarching goal of the research can be very helpful for reviewers to visualize what you are thinking, so that they can get into the nitty-gritty of the methods without losing sight of the big picture. It can also serve as an easy informational source that they can refer back to as they move through the more mundane (and often painful) methodological details.

One thing to consider including at this point in the application is a short overview of the research team that you have assembled to do the work. Since these individuals will be critical to completing the study, providing some context as to everyone's expertise and their specific roles in the effort can be very helpful. It is true that all of this information will be included in the other pieces of the application (e.g., biosketches/curriculum vitae, etc.), but having this information here again can help solidify their actual roles.

Next, it is good get some of the general methodological considerations out of the way. This could include measurement techniques, animal or human or cell populations to be studied, and reagents to be used, that may be applicable to all the aims of the grant. These sections can be filled with references as needed to help keep things crisp and succinct. But be careful about leaving out too much. While you don't want to bore the reviewer with excessive detail, you don't want to exclude so much that the application becomes hard to follow.

Once you have provided this foundation, you are probably ready to get into the specifics of each aim. I think restating the aim again (yes, this would be the third time in the body of the grant) and the specific experimental plan, in temporal, sequential order, as applicable to each aim is a very straightforward way of doing this. Imagine you are actually doing all the experiments or collecting all the data. What happens, in what order? Tell it like a story. It might not be a very exciting story, but it is a story nevertheless. How will you go about the data collection? From where will the patients be recruited? Where will the study activities take place? How will you generate the animal or cell lines?

In some respects, writing these details is very straightforward, but you will likely also start to stumble in certain places since you may not have fully thought through some of the experimental details up to this point. You will likely also realize that there are some problems with the plan that you hadn't quite realized until you actually starting writing it down in painful detail. For example, perhaps you really need an additional control population or perhaps as you start looking up some technical method, you realize that there is more than one way to do things, and you may need to choose between two techniques that both seem reasonable. For the simple issues, try to deal with them right there and then modify the plan to accommodate them. For the more recalcitrant problems, don't think you have to necessarily switch around your plan. Simply make a note of it and move on. You may want to just deal with this later in your dedicated section on potential problems and pitfalls, and what I like to call "risk mitigation." You simply cannot identify definitively ahead of time the best way of pursuing the research you want to pursue to answer the question that you want to answer. So realize that whatever you are putting forward is basically your best guess. Fortunately, grant applications allow you to have a flexible clause, allowing for changes in course as the research progresses. Remember, if funded, most grants have considerable flexibility in how you actually carry out the plan you have described. And while you need to try to do what you say you'll do, you can still change things as the project progresses. The point is not to stick to the path you have described, but to achieve the ultimate goals of your study.

Again, diagrams and figures can help here. By including a flow chart showing the experimental procedures for one or more aims you may be able to convey the essence of what you are trying to do without making the reader plod through thickets of often very tedious text. Recall that many (frankly, I'd say MOST) reviewers will not have the time or patience to work through all the details. There is also a fairly good chance that some of the reviewers are not especially well versed in the specific area of research that you are describing. So anything you can do to make their job easier and streamlined can go a long way to helping your grant be a more pleasant experience for them, which will hopefully translate in a higher score for you. For example, in addition to flow charts, strongly consider frequent paragraph breaks or the use of bold font face with strong title headings/topic sentences to help the reader jump easily from one paragraph to the next without reading every single word. The basic idea is that you need to make sure all the information is there for those readers who demand it but that there is an obvious "path" through the thicket that will provide a means for the less-scrutinizing or detail-oriented reviewers to easily pass through without getting bruised or injured.

For each of the methods section, you will likely require some kind of data analysis section. The data analysis sections should follow directly from the experiments and planned out comes that you will obtain. While some data analyses are relatively straightforward to describe, since they are standard, others may be more challenging to write since there may be some unusual aspects to them. It is always worth, at the very least, writing a detailed outline of the data analysis section, always keeping in mind that you want to actually answer the specific questions that you set out to answer.

Biostatisticians and data analysis sections. Depending upon exactly what you are proposing to research, having the input of an experienced biostatistician can be a huge asset when writing a grant. A thoughtful biostatistician will add language that will not only tighten and strengthen the plan, but it will also *sound* good. It is usually pretty easy to tell grant applications that were not written with the dedicated input and interest of a biostatistician. These can succeed if the analyses are straightforwards, but if the outcomes are anything less than straightforward or the statistics involved go beyond simply simple parametric or non-parametric testing (e.g., *t*-tests, Mann-Whitney tests, Pearson and Spearman correlations) you may find yourself taking on a little more than you have planned, unless you yourself are quite familiar with statistical terminology.

But just because you ask a biostatistician to help does not ensure success or, in fact, even a good data analysis section. I have worked with a number of biostatisticians over the years and they come in all shapes and sizes. You will find the biostatisticians who are very eager to help you, to roll up their sleeves and get involved in the product of the work because they are excited to make a great product (the application) and do some great work if it gets funded. They are scientifically curious about the work that you are doing and are hopeful that they will be able to add significantly to it. In contrast, there are those biostatisticians who pretty much consider themselves hired guns. They are not really interested in what you are doing but will provide text and language on a fee-for-service basis. They will help and hopefully provide some good text that you can use, but the whole experience may be relatively unsatisfying and you will read through what they have provided and realize that it is missing key analyses or ideas, simply because they did not spend the time or effort that was really needed to make the analysis section top-notch. Then when you go back to them concerned/confused and asking for additional help, you feel more like a supplicant than the principal investigator. While unpleasant, with effort and persistence, the resulting product can still be quite good.

Thus, my recommendation is that you obtain at least some biostatistical input to help with the data analysis (and also the sample size estimation section—see below) to help ensure that what you are proposing makes sense and that the section has sufficient "shine" to make it convincing and appealing to the reviewers.

Sample size estimation/justification. Along with the data analysis section, you will probably also want to include a sample size estimation or power analysis. Whereas such sections once upon a time were only expected for human studies, where recruitment is likely to be a concern and that proving out that you could succeed with a certain number of patients was critical, most review sections are now expecting to see at least some kind of sample size estimation for animal sections as well. This is not unreasonable, but it is also worth considering that, unlike in human studies, "recruitment" of animals, even with unusual diseases is fairly straightforward so to prove out that there is still a good chance of finding an effect even with a relatively small number of animals is probably unnecessary, unless you are dealing with larger species (e.g., pigs or primates).

I will not delve into the technical details of creating sample size estimations. But here is one critical fact: you have to have at least some preliminary data or perhaps previously published data before you can attempt one of these. Now, you do not necessarily need a sample size estimation section for every single analysis plan for each aim (though you might, if they are all very different). But it underscores the need to ensure that you have sufficient initial preliminary data even before considering submitting an application. In order to calculate a sample size, you must have some idea of the "effect size" or the magnitude of the response to an intervention or sensitivity of a technique to a specific measure.

Most people feel pretty uncomfortable writing these, unless they have had some previous experience in how they work. The truth of the matter is the actual calculations are not that difficult. In fact, there are online calculators, so if you do have sufficient preliminary data and understand the statistical tests that you are trying to apply, it is actually not that difficult to do on your own. However, this is definitely a place for a biostatistician's help. This is usually very easy and quick for them and should not be a big deal to complete, unless there is a real dearth of preliminary data or the analysis plans are murky.

Potential pitfalls/problems and risk mitigation. No experimental plan is complete without this section. You can include this as a separate small section in each aim or as a single larger section at the end of all the aims. This section is your opportunity to show that you are self-critical and not Pollyannaish in your expectations that all will work out storybook-like in the end. You have also likely identified some potential problems along the way. Again, this is your opportunity to pre-empt your critics, showing that you have identified potential problems and how to deal with them.

So in this section, carefully itemize your potential problems and come up with detours around them and show that they you may still be able to succeed in the overarching aims of the research even if some of the smaller pieces don't quite go as well as you were hoping. Importantly, *this is not a section for denial*. In other words, don't list a concern and then simply say, "this is not a concern." Rather provide evidence that for any given concern you can find your way around it, either through a different set of experiments or with a different approach to the data analysis. If one of your potential pitfalls is, for example, that you and your co-investigators do not have sufficient expertise to complete a specific part of the project, then you can make some arguments as to how you will obtain that expertise or utilize other resources. If there is a potential concern that one major part of the grant will rely on positive results obtained in an earlier part of the study, try to argue that point by showing that even completely negative results will not impact your ability to complete the aim that superficially appears to be depend upon it.

Remember, this section should not be used to argue about the potential overall significance or innovation of the project. You should have made that clear in the earlier sections. By the time the reviewers get to this point in the application, they are not thinking about why you are doing the research, just how you are doing it and looking for how you plan to navigate past anticipated potential challenges.

Timeline. Depending on your funding agency, you will probably have to include some kind of timeline explaining how you plan to do all this work in the allotted period of time of the grant. For most institutions, including NIH, a short Gantt chart generally does the job here, with each specific aim and its period of time pictured.

Most of the reviewers will simply glance at this and move on—this is pro forma but an important step. On the other hand other organizations may demand a far more comprehensive timeline and even potentially a statement of work that specifically outlines which tasks will be completed during exactly which months of the funding period. Department of Defense grants have such a form (which is a document separate from the body of the grant application), but because they are fussy about this aspect of the application, including some brief outline of your planned timeline in the experimental plan is still not a bad idea.

Future plans/additional steps/conclusion. While these sections are not specifically requested, after guiding your readers meticulously through pages and pages of text and figures, it is only fair to them that you tie it up all neatly at the end and add a final sense of excitement. This section could just be about 1/3rd of a page or even less if you are limited for space, but it is valuable to include future ramifications of the work and potential follow-on studies. You don't want the completion of this work to just seem like an end. Rather it should seem like a beginning to something greater and grander. If it is basic or animal work that you are doing, so show how the next step will lead to human studies. If it is an early human study, show how the next step could lead to an initial Phase 2 clinical trial. If it is a Phase 2 clinical trial, show how it will lead to a Phase 3 clinical trial. Or show how learning the molecular mechanisms proposed here will lead to a new set of studies with a far wider reach than you have proposed here. Or if it is an engineering or device issue, show how the work here will ultimately lead to a product. Also understand that there is nothing wrong in saying that what you are ultimately aiming for is to have your idea commercialized in some form to make it more widely available. In fact, to say that a pharmaceutical company may be interested or a start-up company will be built around it with funding through small business grants should be considered a strength of the application, not a weakness. We live in a capitalist society, so don't try to make academia the ultimate home of all your work. For something to truly succeed and reach the largest number of people possible, you may need to see the way to its commercialization.

Supplemental sections of the grant application. Once you have completed your experimental plan, it would be nice to feel that you are close to being done with the application, but depending on to which organization you are applying, you may still have a great deal of work remaining, unfortunately. For most governmental grant applications there are a bevy of additional sections, including human subjects, animal research, the budget and budget justification, resource sharing, select agent, etc. These sections are important and need to be completed as fully as possible. But one word of caution: don't necessarily rely on them to convey information that could also be placed in the body of the grant application. Two specific examples come to mind, that I have personally been punished for before: recruitment and power analyses. If you look at the instructions for NIH and Department of Defense grants, you will see comments saying that you should justify your animal or human numbers in the animal or human subjects sections, respectively. While the instructions may say this, there is a fairly good chance the reviewers will skim over those sections or perhaps not even look at them and then criticize your application for leaving out critical power calculations and recruitment strategies. My suggestion is thus that you specifically include at least a brief summary of this in the body of the experimental plan and then refer to the details as being in the appropriate separate section, should any reviewer care to look at it.

For most of the other sections, I suggest you ask a colleague to look at one of their previous applications and then follow the instructions very, very carefully to make sure you have filled in all of the parts. These sections are really not places to be creative for the most part—but simply to show that you have given everything careful consideration and that you are not neglecting some minor point that could lead to the sinking of the entire effort. There is one exception to this: the resource sharing section. This section has taken on greater significance lately as people are moving to open access platforms, not just for the publication of articles but also for the general sharing of data. It is worth thinking through creative ways of sharing all the data that you collect (for human data, removed of all potential identifiers) via the web. This is one section that you could turn into an additional strength, especially if you make reference to it in the main body of the research application.

A cover letter. The cover letter for most grant applications has a fairly limited function. A really, really strong cover letter will almost certainly have no effect on the outcome of a grant review process. However, cover letters, at least for NIH, can be important for several reasons. First, you can direct your application to the best study section that you think that should review it. Sometimes the folks at NIH will take you up on this, but not always. They may have their own ideas, but if your application ends up going to another study section, you should give them a call and discuss it at least. In my experience, however, NIH personnel as a whole have a better sense as to where grant applications will receive the best review than I or my colleagues do.

Second, you can direct it to an institute that you feel would be most likely to fund it. Which one should fund it should be obvious, but not always. For example, you may have a grant on cardiac imaging. Such a grant may be best funded by the National Institute of Heart, Lung, and Blood (NIHLB); but it could also be potentially funded by the National Institute of Biomedical Imaging and Bioengineering (NIBIB). So in your cover letter you can say that you think it should be primarily assigned to NIHLB with secondary assignment to NIBIB. This means that should your grant get scored sufficiently high in review, it would go first to NIHLB for funding. If it is of sufficient interest and within their pay line (in other words, scored high enough), it would get funded by them; on the other hand, if it weren't, then the NIBIB would consider it for funding as well. The institutional assignment, however, has no real relevance to the review process itself.

Finally, you can use the cover letter as a place to include any additional information that may be relevant. One specific one would be request that a specific individual not review a grant application. These kinds of requests are generally considered, but are more likely to be adopted if a clear reason is provided (e.g., our work is overlapping or, better yet, we have irreconcilable philosophical differences making it impossible, we believe, for this person to be able to review the grant fairly). A cover letter with a grant application is mainly there to make sure the grant ends up being processed correctly, or at least according to your wishes, and not to help "sell it," as can be the case when submitting a journal article.

Summary. Writing a large research grant is the most daunting thing that we have to do as academic researchers. It is far more challenging than writing even a large paper as you are not just telling a good story, you also have to sell it. The grant application has to constantly keep the big picture in mind while smoothly being able to delve in excruciating details when needed. It has to be simple enough to be understandable to a reviewer not that well versed in the area and yet complex enough to satisfy the demands of an expert in the field, without ever seeming like it is pandering or patronizing. It requires a level of empathy with your readers that needs to extend far beyond what you may be used to providing in a paper or in a presentation. And worst of all, it is exceedingly important to get this right, since your funding and your actually ability to continue pursuing the research that you love to do will depend on it.

Chapter 19
Grant Budgeting

Grant budgeting is a world unto itself and to fully address it is well beyond the scope of this book. Nonetheless, I will provide a general overview, recognizing that budgeting a grant can be a time-consuming and confusing process and that it is impossible (and would be extraordinarily boring) to cover all possible issues and contingencies. For new grant applicants, it is best to work closely with an experienced mentor and hopefully your grants administrator to help with the budgeting process. Importantly, always recall that the budget is usually a secondary part of the application. At NIH, a grant will not succeed or fail because of the budget. In fact, the budget is only considered after the grant is fully reviewed and scored scientifically. So don't think just because you make a grant cheap it is more likely to be funded. In most circumstances, it will have no influence on the outcome whatsoever.

Basics. First some basic concepts.

1. *Direct versus indirect costs*. As you may recall, we discussed this briefly in Chap. 16 (Funding overview). Just to repeat here: direct costs refer to money used to directly support a specific research project. This is the money that would be available to you, if funded, to support your salary, research assistants' salaries and fringe benefits (e.g., health care), supplies, animal costs, equipment, travel, etc. Indirect costs (also called overhead or facility and administration—or more simply F&A) are those that are received by the institution for supporting your work, including, for example, building costs, maintenance, heat, light, and the standard administrative aspects associated with a research structure in an institution, such as paying the salaries of your research administrators.

Indirect costs may or may not be considered in your overall budget, so you need to pay attention to the instructions closely. Foundations and some governmental grants will give you an overall budget that includes both direct and indirect costs and then tell you the limit that you can spend on direct costs. This can sometimes get a little bit confusing, so I will give a simple example here. Let's say a foundation says that you have a total budget of $100,000 and up to 10 % of funds can be used to support indirect costs. Your institution where you will be performing the research, looking for all it is due, expects you to use the 10 % maximum. So at first glance, the

© Springer Science+Business Media New York 2016
S.B. Rutkove, *Biomedical Research: An Insider's Guide*,
DOI 10.1007/978-1-4939-3655-7_19

math seems pretty straightforward: 10 % of $100,000 is $10,000 dollars for indirect costs and $90,000 for direct costs for you to spend on your research. But this is actually *not* correct. It is 10 % of your direct costs that are at issue, not 10 % of the overall budget. So the equation becomes:

$100,000 = x + 0.1x$, where x is the total direct costs allowed.

This simplifies to $1.1x = $100,000$, and thus $x = $90,909$ of $100,000 — or $90,909 in direct costs and $9891 dollars in indirect costs. This is not exactly a bonanza in unexpected additional money, but you can see if the indirect rates allowed are say up to 20 or 30 % or the total grant is larger, the numbers can get considerably greater. More to the point, this is a readily avoidable arithmetic error.

One other point about indirect cost calculations is that they don't include major equipment. So if you are going to be buying something large as part of the grant, that also will not be "counted against" you in the calculation of the indirect costs. This makes sense because such equipment is not really considered to incur extra expense for the institution (even if it does take up space and uses electricity, both of which are considered in the indirect cost calculation). So in the example above, if you also were planning to buy a $10,000 piece of equipment, your calculations would look more like this:

$x + 0.1x + $10,000 = $100,000$, or $1.1x = $90,000$ or $x = $81,818$. So you would have $81,818 in direct costs to spend on your non-equipment items, $10,000 for your new piece of equipment, and there would be a total of only $8182 indirect costs.

Indirect costs are something you generally should not be too concerned about unless they are impacting your total bottom line, as in the example above. Most of the time, your grants officers will be dealing with these issues separately as you work through your grant submission and you will only see them in the final grant submitted. But do make sure you read the information concerning budgeting closely. A colleague recently had the unpleasant experience of learning that the grant that was carefully budgeted based on the assumption that the total values allotted were for direct costs but were supposed to be inclusive of direct and indirect on the day before the grant was due. After a great deal of panicked scrambling and reconfiguring, the grant was successfully submitted, but it created a huge amount of avoidable headache and stress.

2. *Budget for what you need.* Another point of confusion is that somehow being cheap and not budgeting sufficiently will help you win a grant. This is usually not the case. You should always budget for what you need and never try to cut corners. One reason for this is that many granting agencies, including NIH, will actually cut your proposed budget by 10 % or more if it is awarded, so it doesn't hurt to ask for a little more with the expectation that you will end up losing it in the end. But the best way of budgeting is clearly going through all your expenses and coming up with a total and then sticking with that. If you find yourself exceeding the limit of the grant, you will obviously need to re-budget. Don't be afraid of asking for a lot of money if you need it. Biomedical research is not cheap, and by trying to short-change yourself, you will only help ensure that the work you complete will not be successful, hurting the potential for your future grant applications.

3. *Personnel costs.* As you work through a budget, one of the most obvious things you'll realize is that your largest expense is going to be on salaries for you and your team. These end up eating often the lion's share of your money, so it is worth thinking carefully about how many people you need and how much of your own time you want to budget for a study. Sometimes, I find working through the equipment, supplies, and other costs (ranging from animal housing fees, to volunteer reimbursement for clinical studies, to travel) easier to work through, since they are far more concrete, and then figure out how much additional money you have left over for salaries.

Salaries are usually adjusted for the amount of time a given person is spending on a project. Thus, if someone is working full time on one project they would be giving 100 % effort on that project. NIH a few years ago moved from describing things as percent effort (which is totally comprehensible) to the much more inscrutable concept of "months of effort." If you are working on a project full time, you would be at 12 months; half time, 6 months, etc. It is easy enough to understand but if you are just putting in 5 % effort on a project that turns into a relatively meaningless 0.6 month.

Another odd thing you may come across are grants that do not allow you take any salary for yourself as principal investigator. Frankly, this always seems slightly strange to me since you certainly should not be donating your time freely to any project. I think the idea behind this concept is that PI salaries, especially those PIs with the letters MD after their names, tend to extract higher salaries than any one else on the research team. So the money is perhaps spent less efficiently than the foundation would like. Regardless, this is something to always look out for on a grant application; if it is the case, you really may want to reconsider applying for it, unless you have substantial other support for your salary and this can be viewed mainly as support for your staff, supplies, etc.

There is also the concept of the salary cap. This is a limitation that is placed on the upper limit of a salary that is going to be paid by an organization. For United States federal grants, which are set by Congress the limits are actually fairly high— $185,100 at the time of this writing. They actually were higher than that in 2008 before the financial meltdown and the Great Recession, reaching $199K; overnight they were cut to $179,900 and have since been inching up again. While these values may seem high, recall that many specialties, including the surgical specialties, ophthalmology, and some medical specialties, have salaries considerably in excess of this value (orthopedists rank the highest currently, with a mean income of about $450,000 per year). Thus, you also may now see why investigator-initiated, grant funded research tends be pursued less frequently by surgeons than by individuals in non-procedural specialties or by PhDs and not MDs. When you add in the considerable time and effort involved in applying for grants, the likelihood of not getting them, and then the considerably lower payments once received, there are many disincentives at work actively stymying academic innovation in the surgical specialties, with most of real innovation being generated by industry. This is not meant to be a criticism—it is just the way the world works; or at least the way it works in the United States.

4. *Cost sharing.* While we are on the topic of salaries, you should also be aware of the concept of cost sharing. What this refers to is the fact that your effort (i.e., your time spent) on a project may not be equivalent to the amount of money you are getting paid for it. In that case, your salary for the work has to come from somewhere. Thus, if you are putting in 25 % effort, but only getting paid 20 %, there would be cost sharing from an additional source to cover that 5 %—this could be for example clinical income if you are seeing patients—or it could be institutional salary support or philanthropic money, for example. Regardless of the details, the concept of cost sharing can also be applied to other areas besides salary too, including equipment costs or services to be utilized in a study.

5. *Supplies versus equipment.* This is a fairly murky area. Clearly, some items are supplies; however, some small equipment-like items—such as pipettes or scales or simple medical equipment—may fall into the category of supplies. This is because, rather than judging each item on its own merits, it is far simpler to create a cost cut-off, above which items are considered equipment and below which they are considered supplies. For example, at my institution, if it costs $3000 or more, than the item is considered equipment; below $3000 it is considered a supply. This differs from institution to institution, but it is worth making sure you get this correct. If you are working on a grant that is going to have indirect costs coming out of it, the more you can move into the safe harbor of equipment (since there are no indirect costs associated with it), the more money you will have to spend on other things.

6. *Consultants.* Budgeting for consultants is usually pretty straightforward. You will need a letter of support and then to agree on an hourly rate for a study. In my experience, it is actually pretty rare for a consultant to cash in on their chips. They decide in the end the amount of money gleaned for the effort is not worth it, and they feel better having simply just contributed. Nonetheless, ensuring that you have a reasonable estimate of costs is important, if only to underscore that you have dotted all of your i's and crossed all of your t's. Recently, my institution has further complicated the ability to bring on consultants, requiring any consultant to provide liability insurance to cover their consulting. I am not sure where from where this concept originated, however, most consultants do not have this. So, instead, we have started to bring on consultants with subcontracts—quite a bit more work for someone to provide only minor input on a project, but it appears to be the path of least resistance. I suspect we will see more and more institutions doing this over time.

7. *Modular vs. non-modular budgets.* This is an issue that, as far as I know, is only specific to NIH grant applications. If the total yearly costs are 250K or below (excluding indirect costs), then you can apply for a modular budget. This greatly simplifies the entire grant budgeting since you do not have to explain in detail every person's salary and cost that you are going to include. However, if you go over 250K you will need to complete a full, detailed application. Thus, if it is possible to stay under 250K, you will save both you and your grants administrator a great deal of work; however, I again would argue that you should not under-budget what you are doing. If your work is clearly going to require considerably more than 250K, don't transform your application to make it fit the mold. In truth the full budget

application is not all that much more work, especially since you will probably still need to provide your institution with an itemized budget for internal record keeping regardless.

Summary. Completing a budget should be one of the lower priority activities in preparation for grant submission, and hopefully you will be able to receive considerable assistance from people at your institution who are well versed in the matter. Moreover, a grant will not live or die by a budget; it is really a secondary issue that only becomes important once it is funded. But having a reasonable and complete budget can help ensure reviewers and the funding organization that you know what you are doing and that you have thought through everything thoroughly. And more importantly, it will help ensure that you have the means to complete the research successfully should your application be funded. Although strictly speaking the budget shouldn't impact the "fundability" of a grant application, it may play into the psyche of the reviewers in subtle ways, especially, if it looks like you are way, way over budget and asking for money for unnecessary items. So just be honest and do a reasonable job: this is one part of the application that you should not sweat over excessively.

Chapter 20
Grant Writing: Pearls and Lumps of Coal

First, it is worth remembering that there is a real aspect of luck to the grant application process. A terrific application will get rejected outright since one reviewer has misinterpreted a piece of preliminary data or the grant went to a group of reviewers who are not expert in your area. Inasmuch as things are actually in your control, in this chapter, I review a variety of assorted issues that I may have touched on earlier either simply to reiterate or expound on them in more detail. I've itemized them as dos and don'ts, in no particular order of importance.

Don't wait until the last minute to apply. Putting together even a short grant application will take a couple of weeks and larger ones can take 2–3 months. It is critical to keep coming back to an application to make sure your language is tight and understandable, and the only way to achieve this is by taking breaks from writing it and then returning to it, so that you can get a fresh view of the work each time. As you write it, you may realize that you need additional preliminary data or analyses or need another collaborator with a certain expertise. Or perhaps you need a letter of support from someone for one piece of the study. Regardless, this demands exquisite planning and time away from it. Working on it 1 hour per day for 2 months is far better and more effective than working on it for 12 hours a day beginning 5 days before it is due.

Don't assume the readers have much familiarity with your topic. You need to think of yourself as spoon-feeding your readers a magic potion, so even those with only limited knowledge will end up understanding things the way you do and come to fully endorse your proposal. But at the same time, you can't pander or be patronizing, so that the readers who do have knowledge are ready to fully endorse your work and get behind it. It is a very tough balance and there is no simple recipe as to how to achieve this. One useful approach is to always make sure sections are carefully labeled so that readers who know all the background can skip a section without losing a beat but those who need all the details have them available.

Do make sure all of your figures and tables are virtually self-explanatory and easily legible. Figures should have all the information available right within the figure itself and not even in the text or the figure legend. Use color to your advantage

© Springer Science+Business Media New York 2016
S.B. Rutkove, *Biomedical Research: An Insider's Guide*,
DOI 10.1007/978-1-4939-3655-7_20

(but remember the color-blind issues earlier). Label data points and lines. Make the figures large enough to read without the reviewer having to zoom in, since they probably will not, or in case they print it out on paper (God forbid). This includes the axes. Similarly use flowcharts abundantly and don't make your tables too complex. Try to keep the font no smaller than about 8 point within any figure.

Do not be afraid of repeating yourself. While this could be overdone, some repetition in a grant application is actually a good thing. A reviewer may be asked to evaluate half a dozen applications, and it is very easy to start forgetting which one was which, and sometimes the details of one begins to meld with the details of another. Repetition can help ensure that your most important points stand out and that the reviewers actually remember them by the time they come to writing the critiques and scoring it.

Do use strong topic sentences, subheadings, and highlight in bold font. If at all possible, ensure that these always make a declarative sentence that drives home the point of the material that follows. To some extent, you want to make it possible for a reviewer to almost fully understand the gist of grant application just by reading those sentences. The rest should be supportive material.

Don't assume just because the material is in a supplementary section, the reviewer will have looked at it. There is nothing more frustrating than to have a reviewer criticize your application stating that you have omitted crucial aspects of the application, such as a recruitment plan or power analysis, because you had placed them in a section *where the instructions told you they were supposed to go*. If it is not in the main body of the grant application, or at least mentioned there with a reference to it being elsewhere, you are setting yourself up for a problem.

Taking this issue on step further, some grants ask that you submit a pre-application (usually a 1–2 page summary of what you plan to do). If this is approved, they will ask for a full application. The instructions may state something along the lines of "The reviewers will have access to your pre-application, so do not repeat information or figures included there." I took this advice in one grant application a few years ago. The proposal was rejected. There were two reviewers, and one of them scored it very low because we had omitted basic information which had all been included in the pre-application, which he clearly never even reviewed. In other words, you should always assume the reviewers will not follow the instructions that they are given and that you should plan on telling the whole story from start to finish just in the single main document.

Do have at least some preliminary data before applying for any grant. Some grant applications are specifically created as seed funding and do not ask for your having any preliminary data (usually these are intra-institutional or from foundations). And for these, it is pretty obvious that any kind of preliminary data that you can provide will go a long way to helping its chances of funding, but is not actually necessary. But for most applications, abundant and convincing preliminary data is key to getting funded. So don't even think about applying if you do not have any.

This idea sometimes leads to a Catch-22. You need money to do the research, but you can't get the money without having done the research. And this interpretation is pretty much spot-on. You actually do need to always be thinking about using any current funding sources to slyly collect additional data to support your next grant application. This can be quite challenging and is definitely more difficult in the clinical realm where you can't veer too far away from what you have proposed without getting into trouble (even with IRB approval). But this is where you must inevitably maneuver your resources to ensure that you are thinking far ahead.

As a final corollary to this idea, never say you are going to do a study to collect pilot data, unless the grant solicitation specifically outlines this. Pilot data as a concept is too risky for most reviewers, and even if you make an argument that you will need to do this in order to lead to a bigger and more complete study, the concept of pilot data is essentially a death knell for an application. So avoid it.

Do recall that proposed research is not the real world. If you start writing a grant application constrained by really thinking through what is doable and what is not doable or what is doable but perhaps very challenging, you are probably going to fail. What one needs to do is to actually describe what ideally will happen if you are funded, unencumbered by any sense of reality (though you can certainly add in some points to show that you are not in space and have considered some of the potential problems). In a grant, you may need to idealize how a specific collaboration is going to work or who is going to be responsible for data collection. You will have to describe many details to convince your reviewers that you have thought everything through so that you can tell a convincing story. However, that story may turn out to be partially fiction, if and when the grant gets funded. Perhaps you'll find that you can more cheaply complete an analysis yourself than using a biostatistician for everything. Or perhaps you will realize that one outcome measure you decide to use in the rats actually has been supplanted more recently by something better. *In short, what you say you will do in a grant application and what you do and how you do it once it is funded will not be identical*. This is the nature of any endeavor that you undertake. Whatever your plans, things will happen to make you change course and do things somewhat differently. So don't let some seemingly challenging organizational aspect of your planned research stand in the way of the application. Just make your best guess as to how you are going to get it done and then deal with reality if and when the time ever comes. Of course, you need to make sure the reviewers are sufficiently convinced as well.

Do recall that grant writing gets easier the more you do it. Well, I would say that grant writing never gets to be painless, but it does become faster as you learn the tricks to putting together a good application and getting your points across. And some applications may actually be fun to write—it is one opportunity to be creative and you may find yourself getting carried away with your ideas. On the other hand, others may just be a burden since the ideas just don't want to flow easily or logically.

Do apply early and apply often. A phrase used to describe corrupting voting (vote early and vote often) actually applies very accurately to grants. The more you apply, the more likely you will eventually be funded. It is really just the time and effort needed that makes this idea so challenging to implement. But don't be afraid of submitting several nearly identical grant applications to different organizations. If you are funded by more than one, you may have to give one up, but, as mentioned earlier, if you subtly alter the grants so that there is little to no overlap in their proposed work (even though they are on similar topics), you may be able to keep all the money should both applications be funded.

Do recycle and reuse parts of an application whenever possible. You may have a methods section that you have written from an earlier application or a human subject or animal section from another. By all means, you should delve into your earlier applications to take advantage of what you have already rewritten and reuse it. For example, I created a data and safety monitoring plan for a grant application some 10 years ago. I have used that same basic plan for innumerable applications since then—always altering what was necessary to make it specific to that application. But I would say 90 % of the text remains unchanged with each application. Whereas self-plagiarism in publishing is forbidden, in the realm of grant applications, it is allowed (since these are not being published with someone else holding the copyright) and should be fully capitalized upon.

Summary. It is impossible to complete a full list of dos and don'ts for a grant application. There are many tricks to writing and effectively communicating your ideas that will only develop over time as you become a more experienced grant writer. However, hopefully you will have a mentor or colleague who will work closely with you to shape and reshape your grant until it has the necessary bright sheen to make it attractive to reviewers and receive the funding that it deserves.

Chapter 21
Research Training, Fellowship, and Career Grants

These categories of grants represent a special group of opportunities that are generally (although not universally) geared to providing junior researchers a prospect to get their foot in the door and obtain their first funding for a project. They are somewhat different than the standard project grant applications since the evaluation of the grant also includes a detailed evaluation of the person applying for the grant and her likelihood of success long term. These grants come in many shapes and sizes, and we will focus on some of the more common ones here.

NIH career grants. Career grants and fellowships at NIH usually are identified by the fact that their numbers begin with the letters F, T, or K, and each is somewhat different.

Both F and T grants are fellowship-type grants and are generally smaller in monetary amounts and last only 1–2 years. K awards, in contrast, are much larger, last 5 years, and are meant to serve as a clear next step that should prepare you for applying and hopefully obtaining an independent research grant, i.e., an R-type grant (e.g., R01 or R21). F grants (also called National Research Service Award or NRSA) are for individual applicants and are a great way to get some initial funding for 1–2 years of additional paid training. While strictly speaking NIH considers you a fellow when you have one of these, you can move into a faculty position as long as you abide by the rules of the grant. They are available for both clinical and basic research.

T grants, by contrast, are training grants given to your institution. In other words, you would not apply for them individually, but the institution would apply and then this becomes available for fellows each year to do additional training. T grants are something to ask your department about and not something that you should start researching how to apply for. If your department or institution has one, you can see whether or not you would be eligible to apply to participate. Usually there is an internal process at an institution that has received one of these to help decide who should receive funding. But do check—they are a great way of starting to do grant-funded research without your having to do the really heavy lifting of finding funding from scratch.

© Springer Science+Business Media New York 2016
S.B. Rutkove, *Biomedical Research: An Insider's Guide*,
DOI 10.1007/978-1-4939-3655-7_21

K awards are considered "career grants" in that they are much larger and are, not surprisingly, considerably more challenging to apply for. There are several of these. The K01 is intended for individuals in the biomedical sciences who do not have a clinical degree and want to pursue a career in basic research. The K08 grant is mainly focused on laboratory science but is mainly intended for people who have clinical degrees, helping them get back into the lab after a period of training (e.g., for MDs after having completed their residency training); in contrast, the K23 is mainly focused on patient-oriented research (i.e., research in which the data is gathered directly from live human beings). Another, the K25, is focused on people with basic quantitative science degrees (e.g., engineering and imaging) helping them apply their skills to biomedical research. Thus, both MDs and PhDs can apply for K08s and K23s, but K01s and K25s are probably mostly relevant to PhDs only. K99-R00s are a special kind of hybrid grant that allows postdocs to initially still be mentored for the first couple of years of the grant before beginning the junior faculty R00 phase. Usually the K99 is completed under a PI, and the grantee then moves to an independent faculty position and is supported by the R00 part for 3 additional years. Academic institutions appreciate these since the person they are hiring will already have 3 years of funding, allowing them an opportunity to obtain their first truly independent R01. Other K mechanisms are also available, so make sure to look carefully at the NIH websites to see rules/requirements and changes to any of these programs.

Grants from foundations. Many foundations offer funding opportunities for fellowships often ranging anywhere from one to several years. Again, the goal of the foundations is to get promising young investigators interested in the specific disease they support. These grants can be fairly generous since they are not only supporting the laboratory/clinical research but also provide some salary. It is always a good idea to talk (by phone or in person at a meeting) to people at the specific foundation to make sure that you are a potentially good candidate and so that you can understand what they are after that is not stated explicitly in the grant information provided. In my experience, many of the foundations are often focused on real disease mechanisms and potential therapies and less on ancillary questions such as testing out a new biomarker or a remote, secondary effect of the disease on another body system. In other words, they really want you to focus on meaningful disease questions not side issues, since the goal is to encourage you to pursue work in that specific disorder and potentially to dedicate your career, at least partially, to it.

General Concepts in Putting Together Career Research Grants

The applicant is being judged more than the research project. There is a saying, "Bet on the jockey, not on the horse." And to some extent, that is exactly how these grants are going to be reviewed. The reviewers will want to see evidence of commitment from the applicant and an appropriate level of achievement for their level of study. In other words, a person applying for a fellowship probably will not be expected to have any previous grants or funding but perhaps should have a paper or two and evidence of having pursued research previously. A person applying for a career award (e.g., a K award) should have several substantial publications under their belt and preferably some grant support as well. In some respects, applying for these awards is much like obtaining a credit card. Without any evidence of previously using credit, it can be hard to get one. Once you have established something of a credit history (and a good one at that), it is much easier to obtain additional credit. In other words, you have to demonstrate your own commitment to get a commitment from a funder. So any way in which you can play up that sense of past and ongoing effort and to give the impression that you are in it for the long run, the better your chances of receiving funding.

Really strong letters of recommendation and support. Recommendations, letters of support from a mentor, and a letter of support from the institution (which are required in many of these applications) can't just be boilerplate, perfunctory statements. They have to be over the top, detailed, and lengthy. Reviewers actually do read these, and when letters provide only lukewarm or moderately enthusiastic statements, those will serve as death knells for the application. Instead, they need to be specific for the applicant showing that the author has really thought about this and spent time and effort in drafting up a powerful letter.

In truth, many recommenders, including your mentor, may actually ask you to draft up an initial version of the letter, which you can then provide to them to modify as they see fit. If this ends up being the case, it can seem fairly awkward. After all, you may not feel exactly comfortable writing a letter glorifying yourself, your accomplishments to date, or your future potential. But you need to. This is not a time to be demure or bashful. You need to spell out everything you have done in exquisite detail and why you are so, so, so deserving of this award. And if your recommender writes a letter of his or her own, it is probably a good idea for you to review it and make sure they have not forgotten anything, unless it needs to be submitted separately.

Remember, you are not applying for a job here. These letters are absolutely NOT the place to be putting any minor concerns that a recommender might include in a letter of recommendation for a job or other position. So if a recommender is reluctant to share a letter of recommendation with you (which for many grant applications are actually included in the body of the grant so that you have full access to them), you should be concerned. There should be nothing with an even subtle critical tone in these letters. In some sense, these are not even really letters of recommendation but rather lengthy testimonials as to how incredible you are.

A mentor with a proven track record. Not all applications will care that much about your mentor, but some may. Having a strong mentor with a history of successful mentoring can be a real positive to one of these applications. A mentor who can point to a number of individuals who had worked with her and are now striking out successfully on their own in the field of biomedical research can be a real plus. If a separate mentor letter needs to be included in the application (which they usually are), then the mentor's skill set should also be highlighted, providing support that he will be able to do a great job with this mentee as he has done with others in the past.

Evidence of a research plan that fits and extends the applicant's skills. The research plan that is provided must not stand in isolation from the rest of the application. Rather it needs to really be considered integral to the development of the entire application. While the research plan needs to do something useful and important, it must serve as a conveyance to further develop the applicant's capabilities. In truth, you can pretty much do this with any research plan, but it is important to highlight how the research will achieve this. This could include learning new procedures, studying a new related field of science, experimenting with new types of data analysis, working with a different animal species or type of cell line or disease model, or having an experience with a different study design. As much as is possible, everything should be portrayed as providing an education for the mentee, such that two things are being achieved at once: the research itself and the further development of the applicant. Of course, not everything needs to be new or different providing a novel educational experience, so, for those aspects of the grant that are clearly well established already, you can also point out that the data being collected can serve as potential preliminary data for use in future applications.

Evidence for continued training and educational plan. Providing proof of a dedicated mentor and a solid research plan may not be sufficient for many applications. You may also need to show some kind of ongoing additional training and education. These can take many forms, and it is definitely better to go over the top on showing the potential things that you will be doing than identifying too few. Usually, this is not especially difficult to do, as long as you are being creative and thinking about all possibilities. For example, you will likely be at an institution that offers many educational opportunities, from undergraduate or graduate classes to short directed courses. Hunt through your institution's website and simply see what you can find. Most institutions recognize the importance of having a plethora of formalized educational opportunities available, in part exactly for this reason. Neighboring institutions or other sections within your own institutions may also offer valuable educational opportunities, so consider exploring these as well.

In addition to this, there are many national and international several-day or weeklong courses available to people wanting to improve a specific skill set. So don't confine yourself just to your university's opportunities—look outside for other opportunities and clearly delineate them in your application. The more intense and directed the course or workshop, the better.

Finally, you should also think about how you can delineate something of an auto-tutorial or mentor-directed educational plan as well. In fact, some applications will specifically ask for those, showing how, over the period of the grant, you will gradually educate yourself in a step-by-step fashion. Of course, most of what happens in the end is never so structured as anything you will put in the application, but that is OK. Recall once again that what goes into the application does not need to be the real world, but rather an idealized view of that world. So just do your best and come up with something that is believable and don't sweat the details as to how it will get done. I think the reviewers themselves usually recognize that these kinds of self-teaching programs are more perceived than real.

Evidence that their direction will become separate and unique from their mentor (especially for K award applicants). This is only the case mostly for career grant award applicants, since fellowships are more geared toward learning the basics in a research area. But for people who are already at a level of training that they are applying for awards that lead up directly to independent research, ensuring that you are on a path toward independence is really critical. If you seem to only be doing your mentor's bidding, that is a recipe for disaster. So both you and your mentor need to be careful and think through how, it needs to gradually show increasing independence until the point that you are working on a clearly different project. The key here is to really work backward and think about what you want to be investigating when all is said and done and in what direction your first independent grant may go. Of course, this is years away, so it is nothing more than an educated guess at best, but that is absolutely fine. As long as you can show that you are thinking about the long term and that this new direction of research has at least some potential of being significant, you will probably be in good shape.

New and early investigator grants. Finally, it is useful to also realize that when you get out on your own, many granting agencies will play nice with you the first time you are applying for grants. That means they are willing to give you a little bump in terms of your numbers: a grant that may receive a score that would not be officially fundable if you were veteran investigator will be funded. The bump is actually considerable and can make all the difference in the world when you are starting out. NIH defines a new investigator as any investigator (age independent) who has not successfully competed for a standard NIH award, such as an R01 or R21 or similar. Of note, the R00, included above, does not count. In other words, if you have received a K99-R00, you are still considered a new investigator when applying for an R01. You only lose the status of a new investigator, once you receive your first legitimate R01 or R21 award.

The early-stage investigator is a new investigator who is specifically within 10 years of completing her terminal research degree or within 10 years of completing her medical residency at the time she applies for R01 grants. The point of this added definition is to help ensure that the time between finishing training and getting full NIH grant support is reduced. Sadly, despite these efforts of NIH in helping to speed the attainment of independent research status, the average age that a researcher achieves her first independent R01 is 42 years. The problem may be less with NIH and the highly competitive nature of the grant process (which certainly does not help), but also the extended training periods that need to be endured by most people entering the biomedical research field. It is perhaps no surprise then that many people receiving their first R01 are already presbyopic and gray haired by the time they finally receive their first truly independent award.

Summary. There are a variety of fellowship and career grant awards that are available to people starting out on a career in biomedical research. While they are meant to make the path a bit easier, they are still competitive. Nonetheless, they are a good opportunity to learn about the grant application process, both its frustrations and rewards. If you can't handle the headaches involved in the grant process, it is better to learn early than later. But if you can handle the application processes, they can be a great way of finding funding and achieving meaningful work. Moreover, success in these early grants can definitely help begin your building a portfolio of success, such that it becomes easier to obtain funding in the future. So definitely thoroughly research and take advantage of these opportunities whenever they are available.

Chapter 22
Grant Review from the Inside

Surrounding a group of tables set in a large rectangle sit 25 people, their eyes focused on their laptops. Next to each sits a jug of water, a microphone, a ceramic coffee cup, and a prominent card displaying each reviewer's name in simple, unadorned black and white. Not far away sit three smaller "satellite" tables, each manned by just a couple of people, also ensconced on their laptops. The room is small—barely capable of fitting the entire group of people—and windowless, but with high ceilings lit entirely by two overly ornate chandeliers, an incongruous touch to an otherwise staid setting. One person is speaking in a baritone-pitched monotone, the words seeming to impress no one. After a few minutes, a balding middle-aged man at one of the narrow ends of the rectangle responds, "Thanks for that thorough review, Mitch. OK, let's see reviewer #2, uh, that's Dr. Shi. What are your thoughts?"

A thin Asian woman sitting near the far corner of the table starts to speak.

"Use the microphone!" a couple of people grumble simultaneously.

The woman stops, reaches across her computer, and pushes a button on the base of the microphone and starts to speak again. "Sorry about that. The previous reviewer covered many of the same concerns that I had about this application. Let's see. In terms of significance, I also felt that the application had a number of strengths. Clearly, if successful, this work could potentially introduce new pathways for potential pharmacologic manipulation and the long-term goal of creating new therapies for the disease. I also thought it was significant that they were going to study in vivo animals models as well as the in vitro work. The biggest weakness in terms of significance was the fact that they do not explain how the RD9 cells were going to be relevant to their long-term work. It almost seemed like an aside. Also, while it is clear that new pathways might be identified, one wondered whether or not they were simply going on a fishing expedition of sorts in some of their proposed experiments. The rationale did not always seem thoroughly considered. In terms of innovation, I...."

© Springer Science+Business Media New York 2016
S.B. Rutkove, *Biomedical Research: An Insider's Guide*,
DOI 10.1007/978-1-4939-3655-7_22

And in the room next door, a similar session was underway and in the room next to that yet another, and another group of sessions in the hotel right down the street in Bethesda, Maryland and 3000 miles away in San Francisco, other meetings were underway as well.

It is grant review season at NIH, and the effort and time to organize the events and ensure that they run smoothly across all the branches of NIH and across all the review sessions is nothing short of monumental.

Peer review is critical to the success of the NIH effort to foster medical science in the United States and throughout the world (by the way, you don't need to be working in the United States or even to be an American citizen to apply for many NIH grants). The individuals doing the reviews are researchers, pulled from both academia and industry, to help provide well-rounded assessments and ultimately scoring of the grant applications. They each are giving up often considerable time and energy to undertake the process, including potentially reviewing up to a dozen grant applications each, writing critiques, and then flying down to Washington, DC (or to a West Coast venue), and sitting in a hotel conference room working through a long list of applications. Their recompense is a several hundred dollars in reimbursement, travel expenses, and per diem living expenses covered for 1–3 days.

As you can probably tell from this brief vignette, the people doing NIH reviews are not generally an especially joyful lot. They have put aside their own research programs, grant writing, data analysis, patient care, teaching, administrative, and home/family responsibilities to spend a couple of days with a group of people, most of whom they do not know, working through challenging science and attempting to make intelligent judgments on work that is often not exactly in their field of expertise. They want to be thorough, to do a good job, to work constructively with their fellow reviewers, to ensure that the NIH staff that are present (sitting at those satellite tables in the room) know that they have taken their review tasks seriously, to seem attentive, and to get their points across without being overly aggressive or too demure. It is not an easy task, and after sitting in this room for 9 hours, with only a 1 hour break for lunch, most people are ready to hit the bar or collapse when the end of the day finally arrives.

NIH grant reviews are the gold standard by which most other foundations and organizations create their review models. Face-to-face meetings are still the norm, although many organizations, including NIH, do perform some meetings entirely by web or telephone conference and even fewer by just email (generally for small grants, such as those to fund a meeting). But regardless of the exact mechanism by which the reviews take place, this is not a simple or painless process.

Timeline for a Reviewer: Leading up to the Review Session

Taken from the reviewer's perspective, things generally play out as follows. Several months before a grant review session (at NIH the season for grant review is thrice yearly, once in March–April, then in June–July, and then in October–November), a scientific review administrator (SRA) will send an email to you asking whether you might be able to serve on a review session. The requests are always polite and never demanding. You are allowed to say "no" of course, although most individuals are reluctant to do so, since they feel a tremendous obligation to the organization that has funded their own work so generously. Moreover, of course, they want to stay in good terms with NIH, and to repeatedly turn down requests to participate in grant reviews might be seen as bad form. Shortly thereafter, a variety of electronic forms need to be signed, including conflict of interest statements. A list of potential grants is provided to ensure that there are no unrecognized conflicts (e.g., they are collaborators in other work with the applicants or they work at the same institution). Then there is generally a period of quiet up until about 6–8 weeks before the review sessions when the reviewer is provided the full applications to read over the Internet. If they are standard R01 grant applications, they are 13 pages for the basic pieces and then another 100–200 pages of associated documents and information. If they are R21 or other smaller grants, they are seven pages long. And if they are a program project or partnership grants, they can each have literally 30–50 pages of intense, detailed scientific writing and huge additional supplementary materials. Fortunately, the Scientific Review Administrator (SRA) from NIH will be looking out for you to some extent. They do not want to overwhelm you, and they try to provide you with grants that are reasonably within your area of expertise, although some may be somewhat far afield nevertheless. You will also be assigned as primary reviewer 1, primary reviewer 2, or a secondary reviewer. The basic idea is that the primary reviewers really need to do a thorough job, whereas the secondary reviewers can take a slightly looser approach. But this doesn't always hold; I've seen secondary reviewers go over the top in the review of an application and be far more involved than either primary reviewer.

Then, over the ensuing several weeks, you need to read through each of these carefully and gradually answer a series of questions (the review criteria) that are outlined by NIH—an approach aimed at making the review process simpler and more uniform. For each of these, you then need to list the strengths and the weaknesses. For NIH, these include the significance, innovation, and approach sections (the three major sections), as well as the environment and investigator sections (the two minor sections). There are also a number of additional criteria that need to be considered including human subjects or animal concerns, resource sharing (i.e., ensuring that the results of the work are sufficiently disseminated), women, children, and minorities, and, finally, the budget.

The reviewer has to carefully wade through and understand the application and then provide a written critique that addresses each of the points. When a reviewer has done that and has figured out the gist of the entire application, he is then forced to grade the application on a 1–9 scale, 1 being the best and 9 being the worst. NIH provides helpful guidelines to appropriately score each part of the application (significance, approach, innovation, investigators, environment), with 1 being almost perfect with no or just a couple of minor weakness and 9 being full of many major weakness and little redeeming value. A 5, the middle value, is an application with a couple of major weaknesses and several minor ones. In general, most individual sections of an application get scored in the 1–6 or 7 range. I am not sure I have ever seen even a single section get an 8 or 9. Then the reviewer is forced to choose an overall score for the entire application. This score is not supposed to be an average of the individual section values, but rather what the reviewer believes best reflects the overall take on the application.

Once the reviewer has worked through the multitude of applications on her plate, she then needs to upload the reviews and preliminary scores on the NIH website. This usually needs to be completed about 5 or 6 days before the actual meeting begins. Then about 4 days before the meeting, the "reading period" begins. At this time, all the reviews and scores by the reviewers are uploaded and should be read by the other reviewers. There is no opportunity to change your scores and you don't know who reviewed what. In other words, you will have a list of the 2 or 3 dozen reviewers, but you won't know which others were assigned to read the application you read. At any rate, by the end of the reading period, you should have a general sense as to what the other reviewers had to say and their views. You will also get a sense as to whether there is good convergence—i.e., everyone kind of agrees on the score and the value of the work—or extreme divergence, in which some reviewers love the application and others hate it. This reading period is always interesting since you may discover that your concerns were actually everyone's concerns and that your inability to understand some aspect of it was actually shared by all. On the other hand, you may find yourself amazed to discover that all the other reviewers overlooked an obvious flaw in the application and for which you gave it a low score. Or perhaps, you are the only person to have scored something very highly, and all the other reviewers were quite critical. One has to take a deep breath before reading the other reviewer's comments and bracing for the silent conflict or agreement that follows.

The Review Session

The review sessions begin with standard introductions by the NIH officials, including the SRA who is to serve as the main point of contact for all the reviewers during the review session. When you are there, you are likely to see other NIH program officials that you have come to know, often including in your own program officer since the study section is probably closely aligned with your own work.

After the reviewers are all given an opportunity to introduce themselves and the NIH officials have introduced themselves as well, the rules of the review session are spelled out, the meaning of the scoring discussed, the agreement that no one is to speak of the goings-on at the review session outside of the session itself is laid down, and procedures for reimbursement are presented. The SRA then introduces the reviewer who is going to act as a chairperson for the session. This person is someone like you—another investigator at another academic institution–and occasionally needs to be reminded of the various rules throughout the proceedings by the SRA. But the system generally works and the people selected tend to be fair and consistent.

Then the entire list of applications that were sent out for review for which detailed critiques were written and scores provided is reviewed. Usually, this is provided as a separate list now sorted according to overall score, with the lowest (i.e., best) applications listed at the top working on down to the lowest scored (worst). There may be 50 or even 60 applications—a huge number by any means—depending on the specific nature of the review session. Thus, the first order of business is to triage the poorest scoring applications. The goal is that the reviewers will spend their time on top 50 % of applications and so cordon off the rest to be simply returned to the applicants with the written reviews from each of the reviewers. These "triaged" applications will not actually receive a numerical score—the applicants will only see a "not discussed" comment on their NIH webpage for the grant.

Misery loves company; it is always good to remind yourself if you end up in this group of not discussed applications, you have plenty of bedfellows, even if you don't know who they are. The good news is that you will still get a review and that if you choose to reapply, you can address the concerns of the reviewers and try again. Or you perhaps will also get a sense that the application was just ill conceived to begin with and better tossed aside. Remind yourself that the only thing that would be worse than being rejected and receiving a critical commentary is to be rejected with no commentary. This is not the way that NIH does things, but some foundations unfortunately do this, and it can be frustrating since you really don't know or understand why your work is being scorned.

However, prior to assigning the bottom 50 % to the junk heap, each application is briefly stated and the opportunity for any reviewer who wants to discuss it can ask for it to be discussed. Most of the time the reviewers remain silent at this point, but occasionally there are some applications that have widely disparate scores (e.g., a couple of reviewers giving it 1s and 2s and others giving it 5s and 6s). In these situations, a reviewer may ask for it to be included in the discussion. That is all that needs to happen for it to be discussed. In my experience, these applications rarely get scored very highly, but occasionally a major error in a reviewer's thinking is disclosed. Of course, most reviewers remain entirely silent during this triaging period, similarly wanting to focus on the best applications and hoping to make the couple of intense days ahead as focused as possible.

Of course, since you yourself have only reviewed a small subset of the total number of grants (perhaps only 3–7), it is possible that every one of the grants you have reviewed is triaged. If that happens, your input on the review session will be very limited, although, as described below, you will have opportunities to vote on all the applications to be discussed. But usually, there will be at least one or two that you have reviewed in some fashion that will end up being discussed.

Then the reviewers get to work considering each individual application. The first application is announced (often alphabetically by PI last name), and the chairperson asks the reviewers to state their overall scores. These will usually be in the range from 1 to 4 or 5, since almost all applications below that level were triaged. When all four reviewers provide numbers that are within 1 point—in other words there is good a priori agreement—the review process will move very swiftly. However, when the values are fairly dispersed, you can be certain that there may be a long discussion. The goal of the discussion is obviously to discuss the merits and problems with each grant and see if all the reviewers can reach something approaching agreement.

The chairperson is hoping that by the end of the discussion, the overall scores are within a close range, thus showing consistency among the reviewers.

And then the discussion begins in earnest, with each reviewer briefly stating the weakness and strengths of the application, going by significance, innovation, approach, investigators, and environment. Generally, the investigators and environment (i.e., the institutions involved and collaborators) are scored fairly high. Occasionally, someone junior or a person with a mixed publication record may be criticized, but it is rare that any investigator ends up scoring low since generally the investigators are experts in their fields to begin with. And most institutions are reasonably high functioning. Thus, the real criticisms in the application generally boil down to problems in the significance, innovation, and approach. Of the three, innovation is generally considered least important. As noted earlier in the section on grant writing, if you are doing important work and it is well done, even if the innovation gets mediocre scores, your application may still score well. Thus, to some extent the significance and approach are the two biggest opportunities and two biggest minefields for every application.

Criticisms of significance can be pretty broad. You can imagine that if one is studying a very rare disease, the significance of the application may be downgraded. However, in my experience, applications rarely get overly criticized if the disease is very rare, since the goal of research is to find treatment for all diseases, regardless of their prevalence. But if the investigator can couch the study of this work in terms of broader meaning (i.e., other diseases with similar mechanisms), the significance will increase. However, applications that come from clinicians' writing grants generally have a stronger significance section than those from nonclinicians, just given the former's ability to more deeply understand the wider application of the work. NIH is funding health-related research, and if an investigator is very deeply buried in disease mechanisms, he may have a more challenging time seeing the forest for the trees or communicating the importance of the research that he is doing.

But if any section is the real target for criticism, it is generally the approach section. Scoring well on the approach section is very challenging especially the first time an application is reviewed. The problem here is that it is very easy for reviewers to have very different perspectives on how to answer the questions posed in a study. They may disagree with the animal model choices, the exclusion/inclusion criteria for a patient population, or the choice of analyses to perform. All four reviewers may have a different set of concerns or see what they each consider better ways for doing the same work. On the other hand, common concerns being voiced by the reviewers probably means there was a real weakness or lack of clarity in some aspect of the research plan.

The Other Sections

After the major sections are discussed, the reviewers then deal with the more secondary sections. These include the human subjects and animal concerns, minorities, etc. The only section here that usually gets people into trouble is the human subject section. If the work is considered at all dangerous or if some of the concerns were not fully discussed, then a criticism here can immediately kill an application. It is rare for an application to founder on racial or sex biases, but this must occasionally happen. If a study can only be performed in men or only women, that is fine, of course. It just needs to be explained and justified.

It is rare for animal concerns to be raised of sufficient worry unless the investigators are working with nonhuman primates. Rodent studies are rarely thought about twice. Similarly safety concerns regarding potentially virulent pathogens or toxic chemicals are readily dealt with and generally do not cause issues unless the sections are completely poorly or entirely ignored (which does happen with remarkable frequency).

Revisiting the Scores

After all the reviewers have had their opportunity to present their scores, the grant application is opened up to broader discussion among the entire group of reviewers. Remember, only about four or five people may have reviewed the application initially, and there may two dozen people sitting around the circle of tables, but now any of those additional people can chime in with concerns, questions, ideas, or accolades. Whereas the SRA may have delegated the primary review tasks to a group of people who should have been very capable in dealing with the application, the assignments may not always be ideal, and there may be someone else in the group with a superb perspective on the entire question that can greatly influence the discussion. Generally, though most people are pretty unfamiliar with the details of the application, having only skimmed it before or even during the meeting, and aren't in a position to take an especially strong view about any aspect of it. Still, I have seen many applications get helped or hurt from comments by one of the people who have not reviewed the application. But much of this open discussion is still between the groups of primary reviewers since they finally have the opportunity to actually discuss an application's strengths and weakness face to face and iron out differences in their views.

At the conclusion of the open discussion, which can last anywhere from 5 to 30 min, the chairman revisits the scores provided by the initial reviewers. The hope of course is that there is now greater consensus than at the beginning. If the scores were fairly tight to begin with, they still might be quite tight, unless some major discovery was made during the discussion. On the other hand, if the scores were really disparate, you'll probably see some movement toward the center or one extreme depending upon which reviewer was most persuasive. Most of the time, people tend not to change their scores too much, I think, because there is a sense of losing face. This obviously should not play into the review process, but probably does nevertheless.

Once all the primary reviewers have stated their scores, then all the other people on the committee silently grade the application on their computers. The score chosen needs to fall within the range of that of the original reviewers. So if everyone gave scores in the 1–2 range, you can only choose a 1 or 2; however, if the range is 2–6, you'll have a wide range from which to choose. A non-primary reviewer is free to choose a score outside the range as well; however, this requires his announcing to the entire group the score he is going to give and the reason for doing so. This happens mainly when the discussion has been a little contentious or if there is a general sense that the range is excessively lenient or severe—but again here, in my experience, I'd say most of the time, people will vote outside the range only if they think the scoring has been too positive only, not too critical.

The F Word

One of the earliest mistakes I made when submitting grant applications was to think that the budget somehow influenced ones likelihood of being funded. I had intentionally budgeted a grant low thinking that it would help get it funded. In fact, according to NIH review rules, funding is the "F word" in a review session. It is not to be said aloud at any point. As discussed previously in this book, the reason for this is that grants are to be judged on their scientific merit only, not on cost. The budget is only discussed after the scores are all recorded. Any budget concerns are addressed at that point and commented on. There is no specific score that is provided on the budget. If the reviewers are very critical of the budget, it will be included, and if the application is funded, the budget may be cut accordingly. At no point during the review session are you to say anything about the budget until the budget itself is discussed and at no point can you "recommend a grant for funding." You are simply scoring the science and leave the funding decision itself to the officials at NIH.

One caveat. While funding is not strictly discussed and should not be included in the scientific evaluation of a study, it can come to play in subtler ways. For example, you may be part of a study section that is reviewing a number of grant applications for a specific RFA (request for applications). In such a situation, the total amount of money may be stated up front, and you can quickly add up based on the budgets of each application how many grants can be funded through this single mechanism. Sometimes this can come into play since you may find yourself very unenthusiastic about one huge application in lieu of a couple of smaller projects. While strictly speaking this should not come into the discussion, it may still influence the reviewers' thinking to some extent, consciously or unconsciously.

The End of the Day

At some point late that afternoon or perhaps in the early afternoon of the subsequent day, you will have worked through the last of the applications and after a few "thank you's" from the NIH staff, you will be released. You and your fellow reviewers will chat for a bit as you pack your computers, put on your coats, and call a taxi or Uber or perhaps take DC's Metro back to Reagan Airport for your flight home. Usually, everyone feels exhausted and drained and is ready to return to the real world and sunlight. But there is generally a sense of accomplishment and camaraderie, and not a few friendships and new collaborations begin after these meetings come to an end. So while I think everyone is relieved, they are also happy to spend time with people they may not know well from a variety of institutions across the United States.

Post-review Session

After spending all that time reviewing the grants, writing critiques, possibly traveling to Washington DC, and spending two high-stress days reviewing the applications, your work is still not quite over. While the NIH SRA will put together a summary of the discussion and complete the entire review results for each application, you are still asked to go back to your own critiques and revise them according to the discussion. In my own experience, many reviewers are just burned out by this point and are not that interested in making further revisions to their commentaries. They need to get back to their own research endeavors and patients and families. After the meeting, the review session is mostly out of sight and out of mind. This is unfortunate, since on many occasions, criticisms may be found in an a reviewer's commentary that are not necessarily reflective of that reviewer's take after the discussion is complete and, in fact, may be contradictory to some of the discussion summary comments. This can leave the applicant quite confused. He will see a rather critical summary statement and then rather positive individual reviews—things not seeming to add up. But such are the vagaries of the review process, and for better or worse, one must read between the lines. See the next chapter for a full discussion of interpreting your scores and comments.

After signing an online post-meeting conflict of interest statement and deleting their files, the reviewers have then officially completed their review activities.

Grant Review Sessions/Meetings Beyond NIH

Grant review can take many forms and shapes beyond that which I have described here, even though NIH study sections remain, I believe, the gold standard in terms of providing thoughtful and comprehensive reviews. As I mentioned, many NIH review sessions now occur online and some even by email.

Many foundations will simply ask the reviewers to provide a written critique followed by a conference call in which all the applications are discussed. In other cases, there will still be a face-to-face meeting to discuss all the applications. In most cases, a written critique will be provided, even if they are short and telegraphic in nature. Some foundations will simply review applications internally with one or more scientific advisors and not involve any outside adjudicators. Regardless of the mechanism, most well-established foundations will provide a critique. Some foundations will also go a step further and ask you to revise the grant along certain lines that the reviewers have suggested, hoping to fund it if you can satisfy their concerns and needs. Since they are smaller, they can be more flexible than NIH, helping shepherd the application through to funding so that they can further their mission.

Summary

The peer-review process is a complex but an extremely important activity. An NIH study section review, described here, provides a case in point about how carefully considered and effortful the entire process is. It is important to remember this when you are on the other side receiving the reviews since you need to simply accept the fact that mistakes and oversights can and do happen. That is why the application needs to be crystal clear and as easy reading as possible. The reviewers are charged with a complex task, and juggling the review of a number of applications simultaneously can be exhausting and confusing, especially when added on to your regular work life. On top of that, the logistics and time spent traveling to and from the meeting venue and dealing with the online review process and associated forms also take a toll. So perhaps it is not surprising that every application does not receive its "ideal" vetting. But the process does work fairly most of the time, and for that, we researchers should be very, very thankful.

Chapter 23
Interpreting Your Reviews

I remember all too well sitting in a large lecture hall in college, anxiously awaiting my midterm exam to be returned. The teaching assistants would gradually wend their way through the classroom, my heart beating ever more strongly. And then one would approach and place the exam face down on the little table that extended from the arm of my lecture room chair. There it lay: several seemingly innocuous pages of paper stapled together. Before daring to turn it over, I would try to read the assistant's facial expression. Was it stone cold? Was there a hint of a smile? Did he just slightly nod his head in silent approval? And I, taking in a deep breath, usually without another moment's hesitation, desperately wanting to end the misery as quickly as possible, would flip over the document and read the red scrawl. When an A was bestowed, a sense of jubilation immediately erupted within me. To have achieved such greatness! I was brilliant, the best! But when it was a C, my heart sank and I could feel this sudden warmth of shame immediately envelop me. I was an idiot, a goofball. What in the world gave me the right to even think I belonged at this fine institution or even more could one day go to medical school and pursue a career as a physician?

After we finish college, many of us have recurrent dreams—or rather nightmares—about being back in school, being late for a test, forgetting to dress for class, or discovering that you had failed a course. Awaiting and finally looking at your score on a grant application conjures up all of those feelings of anxiety, inadequacy, ambivalence, and uncertainty. Of course, no one is going to be hand-delivering you the news and you can at least look at the results in the privacy of your office or bedroom (or perhaps bathroom for those who are prepared for especially bad news). But there is an icy, impersonal aspect to receiving the information that is just as removed as when high school students receive their SAT results or college students learn of their MCAT, LSAT, or GRE grades. For foundations or other funding sources, it is usually a brief email from the organization that suddenly pops up in your inbox in between a message from your mom and a piece of junk mail that did not filter out properly. For government sources such as NIH, you will also

© Springer Science+Business Media New York 2016
S.B. Rutkove, *Biomedical Research: An Insider's Guide*,
DOI 10.1007/978-1-4939-3655-7_23

receive an email, but this email only informs you that your grant has been scored and that you should go to your "personal" NIH webpage to look up the results.

So my first suggestion is to psychologically prepare to look at your scores, days or weeks before you anticipate receiving them. Specifically, you should choose the timing and location where you think you will be in the best headspace. Just because you know it has returned does not mean you need to look at it that instant. Go home, have something to eat and try to get in the right mindset before taking the plunge. After all, it may be that this grant application's score *is* more important than that midterm test grade in organic chemistry—since it may actually be providing you substantial income and research support for the next 5 years of your life. And it could also influence your ability to obtain future funding. Unlike your organic chemistry midterm though, which only happens once or twice, you do have the power to reduce the significance of this application—just by applying for grants again and again and again. The more you apply, the less important any one score becomes and the more relaxed you can be when you read your score.

I suppose if there is any one positive aspect that I enjoy about the process of getting my "grant grade" is that it does make me feel like I am still young in some way. It is as if 30 years have not really passed since leaving the hallowed halls of Cornell University or even if they have, I'm just as versatile and ready to roll with the punches as I was as a newly minted 20-year-old. The fact that one can put oneself through repeated external evaluation on a regular basis and survive (and occasionally even thrive) does say something positive about an individual's grit and determination and ability to roll with the punches that is often thought as an important part of being young.

And with that preamble out of the way, I will start by discussing the current-day NIH scoring system in some more detail than I did in earlier chapters and then briefly discuss scoring approaches of foundations, since they vary widely. In the section following that, I will review interpreting the critiques; finally, I will conclude with strategizing for a resubmission.

Interpreting the Score

First, if your NIH application was not discussed (i.e., was approximately in the lower half of the applications reviewed), it will not receive an overall numerical score that you will see on the NIH website. But you will still be able to see the individual scores from each of the reviewers when you receive your summary statement several weeks later, including the individual scores that each gave it on the sections reviewed (significance, innovation, investigator, etc.). Thus, if you want to approximate an overall score, you'd probably have to average the numbers in some fashion, recognizing that the approach and significance sections probably hold the most weight for each individual reviewer; you won't get an overall score from each reviewer, just a score from each of the sections. But remember that even if it wasn't reviewed at the meeting, you will have obtained detailed written critiques that you can then specifically address—more on that later.

Now, if your application was discussed, you'll have some additional numbers to look at and interpret. We reviewed the numerical meaning of the scores from NIH in the previous chapter: a 1 is perfect and a 9 is terrible in the initial scoring during grant review. For some reason, NIH multiplies these values by 10, and the final "impact score" will represent an average of all the overall scores from the study section (the primary reviewers and everyone else who graded your application). So if the average among the 25 reviewers was 3.8, you'll receive an impact score of 38. But in addition to this, you may (but not always) receive a percentile ranking. In many respects, the percentile is more important than the score itself. This percentile places your application among the others that were reviewed by that study section, or related study sections, averaging across several grant cycles, including the present one; this averaging across grant cycles helps reduce some of the fluctuations that may be seen from one cycle to the next. The lower the percentile the better, but remember that probably more than 50 % of the applications were never even reviewed in the first place, so you'll probably never see a percentile greater than about 50 %. And to be really competitive for funding, you need to be under 20 % and possibly under 10 or 15 %, depending on the institution and the current NIH funding situation, as determined by Congress and the president.

Generally the impact score and percentile follow each other—the lower both are, the better. But there is considerable variability across NIH study sections, and thus an impact score of 29 could mean a percentile of 8 % in one study section, whereas an impact score of 29 could mean a percentile of 18 % in another. Ultimately, it is the percentile that will tell you the likelihood of getting funded; generally, NIH institutes will publish their "pay lines"—that percentage you need to be at or under in order to be funded. Thus, you can do a quick calculation to see whether or not you are probably going to be funded or not. Of course, there are exceptions for young or early-stage investigators where these numbers don't quite hold. Both types of investigators are allowed to have scores that are several points higher and still be funded.

For a variety of reasons, however, not all NIH summary statements that provide impact scores also provide percentiles. This may be because the type of application you have submitted is not that common or is being reviewed in a special panel, and there would be no clear way to generate a percentile. In this situation, you may have a hard time knowing exactly what is going to happen. The thing to do is to call your program officer to try to get a sense of things, but he or she may not know either, though generally if your impact score is below 30, you have at least a fighting chance of getting funded and under 20 you will almost definitely be set.

Foundations, in contrast to NIH's relatively uniform approach, have a variety of means for providing scores. Many in fact, don't give any—all you get is a simple thumbs up or thumbs down for funding—or perhaps an opportunity to immediately revise according to the reviewers' criticisms and resubmit. Others may follow something akin to an NIH approach. Obviously, if it is unclear, you should simply talk to the foundation's research officer to help you better interpret the score, if provided.

Reading the Critiques

We all have our own way of going about this, and the focus needs to be on interpreting the criticisms while trying not to get excessively angry or annoyed. Let me tell you about how I go about doing this. First, it depends on exactly how I scored. If the score was really high, and it looks like it is going to be definitely in the fundable range, I will read through the reviews very carefully from the outset, since I know most of the comments will be positive, and even if there are some negative ones, I'll be able to read them without getting too peeved. On the other hand, if the score is mediocre or the application did not get discussed (and hence there is no overall score), I will generally read through the document quickly to get a sense of the concerns. Is this going to be something that I am going to be able to revise and resubmit or is it dead in the water? My goal is not to troubleshoot or solve then and there but rather to get a gestalt as to whether the application can be resuscitated and possibly still give birth to a funded grant. I forward the critiques to my collaborators immediately by email, send a note with my overall sense of things, and generally put it aside for several weeks as I digest the score, the overall comments, and strategies.

When I am then ready to really dig into the critiques, I will start by carefully reading the summary comments. If this was an NIH grant and it was discussed, you'll receive a summary of that discussion; generally this is the single most important part of the critique, since issues may have been brought forth or highlighted during the discussions that were not included or emphasized in the specific comments of the reviewers. Remember also that the individual reviewers made their comments before the discussion and may not have gone back and revised their reviews to reflect the discussion, so there may be a disconnection between the two parts of the critique. If there is any inconsistency, the comments from the discussion should hold sway as you think through the prospects of revising, since this represents a group opinion.

I then begin to itemize the concerns. One of the most important issues to consider in whether to resubmit an application is the consistency of the comments. If each reviewer is bringing up similar concerns, and those are addressable concerns, you are in much better shape than if all the reviewers have an entirely different set of issues. So, inasmuch as you can, try to group the concerns together. If and when you decide to resubmit, you will only have a single page to rebut, so the more you can group the comments, even if they are not identical, the better. It will also help you get your work through the resubmission process more effectively.

Once you have dealt with the concerns, you can then sketch out a general plan for your next steps. Do you need to do more experiments and collect preliminary data? Did you not get a point across clearly enough? Is one of the aims really bad? Do they think the study is too ambitious and that you actually need to cut down the number of studies? Or perhaps you were not ambitious enough and the study just didn't excite the reviewers. Talk to your collaborators and mentors and get their opinion of the reviews. And finally, talk to your program officer. He can help you get a general sense of what is going on and how best to proceed at this point. They will not be able to offer you specific suggestions, of course, nor will they be able to help your application get funded, unless your score is in a borderline territory—in which case their involvement and endorsement can become very important. More on that later.

For foundation applications, the same general rules apply. Unfortunately, many foundations may only have annual cycles, so a rejection or poor score may mean that the project is grounded for a while. On the other hand, you may be able to learn from the comments and improve your research plan and possibly apply to a different funding source in the meantime with a greatly strengthened application.

Funding and Council: What Happens at NIH After You Get the Scores

Of course, your receipt of the scores, even if they are good, does not imply an immediate deposit of a large sum of money in your name at your institution. In fact, it can take many months and possibly even up to a year before you learn whether your grant has been funded. Naturally, the better your priority score, the greater your likelihood of getting funded and the greater your chance of learning about that sooner. Regardless if your score is sufficiently good, you will be asked to submit JIT or "just-in-time" information, which includes an update on all the investigators' current grant support as well as human subjects or animal approvals. Very low (in other words extremely good) scores may result in an email from your program officer just a few weeks later saying that your grant is going to be funded and that they need that JIT information immediately. But if your grant scored well but not really well—for example, close or even slightly above the pay line—you might end up eventually being funded—it is just that you will not find out very soon. It may only be close to the end of fiscal year, when the NIH institution's administrators have a sense as to how much money is left in their coffers that they are willing to say, OK, you are going to get the dough. Or it may end up getting funded in the next fiscal year after the pay line is set, depending on which NIH grant cycle you applied in. There are many variables, and the sands are constantly shifting, so it is impossible to describe every potential scenario that may arise.

And the flip side is also true—you may learn about your great score and that you will likely be funded only to wait and wait for no obvious reason. This may because there are still funding decisions to be made more globally in the NIH institute or other granting source. These kinds of decisions will not be made until after the institution's "council" meeting is complete. This is a time when an NIH institute's administrators all meet to discuss funding priorities. Generally, grants that scored at or below the pay line will get funded, but a number above the pay line will also get funded—those that the institution has deemed higher priority. Council occurs three times a year in sync with the standard NIH funding cycles.

And now a word about federal budgets and funding. For all federal grants, from NIH to DoD to NSF to NASA, the funding of the yearly federal budget is key to determining your likelihood of being funded. It sometimes seems hard to believe, but the news that you read online or hear about on television about disagreements between Congress and the president on budget priorities actually can affect you personally in a really deep way. If Congress cannot approve a budget by October 1 or they only pass continuing resolutions, all granting agencies have to respond accordingly, often by reducing the number of grants they can fund, at least until a final budget is passed and the money fully appropriated. This means that while you may have obtained a "fundable" score on your grant, you'll suddenly discover, much to your horror, that your grant is no longer funded, or at least not yet. You will be forced to keep applying, only potentially to learn that your grant is funded, but several months later than you had anticipated. When I have a grant that scored well, but not really, really well, and its funding is going to be decided in the fall, I usually know I am in for a tough ride. But like all things, you kind of get used to not knowing and being subject to the whims and fancies of Congress.

Foundation funding decisions, in contrast to NIH, are often far more fluid and faster. After the grant application process is complete, most foundations move quickly to solidify their decisions and try to get the money to the investigators so that the work can get underway. It is important for foundations to speed things along since they, unlike NIH, which is funded by the government every year, are in a perennial state of money raising. They want to announce those grants to help generate more donations. So if you don't understand your scores from a foundation or the meaning of a letter, you should definitely contact the organization's scientific director and try to get the straight story. At the very least, you will learn about the foundation's attitude and ideas and how to make your work perhaps better fit with their funding mission in a future grant application. Having the people who make the funding decisions get to know you a bit better is never a bad thing.

Summary. Receiving and assimilating grant review scores is usually a lonely and often unpleasant experience. You can't commiserate with your classmates who also didn't score well because one of the questions was "unfair" or because the test was too long for the allotted period of time. Remember though that, unlike high school, college, medical school, or graduate school, there is really no limit to the number of opportunities that you will have to apply—it all depends on your time, effort and commitment, and, of course, your imagination and resilience. But use your receipt of scores as an opportunity to reflect on where you have been and in what direction you should be moving. Perhaps the line of research you have been considering really is simply not that important and you should cut bait. Or perhaps you are somehow not getting your message clearly across, even though it seems entirely lucid to you. But if you have scored well—make sure to celebrate your accomplishment.

Chapter 24
To Resubmit or Not Resubmit and How to Do It

First the good news: the resubmission of a grant application that was not funded, whether to NIH or a private foundation, is often considerably easier than submitting the application the first time. In fact, it is much, much easier, and it is one reason to strongly consider resubmitting every single grant that fails, even if it requires dramatic reformatting. For NIH, this is due to a recent change in NIH policy, namely, that you can keep resubmitting a grant application even after it fails its "two strikes" policy. It will be judged as a new grant application on the third try, but with each successive application, it will likely continue to improve and hopefully, eventually, reach the point of funding. So let me repeat myself: regardless of the specific grant mechanism, strongly consider a resubmission if your first application did not succeed. It won't seem nearly as daunting as putting it together the first time around.

But also realize that a resubmission may require a great deal of thought and creativity to get it into a position where it has a fighting chance of being funded. And sometimes, if the criticisms are really deep and severe and broad (i.e., multiple sections of the application are knocked down), it may be better to drop the application entirely and start anew.

Usually, though the concerns are mainly over one or two specific sections or aspects of the grant. For instance, sometimes the concerns are really focused on the significance; perhaps you did not clearly state how important this work actually is. Or the approach section, which is most open to criticism, since every reviewer may have her own set of concerns and ideas for performing the experiments and studies more effectively. Occasionally the innovation plays a major role in the demise of an application. More rarely the investigators and the environment are the application's undoing. Let's deal with these parts of the application, common concerns, and how to address them.

© Springer Science+Business Media New York 2016
S.B. Rutkove, *Biomedical Research: An Insider's Guide*,
DOI 10.1007/978-1-4939-3655-7_24

Limited Significance

If a major concern of the application is limited significance, you may simply need to focus on improving your messaging. Getting the idea of the importance of your proposed work in a grant application can require a great deal of effort. Many PhDs and MDs are not used to saying how great or important their work may be. In fact, research does not need to focus on the most common maladies—heart disease or cancer—but can focus on some of the most obscure and rare diseases and still be considered of great significance. As I have mentioned in other parts of this book, the key to making sure the significance is understood is to *generalize the concepts that you are evaluating such that they have wide applicability outside your one area of study*. For example, if you are studying a rare genetic form of lung disease, explain how the mechanisms underlying the development of pathology in that disease are mirrored in more common conditions (e.g., asthma or pulmonary fibrosis) and how identifying the mechanism or pathway of injury in such a rare genetic disease could lead to important new therapies in other diseases. Don't just list the statistics for your one rare disease that effects only 2000 people on the planet; rather focus on the broader implications and the millions who could eventually be impacted by under-standing the pathway better. Or perhaps you are putting together a clinical trial in another orphan (i.e., rare) disease. The trial may not only test the drug in the disease, but it may also allow you to develop better outcome parameters and biomarkers that can be applied to future trials in that disease.

Another way of hitting a home run in the significance section is by making the story simple and clear—really read through what you wrote in the original with fresh eyes. Give it to friends and colleagues to read. The significance should hit them over the head with its obviousness. Use flow charts or enticing figures/graphics to also help get the point across. Simplicity, clarity, and inclusivity are perhaps the most important things to try to get across. If you are not particularly convinced of the significance yourself, neither will be your audience. Once you are convinced, it becomes much easier to tell a simple story that can convince everyone else as to why this work has the potential to be so important.

And of course scrutinize the reviews in detail. Maybe one of the reviewers mis-understood population of people you were proposing to study. Maybe another had made a specific suggestion for improving the significance—e.g., to look at the mechanisms more broadly or to utilize a specific laboratory technique. Where possible, always try to identify their concerns and try to deal with them explicitly.

One of the worst criticisms for an application is for it to be called "incremental." This suggests that while the research is potentially important ultimately, the proposal is only taking one small step toward that goal. Or it could mean that the technique/procedure/science is already mature and that the proposed work will not add much beyond what is currently available. In responding to the incremental criticism, it is a good idea to take a step back and ask if there was a way of making your idea seem grander and more exciting. Perhaps you do need to be a bit more daring in your aims—sometimes being a little audacious (with the appropriate caveats added in afterward) is not crazy. It may then capture one or two reviewers' imagination, which can help your case immensely. In short, you made need to take greater risks in describing your significance and your actual research plans. If you are being too staid in your assessments, you may bore the reviewers, and then your application is doomed from the outset. If you think about making your application exciting, it will help your efforts a great deal.

The Approach Is Problematical

As already stated, the approach section is often the part of the application that is most open to criticism, in part because if you have a significant idea, no two people may agree on the best way of studying it. Thus, broadly speaking, after digesting the criticisms, you first need to decide what you need to keep and what you need to let go. It is important to realize that the reviewers are given the mission to critique your plans and not necessarily to suggest alternative ones. This means that it may not always be clear what the reviewers are suggesting you do as an alternative to the plan you suggest. On the other hand, if a reviewer does make concrete suggestions as to alternative plans, if they make sense to you, you may want to try to incorporate them.

One common reason that the approach section is struck down is because you don't have enough strong preliminary data to support what you are contending. For that reason, any additional new preliminary data you can bring to bear on the question may help support your approach section. Of course, if you cannot dig up that evidence, then you may really have to go back to the drawing board and try to utilize different preliminary data to support a somewhat altered approach.

As you think through the criticisms, you'll need to decide which are killing the application and which are just needing to be tweaked or clarified. It is not uncommon for a reviewer to not really understand the intrinsic details of a plan, so sometimes rethinking its presentation can also be helpful.

Once again, getting an outside set of eyes on an approach section from an experienced person can be incredibly helpful. Not uncommonly, you may simply not understand a criticism that a reviewer has leveled at the proposal. It may seem like he somehow misinterpreted what you were saying and that the comment is coming from left field. Spend some time reading and rereading these; very often it is simply the phraseology that is not clear and there is often some underlying truth to the comment that can be addressed. Having a second or third person familiar with your work read the criticism may also help you getting to the heart of the issue that has been raised. Remember, don't just assume the reviewer is an idiot or mean-spirited or didn't give the grant proper attention. More likely than not, you are at least partially to blame if some aspect of the grant was misinterpreted or a criticism seems far off mark.

In short, it is challenging for me to give specific suggestions as to how to improve an approach section that gets scored poorly, since the criticisms can vary widely. As you revise, however, try to focus on the specific points of each reviewer—addressing each individually—think about how to buff up your preliminary data to make sure it supports what you are trying to do, and finally, think about improving the general readability and accessibility of the approach. Flow charts, simple tables, and eye-catching figures may help the next set of reviewers feel more positive about the section even if they continue to have some qualms about it.

Not Sufficiently Innovative/Exciting

The innovation limitations may also parallel concerns in the significance. But innovation is a little different in that you don't have to be very innovative to have a very significant and highly scored proposal. And just because a proposal is innovative does not necessarily make it significant. But generally, if you can frame your proposed work as innovative, it will also help buoy up your significance as well. Remember also that of all the sections, innovation, by itself, is probably the least important. If a project is not inherently innovative, it is tough to portray it as such since you simply cannot reinvent it. However, it is always worth pulling out small innovative pieces to something even if the work is not especially novel.

I've also been impressed by how often different reviewers will read the innovation section and come across with totally different conclusions, one stating with certainty that work is new and exciting and the other saying it is nothing more than a logical continuation of what was done before and entirely derivative. Often the proposal may discuss work that has already been published, so it is not unusual if even the most innovative proposal has some work that has already been achieved. This is especially true if you have already published some of your preliminary data. To some extent you only get to be innovative once: from that point onward everything else is derivative.

Bottom line: simply try to cast everything in the most innovative light possible. You'll be surprised how much innovation you may be able to unearth in even the most seemingly mundane of studies if you think creatively about it.

Investigator Concerns

A more important issue arises if there is concern about the investigators. Common issues include the PI being a new investigator or having not published sufficiently in an area. NIH and most organizations try to be supportive of new investigators. In fact, as noted earlier, at NIH, the pay lines are usually higher (i.e., you can score a higher percentage and still get funded if you are young investigator or a new investigator). But because young/new investigators are given an edge up, you can be certain that some reviewers will be suspicious of a new untested PI. For career grants, as discussed in Chap. 21, there is an entire separate set of criteria, so I am not discussing those here. Rather, what I am speaking of is the challenge of applying for say your first R01 or R21. You will be held to the same standards as a seasoned investigator, so it is important that you have had some track record of success, including having completed earlier grants successfully (as coinvestigator or as PI on a career grant), have managed even a small lab team, and have published several articles to show that your efforts have resulted in a real outcome.

If there are criticisms about your (the PIs) experience in the criticisms, your best bet is simply to fight back and show what you have done and continue to do that makes you prepared to serve as PI on a grant. For example, I have seen people be criticized that they were always the first author on a manuscript rather than senior author—implying a persistent junior status on the research team. This seems very unfair since it may reflect the idiosyncrasies of the mentor-mentee relationship more than any ability of the young investigator to take full control of a study. But actions speak louder than words, so anything you can do that shows proof of seniority, experience, and ability to lead a team successfully can be brought to bear on the question. These are things you can add to your biosketch while fighting back vehemently in the introduction to the revised application. Since you must be PI, you should not let this criticism go answered, come swinging back, and fight it aggressively.

There is one other option worth considering to help in this situation: bring on one or more senior co-PIs. If you can bring in someone who greatly enhances the application at the same time providing a new realm of expertise, it could end up improving the application and, even more important, the actual research, markedly. Thus, if it is pointed out that you do not have expertise in area y or z that is included in your application, and adding in this person would help, by all means do so. It would mean a pretty radical rewrite, but it may be worth it, even if you have to share PI-ship: 50 % of something is far better than 100 % of nothing.

Finally, the issue of investigator may not be related to the PI but rather to the absence or inexperience of a coinvestigator who is participating. Obviously, this is much less of a concern than having criticism leveled at the PI. Sometimes this may be more perceived than real—i.e., that person actually does have the expertise, but you didn't make it clear for one reason or another. If so, revise the application accordingly, buffing up the biosketch and all reference to her capabilities in the application. On the other hand, if there is the suggestion that you need more expertise in an area, you may need to add another coinvestigator or possibly a consultant to answer this concern. I recently had this happen in an application. I found an excellent collaborator, and even though he was at an institution 1000 miles away, I brought him on as a coinvestigator; the grant was easily funded on the second try. And in point of fact, having this person on board has helped the data analysis considerably. It was a win-win for both of us, and this was all thanks to the suggestion of one thoughtful reviewer.

Environment Concerns

I have seen this concern arise quite infrequently, and usually people get scored in the 1–2 range on this factor regardless of whether they are in Boston, San Francisco, or Kalamazoo. Usually, by the time you can even consider submitting an R01 application, you have already developed a good infrastructure and your institution is sufficient to support the effort. In the rare case that a concern about the environment is raised, it may just be a matter of improving the relevant sections of your application to support this. Again, including information about how great your institution/situation is in the body of the grant (i.e., research strategy section) can also help get this point across most effectively, rather than just relegating it to the facilities section.

Human Subject Concerns

Concerns stated about human subjects are not to be taken lightly. It is not at all uncommon for human subject concerns to be voiced at a study section. These should be taken seriously and not simply discarded as the reviewers simply "not getting it." Even minor concerns can kill an application, even if it has scored otherwise well. My take on issues with this section is to go over the top in terms of dealing with all potential issues at the time of the initial application. Much of my research has focused on bioengineering issues, and placing new electrical devices on human subjects can be considered potentially harmful. I have always taken the most conservative approach in attempting to ensure human subject safety and to explicitly state every conceivable and foreseeable problem and how I am going to deal with them all. If you feel that you have done this on the initial application and criticisms are voiced in the reviews, just try to deal with them one by one. Again, getting outside input on this can be helpful to help you gain perspective. If necessary, you can create a data and safety monitoring plan to add to the human subject section and obtain a letter of support from your institutional review board.

The human subject concerns are amplified if you are doing a study in children or in other "vulnerable" populations. If you are criticized for this, you need to go over the top to ensure safety and, if necessary and plausible, even doing measurements on adult subjects before considering investigations in children.

One other concern may be that you are planning to study too many (or too few) patients, as interpreted by the reviewers, even if you have presented a complete and convincing power analysis. If this is an issue, you will obviously need to reconsider your recruitment plans and if your interpretation is really accurate. The more preliminary data and complete your sample size estimation, the less likely reviewers will be able to criticize it, so really give this thought and try to revise it to make it bulletproof.

Animal welfare concerns. It is relatively uncommon for reviewers to be very critical of animal welfare if the studies are involving mice, rat, or even less senescent forms of life (e.g., zebrafish or invertebrates). I think I have yet to see a mouse study get scored poorly because of animal concerns.

However, the issue is very different when dealing with larger, more senescent animals such as dogs, pigs, or nonhuman primates (e.g., monkeys). Concerns will need to be meticulously addressed. Again, it is best to try to deal with all of these concerns at the time of initial review. It is better to have to avoid digging yourself out of a hole in terms of how your monkeys are going to be cared for or what kind of food and exercise will be provided to your dog colony. Don't let yourself fall behind the 8-ball on these issues, since there may be a bias toward simply not trusting your application when you try again, as you attempt to explain away concerns that were voiced on the first review. But if you do find yourself in that position, just follow my recommendations for human subjects—go over the top and try to make it bulletproof. A letter from your IACUC at least endorsing your plans can also be helpful to include.

Women, Minorities, and Children

Generally your research should reflect the population of your region if you are studying a problem that affects people of all ages and both sexes similarly. That situation, however, is relatively uncommon, and in most applications, you will need to specify why you are not studying children (the disease doesn't affect them) or why you are only studying them (you are in a pediatric hospital and the disease only affects children). The same is true with women. If the disease only affects men, or affects men twice as frequently as women, you will have a sample enriched with men; your healthy control population, if also included, should then have a similar bias. And a disorder that primarily affects one minority or is rare in a minority will also need to be explained. Clarifying these points can be critical if someone expressed concern the first time around.

Also, allow me to make a short comment about the planned/target enrollment table in NIH applications. This table should reflect the calculation regarding male/female, ethnicity, and race that is described above. It is rare for the table itself to be the object of criticism, but the omission of the table will spell doom for your application the first time around. Make sure you include it and take it seriously in any NIH application that includes human subjects. Also, the difference between race and ethnicity is not something you will generally find in any dictionary, but these are standard grant speak. As of 2016, ethnicity refers only to Hispanic versus non-Hispanic; race captures all other descriptors.

Resource Sharing

Although one of the more minor categories of additional scoring criteria, resource sharing represents an important opportunity to clarify your plans for disseminating the results of the study on which taxpayers may have spent easily more than $1,000,000.

So it is only fair that you provide a detailed accounting of how you will let the world know about your work. Generally, most reviewers will be content with your saying you will publish your results in peer-reviewed journals and present at national and international meetings. But at other times, you may need to be more creative. For example, including web-based data sets and calculators may add value and strengthen the general applicability of your work. Or perhaps a medical society and a nonprofit or other organization will want to help promote your outcomes in broader ways.

Budget

First, if the reviewers were critical of your budget, but you believe they were wrong, you should say so in your revised application and clarify why the budget actually made good sense. Remember NIH is likely going to cut your budget by 12 or 15 % or more automatically from what you requested. So don't give up on your proposed budget too quickly. However, if they were critical of it for good reason, then you should graciously accept the change and modify it accordingly. There is little harm in arguing the point though, except that being too persistent can make the reviewers feel negatively toward your application in a broader way when it comes to the time for rereview. So be flexible, even if it means being a little less ambitious in your work. The next set of reviewers may feel more kindly toward you if you are not rigid in how much money you are asking for. Although the budget is not supposed to be considered in grant scoring by reviewers, I do believe it plays a role unconsciously.

Useful Approaches to the Revised Application Itself

Depending on how you scored (or didn't score) on the initial application, you may have different goals in the revised application. If you scored well, but just didn't quite hit the funding mark, your goal in the revised application should be to make only those changes that are necessary, helping to ensure that the review process is as simple and painless as possible for the reviewers. This means summarizing the problems neatly on the introductory page and then only changing limited areas of text in your application, highlighting them in bold or italics. Making the reviewer's job easy and showing simply how you addressed all the concerns may help your application sneak across the pay line without a huge amount of fuss. No need to fix things that don't need fixing, even if they look less than perfect now. If you start changing other aspects of the application, you will distract the reviewers from criticisms that they brought up. Remember that they want to keep their review jobs simple too, so don't give them additional, unnecessary work. Also, you should recall that this is not a college midterm or grade school spelling test. You are not aiming to get an A+ or 100 %. All you want to achieve is a score that will get to funding; a B+ is fine, if it means that you crossed that threshold.

On the other hand, if your application scored poorly, you may just have to rewrite the whole thing and try again. This means not bothering with italics or bold text and just giving the whole thing a fresh once over. You'll need to make the reviewers look at the entire document since your changes are likely to be so deep and complicated, working through many paragraphs of altered text may be rather tedious for the reviewers, even those who had read it through the first time.

Revision Grant Review at NIH

Revised applications are generally reviewed along with new applications at a grant review session. However, at least a few of the reviewers who evaluated your first attempt will be asked to look at yours again. This is good news— since they may have made specific comments that you will have now addressed and hopefully answered completely. Even the most critical of reviewers may feel more favorably disposed to your application if you have made a valiant effort to fix the errors that they identified (whether or not in your heart of hearts you believe that they were actual errors). Unfortunately, not all the people reviewing the application may be the same. No two study sections have the exact same composition, and one reviewer, new to the application, may identify a whole new list of concerns. This is where having a champion a review session can make a huge difference. If someone feels strongly about an application, that person may argue that you did make major changes and that it is now much stronger. Only if the new reviewer has truly substantive concerns completely overlooked at the first review session is it likely to have sufficient weight to hurt the application. Generally, though, new reviewers feel like they came in a little late to the game and are willing to bow to the expertise of the people who reviewed the application the first time around. Still, new reviewers to an application can occasionally be vociferous in their opposition, so always try to ensure that you direct your resubmitted application to the exact same study section which reviewed it the first time around. You can help achieve this by making sure it is absolutely clear in the cover letter which section reviewed it initially. If it ends up going to a different section (which you will discover through an automatically generated email from NIH), make sure you make a fuss. Mistakes do occasionally happen, and it is best not to be passive.

One final important point about NIH review. Sometimes your grant may have simply ended up in the "wrong" study section initially. There are many, many study sections and more than one may be able to review your grant, though each has its own set of biases. Sometimes, it makes better sense to try to shift it to a different study section entirely for rereview. This would require talking to the administrators at NIH prior to submission. (This is something that I have not personally ever done, but I have heard of others who have had success with this approach.) Alternatively, you could consider doing a major overhaul on the grant, including retitling it and then submitting it as a new application, that will hopefully land, this time, in a more receptive study section.

Resubmitted Applications and Foundations

Most foundations will allow you to resubmit an application after it has been initially reviewed and not funded. But the approach here may vary widely depending on the foundation. Some may give you feedback and simply say revise according to these concerns and rather than telling you to wait for the next cycle and then send it back out immediately for rereview. Others may say simply not to bother resubmitting. Generally, you should feel free to contact the foundation directly and try to get a sense of things by phone or email. The science director at a foundation will often have their hand deeply in the review process and will likely try to be helpful if you reach out to them personally for advice.

Summary

Ultimately, revising and resubmitting an application is far easier than putting together the initial application. But care must be taken to address every point succinctly yet completely. Making the revisions clean and your message loud and clear is an important part of the revision process. It is also an important opportunity to take stock and a time for self-reflection. If you start revising a poorly scored application and realize that the criticisms were harsh and so deep, it might be better to start over on a new application in a different direction. You can still use pieces of your original application—there is no law against that—but now with an altered slant. Sometimes starting anew is also good psychologically, especially when your initial application was butchered in the review process.

Part IV
Good Presentations, Conferencing, Networking, and Other Useful Tools

Chapter 25
The Art of a Good Research Presentation

Like the chapters on grant and paper writing and revising, there is an entire literature on creating effective presentations with PowerPoint or Keynote, and my goal in
this chapter is not to introduce you to the finer points of navigating those programs
and making beautiful productions. Rather, I would like to instill a more general
philosophy about presentation that I hope you will find useful. I should make it clear
that I have never won any awards for my presentations per se, but having sat through
innumerable grand rounds presentations and having presented at national and international meetings many times, I would like to share some basic rules of success.

Rules #1 and #2. As my friend David Preston, MD, says there are only two
important aspects to giving a successful talk: showing up and finishing on time.
Those two points seem really simple, yet you would be amazed how many people
arrive late or just at the last moment, cutting the timing so tightly that they don't
have an opportunity to set up their presentation and consequently fumble with their
computers and the laser pointer. Or worse yet, they may forget about the about the
talk entirely or be delayed for reasons beyond their control. As obvious as it may
seem, always leave yourself an extra 10–15 min just to get settled in, see the size of
the room, test out your presentation and microphone, and meet and greet some of
the early arrivals. If you are traveling from a great distance to give a talk, make sure
that you plan to arrive hours earlier or perhaps even the day before. By doing so you
will not only de-stress yourself but also the organizers of the conference; the people
running it will always be worried that something is going to interfere with the presentation, so anything you can do to get there early (and possibly also convey to
them by email, phone, or text) that you are on your way will go a long way to winning friends and making for a well-received presentation.

Finishing a talk within the allotted period of time is more of a challenge for most
people than showing up on time. First, always make sure you know how long you
have to speak, planning for at least a short period of questions and answers at the
end. For a one-hour time slot, aim for it to be completed in 45 or 50 min so that there
is sufficient time for interaction and questions at the end. But more importantly, as
I will reiterate below, don't try to cram your talk full to the point where it is busting

© Springer Science+Business Media New York 2016
S.B. Rutkove, *Biomedical Research: An Insider's Guide*,
DOI 10.1007/978-1-4939-3655-7_25

out of at the seams—your presentation is not an opportunity to show off your work and how great you are. You should view it as an opportunity to inform the audience about your work while keeping them engaged and interested. There is no better way of getting a group of people more disengaged and annoyed than by running over your allotted time or realizing that you are so far behind in your talk you are going to have to skip over a series of slides if you are to have a prayer of finishing on time. Not to mention the annoyance the conference organizers may feel if yours is one in a series of talks and now you have set the entire day back by 15 min. Simply put: that should never, never happen. The aim should always be to have your talk completed well within the allotted time slot—either by practicing and timing it or because you know your material and presentation style so well that you can be reasonably certain of finishing well within the time limit.

Another thought: I have never heard anyone complain about a talk being too short, have you? Finishing 5 or 10 min early will seem like a gift to a large section of the audience who will suddenly have some precious unexpected time on their hands, perhaps just to relax for a few minutes before going back to clinic or to grab a cup of coffee. Or if yours is part of a series of lectures in a program, you'll help ensure that the program stays on track or perhaps helps get it back on track if someone else went over (which is virtually inevitable). There is no more effective way of winning the admiration of the audience than by being brief. It shows humility and respect and a basic appreciation that your needs are not primary. But, remarkably, ending a talk early goes against virtually everything we learn. It is as if we feel that we are somehow abrogating an important opportunity to cram in one more piece of critical information that, in actuality, most will forget the moment they walk out the door.

So get there on time and end early. Make the audience like you from the moment you begin until the moment you end and leaving them wanting more. There is no greater accolade than being asked to return to give another talk.

Rule #3: Know your audience. This may be self-evident, but it is extremely important to know to whom you will be speaking. Are they going to be high-level researchers or a more general audience in your area of study? Is the audience going to contain mostly medical students and residents? Are you going to be speaking to people from industry who may also be interested in your work for other reasons beyond simply gaining knowledge? Having some sense of the crowd is critical to understanding the content and speed with which you can present and how "basic" you need to go in an introduction. The most challenging audiences are those in which there are a range of people, from those with great expertise to those who are not familiar with the area of research at all. In those situations, it is good to aim relatively low while simultaneously trying to keep the more knowledgeable audience members engaged by presenting new or unusual data. Knowing your audience will define your content and that is always a very important place to start as you design your presentation.

Rule #4: It is not about you, it is about them. Okay. This is a major point that I would like to make in this chapter and at which I have already hinted. When you are asked to give a presentation, whether it be a research seminar in your own institutions, grand rounds in an institution across town, or a presentation to a group of medical students in a country in sub-Saharan Africa, you should be thinking of your audience front and center. Who are they and what are they going to care most about? But once you have that figured out and know what points you'll plan on covering, you need to think from their perspective and be empathetic. Try to imagine if you knew nothing about the topic and were only being introduced to it the first time: what would you find simple, interesting, or confusing? What would need amplification? What are simply extra details that just add some color but also detract from the story as a whole?

In medical school, one professor made a point that has stayed with me. After you hear a talk, how much do you really remember the next day or the next week or the next month? Generally nearly all the details are gone. Even if the speaker gave a tremendous presentation on a fascinating topic, generally what you end up walking away with and carrying with you is just perhaps one or two small concepts that somehow tugged at you more deeply than any others. And I think that is all you can really hope to achieve as you prepare a presentation: that the members of the audience will take away just a single major point that they can hold with them. Perhaps it is a vague recollection of a new disease mechanism or of a new therapy or a different statistical approach to a common analytical problem.

The point I am trying to make here is that the talk should not be viewed as opportunity to prove how incredible you are — how many grants you have or how much work you have accomplished or how many experiments you have run or how big your lab is or who is funding your work. Your point should be simply to educate as most effectively as possible and to make the audience finish the talk wanting more.

Rule #5: Tell a story. As an undergraduate at Cornell University, I had the opportunity to participate in the senior chemistry lecture series. It was for those people who were pursuing laboratory research and needed to complete a thesis. My research, as I mentioned in the Foreword, had been focused on synthesizing a new chemotherapeutic agent. The person running the seminar, Roald Hoffman, PhD, was one of the discoverers of one of the basic mechanisms of covalent bonding for which he had won the Nobel Prize. Early in the course, he made an important point about being an effective speaker: always tell a story. Try to couch your ideas in the form of a story or narrative rather than a series of seemingly disconnected fragments. If this means taking a short digression or two to fully flesh out the narrative nature of the work, that is fine. The point is that if there is an obvious beginning and an obvious end with perhaps a little climax two thirds of the way through (the classical "golden section"), so much the better and more powerful. We learn stories as children and hearing a talk in the form of a story makes it simultaneously appealing and comforting. It also creates a flow and dynamism simply not possible if you are viewing your presentation only as an opportunity to show sets of disparate data.

Rule #6: It's a performance. Even if acting or theater is virtually alien to you, it is helpful to think of a presentation as a performance. You are going up there to satisfy a group of listeners and ensuring that their 30 minutes or 1 hour is well spent. This harkens back to the idea that the presentation is more about them than about you. To some extent you need to think about subjugating your own concerns to their enjoyment and interest in the presentation, even if that means omitting certain things or becoming so fluid with the material that you can really let your inner self shine through clearly. If you think about it as a play and your taking on a slightly different character, it can make the presentation both more fun and less pedantic.

I like to think about the fact that all nonscientific performances are about the audience too. Even though in our society famous actors have become huge icons and almost bigger than life, the vast majority of performers do work that is relatively modest, and these individuals give their all not only for their greater glory, but rather for your simple enjoyment and pleasure. The act of bowing at the end of a performance is an act of submission of sorts, emanating from the way servants would bow to European royalty in centuries past. We have put on this performance for *their* enjoyment and education, not simply because what we are doing is so cool or interesting. We academics don't bow at the end of a performance, but we should think about it that way. In fact, it is kind of interesting that we do not—considering that there is usually soft, polite applause after a presentation is completed, no matter how small.

So the bottom line: don't be afraid to behave like a performer and rehearse certain lines and aspects of delivery. And even if some of that presentation seems a little unnatural to you, that may be a good thing. But that means also not reading from a script. Even if it is your first big talk, reading from a script will make you sound wooden and scared. There is no better way of turning off an audience than reciting material, even if you have it memorized and can make it sound somewhat natural. Always try to be extemporaneous in your delivery while still having the structure and what you are going to say with each slide well cemented in your head. Now it is true that I have heard a few people give successful talks by having every word memorized—after all our politicians do this routinely, occasionally to good effect, but they have teleprompters which allow them to engage with the audience in a way that is not possible for most of us. In short, if you absolutely have to read from a script, have it so well memorized and rehearsed that your delivery seems virtually natural.

Rule #7: Be excited and enthusiastic, but don't overdo it. I think it is very helpful to convey an air of excitement about the work that you are presenting. Again, this will help keep the audience engaged and awake as compared to if you are speaking in a humdrum monotone. Let your own fascination for the work that you are pursuing shine through. But don't go too far and start getting self-important about it. There is no bigger a turnoff than having the presenter repeatedly convey the brilliance of their insights; even if your work does contain remarkable insights, it is better to not overstate the case. Let them be impressed without your telling them to be impressed. And some gentle enthusiasm is a good way to do that.

Rule #8: Make great slides. Up to this point, I have been focusing entirely on presentation styles and the philosophy of giving a talk. But the truth is that most of your talk is going to probably be based on a series of slides, made in one of the standard programs such as PowerPoint® or Keynote®. And much of your preparation time will be geared toward putting together a clear set of slides to tell your story most effectively. Here is a list of simple dos and don'ts about how to go about this.

Do keep your slide content brief and succinct. Complicated slides are a turnoff. Words are a turnoff. One or two figures per slides with limited text are far more effective than paragraphs of material or long bullet point lists.

Do aim for clarity with every slide. Every slide should be virtually interpretable without an explanation—that means having graphs with axes labeled clearly, the points visible, and different groups of data discernible and identifiable and large enough to read from a distance.

Do vary slide content. Having a series of slides that all look the same, one after another, can be mind-numbing. I see this most typically when a presenter shows one gel after another or endless brain scans of some sort (e.g., functional MRI). People can generally take two or three similar slides in a row, but that should be about it. Varying content is a simple way to keep people engaged. If that seems challenging given your material, then you should really rethink what you are planning to speak about.

Do use figures, videos, and animations to your advantage. I find that if I am really wanting to put the effort into making a powerful presentation, I could spend endless hours doing this. And part of the reason is constructing elaborate and, I believe, eye-opening videos or animations to explain a new concept or dense material simply. Really thinking through the best means of conveying a complex idea means walking people through it one step at a time; animations can be very powerful for this purpose. Moreover, there is no more powerful way of getting a point across than showing a video. I still recall seeing an early video of someone completely recovering from a stroke after being given TPA (tissue plasminogen activator)—the before and after videos were just astounding and even though the evidence was just anecdotal, it made a huge impression on me.

Don't create laundry lists and go through them one item at a time. You may feel that you owe it to your audience to be "complete" and "thorough" but I can tell you that no one in your audience will feel that way. Long bullet point lists are terrible, unless your main purpose is to intentionally produce a sense of being overwhelmed. In other words, you can use these to good effect if your goal is to prove a point, say about the virtues or detractors from a test or perhaps the varied symptoms of a disease. But I would ordinarily avoid them, even if it means being incomplete.

Don't put up slides that are unreadable. So often people will put up slides with huge amounts of information, most of which are entirely illegible, except for a figure or two buried within it. The presenter will often make some comment like, "You probably won't be able to see this if you are in the back of the room…" What? Why would you ever think of presenting something to a large group if it is not visible to a third of the audience? The point of the presentation is to keep people engaged and interested—again remember the "it's not about you, it's about them" philosophy—and if you are lazy enough not to make your slides legible, you are conveying to the audience the idea that you simply don't care.

Do reiterate important points. I think this is something with which many of us could do better. There are certain situations where reiteration is not really justified—perhaps in a paper, but in certain situations, like a presentation or a grant application, a certain amount of reiteration is key since it helps cement basic concepts while also providing an anchor for the listener to fall back upon. As an audience member, you generally feel better about yourself, if you understand what is being discussed and leave feeling like your knowledge base has been enriched in a meaningful way. In order to achieve this, it really is helpful to introduce a basic concept early on and then keep landing back on it during the presentation and then finally reiterating it at the very end. By taking this approach, you can feel pretty certain that it will stick with most people. This anchor can also serve as a useful taking-off point for some of the finer points you are trying to convey, but don't anticipate people remembering them after leaving the room. As I mentioned at the beginning of this chapter, you really can't expect people to remember more than one or two things a week later. So make sure you achieve that one simple goal.

Do leave plenty of time to put together a talk. If I am putting a new presentation together, I will usually leave several weeks to work on it before the date. The reason for this is that each time I come back to it, I'll have some new ideas or realize some flaw in the approach that I had not recognized before. As is true in grant and paper writing, it is critical to not attempt to cram together an entire talk in just a several-minute period. Having repeated time away from a work is critical to gain perspective on it and to keep improving it. Of course, it can become very time-consuming, since in the age of Powerpoint® and the Internet, you can always download an additional photo or improve a figure. So while you should keep a limit on it, lest it become all-consuming, start early.

Don't be pedantic or a know-it-all but try to be at least a little humble and self-effacing. I don't like it when I am talked down to or made to feel like a child. And there are certain people who have a way of presenting in this fashion. This is usually the case when someone is giving a review talk perhaps in a course at an organization's national yearly meeting. "Experts" will be giving presentations on various topics, and since they are "teaching," they feel they have the right to treat you a bit like you are in grade school. However, a good teacher is always respectful and recognizes his own limitations in the understanding of material, allowing himself to be at least occasionally self-effacing. You don't need to prove how smart you are. The fact that you are up there speaking should be evidence enough that you are no slouch. Again, it is not about you, it is about them.

Do practice, practice, practice. As I said at the beginning of this chapter, presentations should be considered performances. And a successful performance, whether you are an actor, musician, or dancer, always requires a huge time investment in presenting the material in a succinct, clear, and powerful way. To just throw some slides together and then start speaking is an insult to the audience. Of course, if you know the material well and have given a variation of the presentation many times, you may not need to practice this new specific presentation at all. However, when just starting out and presenting new work to a new group, practicing with the presentation is critical. You will learn what slides work, which don't, whether the order makes sense, whether you are talking for too long (again, you can never really be too short), and whether there is another variation and a good tempo to keep the talking moving smoothly. Practice also means cutting down on your "uhs." Occasional "uhs" are fine, but when your presentation is jam-packed with them, it can be tiresome. And if you are doing it correctly, you will discover that you are probably never saying the same thing the same way twice—and that is fine since you are hopefully not memorizing a script. On the other hand, there may be a short sentence or phrase that you do want to memorize verbatim since it is critical and is best expressed in a very specific way.

Do practice in front of friends and colleagues. Perhaps the most effective way of ensuring a successful presentation is by practicing in front of trusted colleagues and friends. The feedback you will receive will be undoubtedly unmatched to any self-criticism that you can manage on your own. One effective way of practicing and getting feedback from multiple individuals is by presenting the work to a small group of year peers in a seminar-like forum. As a group they may be able to provide more incisive and constructive feedback than is possible from just a single person.

Do add humor, in limited quantities. There was a time (I believe in the late 1980s through about 2000) when every presentation was filled with a prerequisite Gary Larson *Far Side* cartoon. In many ways, I miss those days, because you could almost go to any talk and virtually expect a few jokes at some point during the presentation—usually one at the beginning, one or two in the middle, and then a final one at the end. But those days seem to have been long forgotten, and it is increasingly rare that there is any humor at all in any presentation. I think people feel virtually compelled to stick to the science and not joke around even for a moment. After all, medicine and biomedical science is a serious business. And, frankly, regimented humor, such as the *Far Side* approach, is not all that appealing.

But I still believe some limited, well-placed unexpected humor can do a great deal in breaking up the intensity of a presentation. Perhaps this goes back to my strong conviction that you are putting on a performance, and part of that performance is providing a break from an intense onslaught of data and concepts—some comic relief of sorts. Breaking up the rhythm of the talk, or rather offering a brief respite, can be immensely effective at reestablishing interest and focus.

Also, humor should not come out of the blue, but rather be intrinsic to the presentation itself. That is not always easy to do and Gary Larson may not be the ideal source from which to draw. Some people may also not feel comfortable delivering humor—it takes practice and doesn't come naturally to all. So if there is an obvious and relevant place to put in either a humorous image or comment or, dare it say it, a cartoon, go for it!

Don't become too smooth. I have been arguing that to a great extent, a successful presentation really can be viewed as a performance of sorts. The more you practice, the more you think about your audience and the more you produce a well-prepared production, the more successful you will be. But it is possible to overdo this. It occurs relatively infrequently, but it is when the presenter ties everything up into a neat little package that seems almost too good to be true. Or is so committed to selling an idea, or drug, or disease mechanism, you start to distrust the presenter. So there is almost a concept of being too smooth, of being too simple and too neat that can sometimes play against you. But as I say, this is definitely an uncommon issue—it is far more likely a presenter will be entirely incomprehensible than present a story that simply sounds so simple that it cannot possibly be genuine.

Do disclose your conflicts. Whether necessary or not, it is always wise to disclose your relevant conflicts of interest at the beginning of the presentation. Doing so will make it clear that you are not only being honest, but that you are also giving the opportunity to the audience to question the truth of what you say because they may "suspect" that you have a conflict but are hiding it. Laying out everything into the brightness of day can help obviate or entirely eliminate those concerns. Now I say "relevant" conflicts because there is also a way of overdoing your disclosures by having a long list of conflicts with only one or two actually being relevant. This ends up being just another form of obfuscation since an audience member can't possibly make a determination in a few seconds as to the relevance of any one item. However, some organizations demand that you do this so that you are complete. But in the end, I just think this is silly. Relevancy to the presentation is all that matters. Hopefully, the presenter can be honest enough with herself to ensure she takes that relevancy seriously. For more on conflicts of interest and disclosure, see Chap. 28.

Do acknowledge. It is really critical to acknowledge all individuals and funders who have made your work possible. Why do this? Well, first it is only fair. You can't simply take credit for all of your work. If one graduate student or postdoc performed most of the research, make sure you point out again and again that they did the work and that you presenting this as their surrogate. But in terms of collaboration, it is important to highlight that all work is a team effort. Don't forget that there is a fairly good likelihood that some of your colleagues sitting in your audience are also collaborators with you. To not see their contribution acknowledged can be frustrating at one level, and if the work is considerable, it can be downright infuriating. We've all been there. I was recently in the audience in which a student, the member of a collaborating lab, presented data that was collected through an NIH-funded research study in which I was the principal investigator. The data that he presented were from patients and healthy subjects that we had enrolled and studied. When the talk concluded, the only person acknowledged was his thesis advisor. A short time later, their thesis advisor, recognizing I was in the audience, and probably seeing my expression of disbelief, came over to me immediately apologizing that we were not acknowledged. I had little choice but to accept his apology. Clearly this was a major faux pas and you may not always be able to seek out the person in the audience offended by your omission. Frankly, it borders on the illegal—many universities, journals, and funding agencies would consider such misappropriation of research data without proper acknowledgment to be equivalent to academic malfeasance. Although I think calling it scientific misconduct would be a bit much, it is moving in that direction.

My bottom line is that you should not take acknowledgments lightly. They may seem like an afterthought in your own work, but to the person being omitted it can represent a major offense.

Another question that comes up is where the best positioning for acknowledgments in a talk is. Most people still put them at the very end. Recently, however, I have seen a number of presentations where they were placed up front, right after the title slide. To some extent this makes more sense—after all they contributed to the work in substantial ways, so it may make sense to acknowledge all your collaborators right at the beginning, as well as reiterating all relevant contributions during the talk itself. I think doing so is also good since it makes the contributors seem less like an afterthought and come across as more intrinsic to the actual work being completed. We will have to see how widely adopted this approach becomes over the next few years.

Thus, as far as acknowledging your collaborators, the analogy to a movie or performance again holds. To have a movie without any titles before or after or a program of play with no names of the individuals who contributed to the effort, including benefactors (in other words the funding agencies), would be essentially unheard of. So you must do the same here. Another way to help ensure that you are complete is by conferring with your lab members. They may recall that someone else contributed that you might have otherwise forgotten.

Summary. As I have said repeatedly in this chapter, it is not about you, it is about the audience. The point that I hope to have conveyed is that the best way to have a successful presentation is to think of your presentation as a gift to your audience. Don't think of it as an opportunity to show off your incredible research or a platform to convince a group of reviewers that your research is worthy of funding or to gripe about past injustices. Think of it as an opportunity to inform and teach, to leave your audience feeling enlightened, enlivened, and, most importantly, wanting more.

Chapter 26
Effective Conferencing

I recall the first medical conference I ever attended. It was the 1993 American Academy of Neurology Meeting held at the Hilton Hotel in New York. I was in my final year of neurology residency and was on elective and received the OK to travel to the Big Apple and attend, even though I was not presenting any work there.

From the moment I walked in the door, I was completely overwhelmed. The halls were packed with well-dressed, unfamiliar people, all talking, walking swiftly, or flipping through their program guides. I stood in amazement, not only at the huge number of neurologists all gathered in one place but also with the odd accouterments—little booths with plastic signs indicating where one can register or pick up packets and bags, stands selling various neurological goods, and a plethora of signs pointing confused attendees to different conference venues.

After a few minutes of disorientation, I eventually figured out which registration booth to visit in order to pick up my own packet of materials. With those in hand, I fumbled around until I eventually figured out in which direction to go to the first course for which I had pre-registered. And over the next couple of days, I vaguely figured out the program, attending a poster session or two, a couple of plenary talks, an awards ceremony, and a few platform sessions. After 2 days, I was ready to get out of there and return to Boston. I felt thoroughly overwhelmed and frankly down-trodden and sad. It seemed that so many people were doing so many different and interesting things that it made me feel that any work I was going to do would hardly amount to anything. That feeling lingered with me for weeks afterward before it gradually dissipated.

My reason for giving this anecdote is that I really, really wish someone had prepared me for the onslaught of a medical or scientific conference. A little psychological preparation can go a long way: from understanding the pace and tempo of these events, to understanding their emotional power, while still keeping their importance in perspective. I will attempt to do that here.

Prepare. Whether you are attending a smaller conference or large national meeting such as the one I described above, preparing for a conference and having a plan of attack are important. Are there any sessions that you absolutely should attend,

© Springer Science+Business Media New York 2016
S.B. Rutkove, *Biomedical Research: An Insider's Guide*,
DOI 10.1007/978-1-4939-3655-7_26

like those in which you are presenting a poster or speaking or where important collaborators or peers are doing so? Once you have identified these, you can then gradually work your way through the program book or online tracker to decide when to arrive and when to leave and how to fill your days. If you have a detailed list of abstracts and have the time to review those in your area(s) of interest before you head there, all the better. Many larger conferences now have convenient apps that can allow you to create a personalized schedule.

But this preparation should include more than just looking at the program guides and creating a list of things to do at the conference—try to read up on the city and venue online. To have a general layout of the hall or convention center cannot only make the experience less confusing; it can actually make it more enjoyable, since you'll have a familiarity with your surroundings before ever walking into the door.

Don't stay too far away, but maybe not too close also. Hotel accommodations at larger conferences are generally not cheap—several hundred dollars per night. And the nicer and more conveniently located to the event, generally the more expensive. (The cost of the hotel also depends markedly on the city. Hotels in smaller, midwestern cities are considerably less expensive than places like New York, Boston, or San Francisco.) Obviously, you should only stay where you can afford, but I do think staying far away from the meeting—as most younger attendees do since the costs are much lower—is actually disadvantageous. It is probably better to share a room with a friend and split the costs if possible and stay closer than to have a room to yourself 3 miles away on the other side or the railroad tracks. Being close lets you interact with friends and colleagues and to more easily attend sessions and meet new people. If you are residing at a distance, you may find yourself missing large swaths of the conference and arriving late or leaving early, perhaps missing some of the best times for one-on-one interactions.

Prepare to be overwhelmed. As you can tell from my personal narrative, the first thing that will happen when attending a large conference or even a medium-sized one is that you are going to feel completely overwhelmed and, well, Lilliputian. There will be hundreds or even thousands of people working in your field ambling about, endless walls of posters, huge halls with hoards of people in the darkness watching one person after another giving talks or receiving this or that award, and multiple sessions on a variety of all topics occurring concurrently. And there may be a colossal exhibit hall with huge displays advertising new drugs or technologies, books, and foundations each with its own agenda.

The sheer size of a larger convention can be daunting, but then when you realize that many of these people are each like you—perhaps doing basic research or seeing patients or some of both—I think it is very hard not to start to feel small and insignificant. How can you ever hope to achieve significance when what you are doing is one small piece in an otherwise huge field? And as a junior person attending one of these conferences, this sense of insignificance is even further amplified.

So it is helpful to psychologically gird yourself for this. It is important to prepare mentally and accept this for what it is: people in many different individual fields all coming together to present their work. The truth is that your work is still significant and important in its own way—it is just that you are not alone. It is also absolutely critical to take breaks and just get away from the crowds, to go for a run or out to a nice lunch or dinner with a couple of friends, or to hide out in your hotel room for a few hours. It is a good idea to reestablish a sense of self in the midst of all of this organized pandemonium.

I have found that with time, I have actually begun to enjoy the crowds and buzz of the whole event. Perhaps it is simply because I know what to expect. Or perhaps it is because I know more people. Or perhaps it is because I know that when I return to work in a few days, I will once again feel significant.

Prepare an effective poster. Unlike research papers, grants, and presentations, I am not going to dedicate an entire chapter to designing and displaying an effective poster. Most organizations will provide a pretty clear template for you to use to show you how to present the data, and for the most part, the posters themselves will get recycled and you'll never look at it again. It's true—many organizations now have an online poster repository where you can upload your poster and have its contents live indefinitely on the web. But for the most part, posters really only provide talking points and are not meant to be the final culmination of a body of work. I say this because it is simply not worth spending an excessive amount of time and effort in creating an eye-catching, all-comprehensive poster. You should be spending your time writing stronger grants and research papers or creating powerful presentations. The idea of "opportunity cost" should be first and foremost in your mind on this point—if you are going to expend a great deal of effort on this, you will be giving up time spent more valuably elsewhere.

But there is one aspect to this that I try to encourage my mentees to pursue: a poster may be able to serve as the beginnings of a research paper, providing the basic introduction, methods, and data analyses that you will ultimately include there. So from that perspective, you may be able to accomplish two things simultaneously, namely, writing the paper and creating the poster. Generally, however, we are often in a position of putting together the poster many months before we are really ready to fully write up a paper, often because data sets are incomplete or analyses unfinished.

A few points about creating an effective poster:

1. **Keep it simple**. Like group presentations, don't try to be comprehensive and include an entire paper on it—bullet point lists and basic figures that convey information in a simple way are best. Posters with incomprehensibly complex figures and microscopic text are generally a turnoff, especially if the viewer is enjoying a bit of wine or beer while reading it (frequent accompaniments to many poster sessions).
2. **If possible make the title declaratory**. If you can capture the conclusion of your work in the title, so much the better, since quick messaging is key. So rather than having a title like, "A review of findings in elderly patients with COPD," try "Elderly patients with COPD have reduced diffusion coefficients."
3. **End with a set of conclusions by bullet point**. Again keep it simple. Many people will look only at the title and then the conclusions before they decide whether they want to read the rest of the poster. Also, make sure the conclusions

are not too low on the poster. People often tend to stick them in the lower right corner; if at all possible, try to keep them closer to eye level.

4. **Acknowledgments are still relevant**. Always include funders and relevant collaborators.
5. **There is no need to include references**. This is not a research paper, so you should just skip these unless they are really critical.

Printing your poster. Posters are bit of a pain. You have to print them out and carry them in awkward tubes that count as second pieces of carry-on luggage when you bring them on a plane. Since you are probably going to recycle it when you are done anyway, I strongly suggest having it delivered directly to the hotel or to the conference. Many conferences now have printing services available, though I think these tend to be overpriced and more expensive than using one of many online commercial services (I have been using Makesigns.com for years and they have always done a remarkably good and reliable job). An alternative I have also tried is creating a fabric poster. These can be thrown in your luggage like clothing. I personally think this is a great option if you plan on reusing it. They tend to be more expensive, however, and always look like they need a good ironing or steaming before displaying.

Poster presentation. Poster sessions vary in how they are organized, but generally the presenter puts up the poster at some point and it is allowed to sit there for several hours as people mill by and read and learn from it. Usually, there is also a time when you are supposed to stand by the poster for about 1–2 hours present the work to interested individuals, and answer questions. In many conferences, these times are also accompanied by coffee and muffins/bagels in the morning and wine/beer and cheese in the evening. It is supposed to be social but also educational. In some situations, a moderator will walk around with a microphone and gradually make her way down the row of posters asking each person to briefly present his work for just about 3 or 4 min. Then there is a brief opportunity to ask questions before the moderator and the associated crowd move on to the next poster.

Regardless of the specific method in which you are presenting the poster, standing by one always feels a little like you own a little shop on Main Street and you are waiting for customers to come by, hoping that someone will come in and actually express interest on what you are "selling." And you need to be prepared for that feeling of people not caring. The vast majority of people will glance at the poster title and simple continue on without even as so much noticing you. A smaller contingent will briefly look at the introduction results, and conclusions, nod their head approvingly, and move on. And an even smaller contingent will stop and actually show genuine interest. They may ask you a specific question after reading the poster for a few minutes or better yet ask, "Could you walk me through this?" Then it will be your opportunity to either give them a quick overview or explain to them in a step-by-step manner what it is about. In many cases, however, the people coming by are just a bit shy and would actually like you to explain it to them, but are reluctant to ask. That is why it is generally good that if someone stops to read it for even just a few moments, you actually ask if he would like you to explain it to him. Most people will ask you to go ahead and will then stop and chat for a short while; occasionally, some will say no thanks and then just move on. But I think being timid in these situations is not helpful it is better to be active and reach out to the people walking by, just as a shop owner on Main Street may try to attract customers with advertising.

Poster sessions can get quite crowded depending on the space allotted, and you will soon realize that actually many people are not even looking at the posters but are rather socializing. And it is definitely true that there is probably more socialization around poster sessions than at any other single venue at a conference. That is good—much of it may be bumping in to someone you haven't seen in years, but it is also an opportunity to make new friends and to network effectively (see more on that in Chap. 27).

At any rate, don't expect any specific outcome from a poster session. Only a few people may show interest and a couple of colleagues who had promised they would come by may never materialize. And you may also feel like you are selling a losing product, standing there alone by your poster in your nice suit or dress, one among many, no one even showing a hint of interest. To make matters worse, perhaps one of your neighboring posters has attracted a continuous large crowd of people, with one person trying to squeeze by another to get a glimpse of what is being presented. It can make you feel like the ugly stepchild. But don't feel bad: your turn will come.

Multiple posters. Sometimes you'll see several posters in a row with the same title formatting and with the same group of authors listed in various orders on each. Usually one lab or research group has several related posters and has created a virtual monopoly in one area of the exhibit hall. But to do this, they had to submit multiple abstracts and may be milking a topic for all it is worth. I am really not sure there is a huge benefit to doing something like this. Certainly don't pursue this simply for the sake of doing it. If you do have multiple things to talk about and it seems most reasonable to have multiple posters, then go for it. But just remember multiple posters means multiple headaches of putting them together and then finding a team to present them all, which can add to costs, etc.

The exhibit hall. One place you will see people flocking to is the exhibit hall. This is the space—often huge if the meeting is large—in which biotechnology companies, laboratory companies, pharmaceutical companies, medical device manufacturers, nonprofit research foundations and associations, publishers, and diagnostic service companies display their offerings and services. Along with large signs displaying the company name and product, some of these booths are often remarkably ornate, adorned with carpeting, comfortable couches, chairs, and stools, where you are invited to sit and linger. There is food too—from candies to cookies to cheese and crackers and generous helpings of cappuccino. Most have a hoard of well-dressed men and women eagerly awaiting your potential interest; even a momentary glance at their display and you may find yourself accosted and asked if you are familiar with their products and would you like to come in and relax and have something to eat or take an interactive tour of their product offerings.

For the most part, the exhibit hall, at least a medical meeting, in my opinion, is a bit silly. Now at a conference like the Consumer Electronics Show where people have an opportunity to play with all sorts of cool new gadgets and want to interact with the staff who can explain them, exhibits make a great deal of sense. You learn about the products, get to experience them first hand, and possibly buy or order a few for friends and family. At a medical conference, in contrast, the goal is generally much more subliminal — they want to get into your head, so that when you are thinking about prescribing the newest and greatest multiple sclerosis drug, you'll choose the one where you had a nice experience with good coffee and an attractive representative who spent a lot of time talking to you and smiling a lot.

Not long ago, the other fun part of these exhibit halls was that they would shower you with all sorts of cheap, irrelevant odd ball gifts with the company's name and logo inscribed all over them. I brought home all sorts of goodies, from radio headphones to beach balls to flashlights. I even once obtained an incredible miniature screwdriver set for use on eyeglasses and such. But those days are long gone now. The companies are forbidden to give anything of value or anything not directly related to the product that they sell. So you will find yourself collecting pens and notepads (and who uses those anymore anyway?), but that is about it. Of course, this all for the better, since the manipulation is bad enough without lugging home a whole bunch of cheaply made, mostly useless products that end up in the back of some drawer in your kitchen only to be forgotten. Though I must admit, I still use that miniature screwdriver set nearly 25 years later.

There are a couple of valuable aspects to the exhibit hall, however. The first is if you are actually in the market for a specific product or service. This is your opportunity to look at the newest systems. For example, if you were thinking about purchasing a new device, this would be a good opportunity to see many at once and compare features and ease of use to determine whether you might want to buy one for your lab or for your practice. The second is that it is a good opportunity to look at new books that may be of interest. Stopping by the publishers is probably worthwhile, since it is nice to browse a whole bunch of titles of potential interest all in one place. While doing so on Amazon is also fine, there is something nice about holding an actual book in your hand as well, even if you just end up purchasing the electronic version.

Platform sessions. Outside of poster sessions, the events at conferences I enjoy the most are platform sessions. These usually consist of a series of short talks (generally 10–20 min) on specific topics of interest. They are held in moderately sized rooms that can often hold a few dozen to a couple of hundred people, depending on the size of the event. There are one or two moderators who sit at a desk at the front of the room on a raised platform and do the introductions and ask questions and generally ensure that everything is running smoothly and on time. Both junior and more senior members will give these talks that usually include the presentation of new research results. It is a great opportunity to float new data out there and to get quick feedback. In fact, heated arguments can erupt when people with very different opinions find themselves publically at odds with one another. Those are often entertaining to watch. But more importantly, it is an opportunity to learn about the uncertainties and questions in a field and possibly to hear some widely differing opinions.

While platform sessions don't offer the same one-on-one interactions possible at poster sessions, they are nevertheless quite valuable. First, they will offer you the opportunity to be among the first to see results of some new drug trial in a disease or to learn of a new genetic mutation. The presentations may provide breaking news and there can be a real excitement in the air when someone is presenting something truly novel and important. Second, they offer you an opportunity to see and recognize many of the leaders in a field since they may attend these and ask questions or may be presenting themselves. Third, it also gives you an opportunity to hone your own skills at interpreting others' data and methods and to see if they pass the sniff test. Not everything presented will be the highest quality or believable in fact. So you will have the opportunity to be a judge on your own and determine whether you believe the work is really worthwhile or not. Finally, you will also have the opportunity to ask questions, and I strongly encourage people to do this. Frankly, I find asking questions in this forum far more unnerving than giving a prepared talk. Since you are likely to be unfamiliar with the material, the question you ask has the potential to be silly—and plenty are—or the answer entirely obvious. But it also allows you to think critically through material and directly ask the authors questions.

If you are the one giving the presentation rather than sitting in the audience, I refer you to the earlier chapter on presentations. But in this setting, try to be especially clear and simple at all costs and don't feel obliged to present every iota of data that you have collected, even if you feel like this may be the only opportunity you will ever have. You won't be able to talk for very long, and if your presentation is placed toward the end of the session, people may be starting to lose interest. So keep it short and sweet and lively. And when answering questions try to be courteous and non-argumentative. Accept criticism, whether accurate or not, and move on. Getting into a heated argument with an audience member is rarely worth it.

After hours. Much of importance at what goes on at a medical conference happens after hours, after the exhibit halls have closed for the day and the formalized talks are over. You will soon find yourself adrift in an unfamiliar city with perhaps only a few people that you know. However, this is a great opportunity to make new friends, cement more tentative relationships, and, yes, believe it or not, actually have a good time. Over the years, I have developed a number of terrific relationships with people who have become both friends and collaborators. Although we only see each other a couple of times a year at conferences, we try to go out for dinner, go for a run, or just spend some time chatting over a cup of coffee. Conferences can get very tiresome and to have some downtime with friends can help you gain perspective.

On the other hand, sometimes it is nice to just get away from everyone and spend time by yourself in your hotel room—maybe even really splurging and being completely antisocial and ordering room service. Whether it is time to work, write emails, settle down with a good book, talk or Skype with your family at home, or just watch television, it is another effective way of getting away from it all. It is easy to feel that you are "on" the entire time you are awake at a conference, so it is definitely important to ensure that you have those moments by yourself to relax and reflect. That will help you recharge for the next day of conferencing.

Summary. Conferences can be overwhelming, and it is very difficult for most of us not to feel at least a little intimidated by them given the sheer volume of data being presented and the number of people who all seem to be doing important work—almost always, it feels, more important than yours. But they are also opportunities to show off your work, learn a great deal, and foster new studies, new collaborations, and new friendships. So don't avoid conferences simply because you find them producing a mixed set of emotions, some of which are not all that welcome. Remember that they are nourishing you at many, many levels and you may actually have some fun while you are at it.

Chapter 27
Networking in the Early Twenty-First Century

The concept of networking is challenging to define. The online Urban Dictionary describes it as "A yuppie euphemism for kissing ass in order to get a job or obtain a raise or promotion. *Regardless of your skills, intelligence, or education, if you are not good at networking you will always earn minimum wage and live in a trailer park.*" And it I think it is true that there is definitely a negative connotation to the concept, as if you are an "operator" and trying to maneuver things to your advantage perhaps to the disadvantage of others. But that is not and should not be the case. In fact, when I talk of networking, what you are doing is not selfish, but rather you are helping to improve the environment and possibilities for all people involved: the whole is greater than the sum of its individual parts. Networking, in my mind, means creating new collaborations for study, new opportunities for discovery, for bringing younger colleagues into the collective and at the same time tapping off the multitude of resources available to more senior individuals. When I speak of networking, I mean taking the steps necessary to initiate and invigorate meaningful connections between people to help advance biomedical science.

Networking can really occur anywhere—in your office, at national conferences, or in the hospital cafeteria. For example, it is always amazing to me to learn of work being completed in a lab just across the hall from mine that could dovetail with my own efforts or how work being completed by a colleague across the country could benefit from my joining in.

In this short chapter, I present a few general rules for a successful networking. I am sure there are more and you will over time likely develop some of your own as well:

1. **Don't be shy**. This may sound silly/obvious, but being timid is the worst thing when it comes to growing your research program. And to not be timid takes a fair bit of effort. For example, at a poster session, don't just walk silently up and down the aisles and ignore the gaze of the presenters. Rather stop, introduce yourself, and then ask them about their work and perhaps tell them about your own. Or after a platform session, if there was a speaker whose work you found interesting or had a question about, go up and talk to her and if you learn vaguely of someone doing

© Springer Science+Business Media New York 2016
S.B. Rutkove, *Biomedical Research: An Insider's Guide*,
DOI 10.1007/978-1-4939-3655-7_27

work in your hospital that might help inform what you are doing, by all means, reach out to him and see if he can help you and perhaps in so doing, you can also help him.

2. **Be trusting—don't be scared about sharing data or ideas**. Now I am not saying tell everyone about your next and best greatest idea, but there is little harm in sharing ideas or data with people (as long as the later is de-identified, of course, if you are dealing with human data). Most people are not going to be interested or as possessive of it as you are, and there is honestly little concern that someone is going to steal a good idea. More likely than not, if they find it interesting, they may want to work with you on it as well. Also, the trust that you show to them will help encourage an honest and effective working relationship going forward. In all my years of doing research, I don't think I know of one situation where someone has stolen one of my ideas, or if they did, they hid it really well. Anyway, whenever you submit a paper for review or a grant application, you are basically making your ideas known to the wider world. That too requires trust, so ultimately you are going to have to share your ideas, so you might as well not be shy or scared, and just go ahead and do it.

There are probably some areas where one does have to be a little cautious about giving away too much information. For example, in the field of genetics where discoveries are still hotly contested and races to identify specific genes can cause friction or arguments that can reach remarkable proportions. So perhaps in that one hot area, you should be cautious.

3. **There is plenty enough to go around for all—don't be selfish**. With everyone competing for research dollars, it is easy to feel that the pie is small, and if you don't grab a piece first, you may be out of luck and go hungry. But that is far from the case. In fact, you should think of the pie as being virtually limitless. Just because someone takes a large piece for himself doesn't mean there isn't plenty more to go round. So don't play your cards close to your chest and look for advantages over others, but rather be generous. Think about ways that you can help improve someone else's chances of success by perhaps offering feedback on a grant application or sharing data that would be useful to them or perhaps offering to lend them a piece of equipment that they need to complete work. While you should not be anticipating a tit or tat response to these small good deeds, such obvious generosity usually only comes back to pay you in spades. And if it doesn't come back to you personally, hopefully they will pay it forward to someone else.

Acknowledge help that you have received. As I mentioned in the chapter on presentations, acknowledging the assistance of colleagues to work completed is absolutely essential. It is only honest and fair to them. But you just don't have to do it at the end of a presentation or in the acknowledgement section of paper, but do it in all of your interactions. Let them know that you are not taking their help for granted or have forgotten what assistance they gave you years ago when you were first setting out. People really do appreciate being recognized for contributing in some way, so don't be miserly with your thanks.

Actively seek to introduce people to one another. One aspect of my job that I find especially enjoyable is being able to introduce like-minded people to one another. Two colleagues in two different fields with whom I work may actually have many things to share together without my involvement. Making those introductions and facilitating collaborations in which I end up not being included is not a bad thing at all. In fact, it is a wonderful gift to the other people.

Don't be afraid to go far afield. In parallel with my discussion in the idea generation chapter, embrace different areas of expertise. If the only people you network with are in your own or closely allied fields, you may find that while you are networking successfully within your own narrow area, your network is not broad enough to generate new compelling ideas or major breakthroughs. Of course, reaching or networking far outside your field is challenging for a variety of reasons, as I have already discussed: you may not speak the same scientific language, you may not find similar things interesting, and you may have different immediate and short- and long-term scientific goals. But that should not stop you from at least trying. I have been consistently impressed by how the personal characteristics of people intent on bettering the world through scientific innovation allow them to work together effectively. As your networks expand into new areas, you may find yourself collaborating in fields that you once thought you would have virtually nothing to do with. Of course, meeting these people can be challenging and may require a "cold" email to get the ball rolling since you came across an article you read or via an Internet search. You are not going to find them at a scientific meeting that you attend or at the lab across the street.

Put considerable effort and thought into "first contact" situations. One of the more challenging aspects of creating new collaborations is your first phone call or face-to-face meeting with a new potential investigator. Perhaps you reached out to her because of an article that you came across or a presentation you attended at a national meeting. These "first contact" presentations remind me of the television show, *Star Trek*, where the officers on the starship *Enterprise* have to be cautious about how they first introduce themselves to a new civilization that does not yet know about the Federation. Great care has to be taken to ensure that the culture/ planet is not freaked out by the presence of all these people traveling via intergalactic spacecraft that they had no knowledge about. Similarly, when reaching out to a new investigator, you don't want to overwhelm him or her with gobs of data or excessive enthusiasm. It is far better to have thoughtful and considered discussions, each party having an opportunity to present their work and considering potential areas in which to work together or how you can inform each others' research. Only over time will such tentative first steps turn into a sustained collaboration.

If the opportunity avails itself, attach yourself to a network "hub." Albert-Laszlo Barabasi in his book on network theories, *Linked*, describes the concepts of people who serve as "hubs." Most individuals know a few dozen people fairly well and perhaps a couple of additional hundred in a fairly limited capacity—perhaps only by attaching a name to a face. But there are certain people who are appropriately considered hubs—people who are associated with many hundreds or even thousands of people. Often, these are people in positions of authority—such as the president of an organization or the editor of a major journal or someone who has been remarkably successful in their own research. These people can help connect up people in different fields and in whom the standard concept of "six degrees of separation" seems to collapse to just two. By knowing one of these hubs, you have indirect access to an innumerable number of other people.

Now these people may not be seeking to do you any favors since they are usually in a position of power and may have many other demands on their time. But they are valuable to get to know since they may make introductions, perhaps even casual ones that can turn into important long-term relationships. And since they are in positions of power, they may reach out to you to and ask you to become involved in a new project. Or perhaps they can make a "warm" introduction to someone across the country or the world, in which you are afraid a cold call will go nowhere.

While this concept may seem a bit more self-serving than some of the other networking ideas I have mentioned, you shouldn't consider it that way. Connecting yourself to one of these hub individuals is something these people expect and enjoy. But more importantly, through this hub, it means that somewhere out there, another person who has not yet met you or even knows about you will be enriched by starting a future collaboration with you.

Put yourself out there. This may seem obvious too, but if you never publish, if you never present posters, and if you never go to national meetings, you will remain isolated. Becoming part of a bigger network means taking risks and being an active member of the larger scientific community. So at all costs you need to become an active and engaged member of that community. Seek out opportunities to serve on committee's in your national organization or to review abstracts. Make yourself available to a journal editor. There are many things you can do to make it known that you want to take part in your research community in a bigger way.

Don't say "no." Someday you may be asked to serve on a committee or take part in writing a review article or a position statement or perhaps to simply review a grant or serve on a study section. Embrace these opportunities. They are a very powerful means of showing to more senior people (generally the people asking you to serve) that you are interested in being a real participant and being a contributor, not just a taker. Not only are you going to make a positive impression on them, but it will also afford you an opportunity to meet new people, some of with whom you may end up finding yourself collaborating. Moreover, these same people will likely be reviewing your own work at some point and having them know you and having a favorable impression of you will only help your efforts succeed. Obviously, when you do say yes and agree to do the work, make sure you do it in a timely and high-quality fashion. While constantly saying yes to every request in the early years of your career can mean you end up taking on more than you may want, remember that at some point, you'll actually be able to start to become selective and turn things down. But even now, I find myself generally reluctant to turn down any opportunity to participate in the greater academic environment as not only do I find it a good opportunity to make new friends and collaborators, but also I believe it is an ethical obligation.

Be social. Perhaps this is entirely obvious, but I will state it here nevertheless. Not everything has to be about work when you are with colleagues. Go out with them, both at home and away, for dinner or to a bar or sporting event. Don't limit your engagements with colleagues to just the formal activities of a conference. The discussions that take place over a beer and chicken wings in the hotel bar at midnight can end up being more important than those of the conference itself.

Recognize that your network is dynamic. I may be giving the false impression that the longer you are in your career, the larger your network of friends and collaborators. But this is probably only partially true. While you will undoubtedly slowly get to know more and more people as the years go by, networks are not stable structures, and collaborations and the intensity of a working relationship will change with time. Some collaborators may move far away and make working together difficult; or perhaps they will leave academia and join industry; or some will inevitably retire or pass away; and, of course, new younger ones will join the field. So you should accept the fact that you may find yourself interacting with one group intensely perhaps for years but then watch the group gradually disband or weaken and your alliances refocus with another group. It is best to accept the transient nature of everything, and a healthy recognition of the natural dynamism and ongoing change within any network is part of that story. See also the early chapter on collaborations for more thoughts on this idea.

Summary. Part of being a successful and happy researcher is having a large contingent of colleagues with whom you work and the sense of your being part of greater structure. This only happens through sustained and considered networking. Having a network of colleagues across the country and even across the world provides a feeling of value that is good not only for one's sense of self, but, more importantly, helps ensure a varied and exciting career. It means having an opportunity to travel, to interact with people at all points in their career, to be part of multicenter or larger studies, and, quite honestly, to feel like you have a group of friends far and near.

Chapter 28
Conflicts of Interest

The recognition and importance tied to conflicts of interest has grown dramatically in the past few decades. And with the increasing weight being placed on these, a variety of policies have been created at most institutions to formalize the reporting of conflicts and a legal or policy structure for identifying them. In this chapter, I will try to provide an overview as to what constitutes a conflict of interest, which types of conflicts are absolute no-no's, those that are softer conflicts, and the various reporting one needs to do to ensure that these are being handled correctly. Since many of these are university or medical school specific, I cannot possibly hope to provide an accurate assessment of all conflicts across the United States or the world and how they would be handled. I also hope not to just recite a litany of legal rules, but rather to explain my views on some of the larger-picture issues concerning conflicts of interest.

We are all conflicted. I must get this point out there right from the beginning. We all want to be correct, we all want to have successful research, we all want to get the big grant, we all want to see our papers published, we all want to move up in academic rank, and we all want to be liked and respected. Conflicts of interest policies are geared mainly toward one thing and one thing only, namely, money. But, in truth, the financial aspect of life is only one small piece of what I believe is a bevy of conflicts that we each must contend with every day. And many of the things that drive us to do what we do also lead to conflicts between doing honest scientific work and being biased toward positive outcomes for nearly everything we do (see more on this in the scientific conduct and misconduct chapter). I sometimes feel that the obsession on monetary-based conflicts of interest has become overstated that we end up losing sight of all the other conflicts we as human beings cannot help but maintain every day as we try to go about our work in an honest and forthright manner. To make this clearer, I feel like every disclosure statement should also include information along the lines, "Dr. X. has an interest in being promoted to the rank of associate professor, he is actively seeking funding in the field from three organizations, and also hopes to have four research articles in the field published within the next 12 months." In many respects, it is quite silly to think that financial gain is the

© Springer Science+Business Media New York 2016
S.B. Rutkove, *Biomedical Research: An Insider's Guide*,
DOI 10.1007/978-1-4939-3655-7_28

sole potential motivator encouraging us to "accentuate the positive and eliminate the negative," as the song goes.

I guess my point in bringing this up first is that I want to make it clear that conflicts of interest policies only focus on the remarkably narrow issue of money and that this obsessive focus sometimes obscures the fact that other conflicts may actually be more pertinent when interpreting the results and conclusions of a scientific study or presentation.

Financial conflicts of interest—the absolute no-no's. Having put the concept out there that we all, in fact, have a multitude of conflicts lets us deal with the financial conflicts of interest that our institutions and employers are focused upon. To start with, almost all academic institutions do not allow or limit your participation in *clinical* research on a technology, which includes everything from chemical compounds (i.e., potential drugs), medical devices, cell lines, or service-related companies, in which you have a financial interest. Let's start with a simple example. If you owned $50,000 dollars worth of stock in a pharmaceutical company (e.g., Pfizer) and you were involved in a clinical trial testing, a new cholesterol-lowering medication produced by one of those companies, that would be viewed as a conflict of interest. Why? Well there is the concern that you would have a financial bias toward having a positive outcome since if the drug were really successful, the stock price might go up and you would make money. While this may not seem huge, since a large company like Pfizer's stock price is going to be affected by more than the value of a single new relatively small drug in its pipeline, let's make it still more obvious.

So instead, now imagine you have substantial equity (stock ownership) in a small, publically traded company that has a potential breakthrough medication for a specific condition, since using the drug/technology in this condition was your idea in some way (and perhaps you helped found the company). You are (inappropriately) participating as a clinical site in the multicenter phase 3 trial in the hope of obtaining FDA approval. If the study is a success, it is likely that the price of the stock value will soar if the study is positive. Moreover, it is not unlikely that there may be a price run-up prior the announcement even being made, which occurs very often. Although you are blinded to whether individuals are on drug or placebo, you end up being somewhat unblinded because about half the people keep complaining about tingling in their feet and that this is a known, reversible but relatively common side effect this medication produces. Not surprisingly, there are a variety of ways in which the fact you own money in this company could be influencing your involvement. For example, perhaps you choose to downplay the complaints of tingling, even though they are very troublesome, because you want the drug to work. Or perhaps you can start to see that those with tingling in their feet are actually having a clinical improvement. Or perhaps someone has a more serious adverse event (e.g., a heart attack). You decide to report it but make it clear that it could not be related to the medication itself. So the conflict not only may make you treat the subjects who are participating differently, but it may also cause you to reinterpret data in ways that could be detrimental to a patient's health. It could, of course, also make you participate in "insider trading" of a sort that is also illegal, not only from an academic medical perspective, but from the Securities and Exchange Commission perspective. You may choose to sell your stock perhaps without knowing the full outcome of the study before it has completed, but with having a pretty strong intuition that that study is going to be completely negative. Or perhaps you have been talking with friends at other hospitals who are also participating in the research and they have been noticing similar findings as you, thus, further compelling you to act in some fashion, in part based on your potential for monetary gain or loss.

So the bottom line is that this is pretty simple: owning stock in a company and doing clinical research on that company's technology is almost always a complete nonstarter. This is true from many angles. The good news is that this is easily avoidable: don't own stock in drug or medical device companies. One exception to this is owning mutual funds that contain some of these companies. This is considered acceptable, since most mutual funds are made up of dozens or hundreds of companies, so it is unlikely that you would be acting in a way that is conflicted in this situation. Not to mention, if mutual funds were included in these kinds of rules, monitoring conflicts would become a more complete nightmare than it already is. A second exception to this rule is if you own just a small amount of stock in the company (the so-called *de minimis* amount). At Harvard, that amount is currently $10,000. So you can actually own up to that amount in a study and still do research on it. But be careful. Stock prices could go up and you may very one day realize you have gone above that amount simply because the price of the stock has increased, even though you have not obtained any more shares.

For privately traded companies, the same rules hold. Now you probably won't have access to a privately traded company unless you are a friend or family member of one of the primary players in the company or because a company has been created around a technology that you have helped develop. But if you find yourself in the position of owning shares in a company, just because it is private and not publically traded, you again have to avoid any clinical research on the technology. In fact, private equity is even more closely scrutinized because it is exactly that—private. That means the Security and Exchange Commission is not involved in oversight of the financial doings of the company and things are more easily hidden or obscured.

Of note, this ability to not do clinical research on a technology in which you have a financial interest extends beyond just doing the research. At some institutions, it may also mean that you are not allowed to publish on it either. For example, if you served as a consultant on a multicenter study in which you were involved in developing the drug, and even if all you did was help guide the research in general ways, you may not be allowed to be included as an author on the paper. This has been the rule at Harvard, but it has recently changed. A researcher with a conflict is now allowed to be included as an author, as long as the conflict is disclosed and the investigator does not have a major position on the paper (i.e., is not one of the primary or senior authors, but rather occupies one of the middle positions in the author list). Again, you need to check into your institution's rules and regulations to fully understand the story. Remember also that those rules and regulations change frequently, so it is also good to recheck the rules or, better yet, talk to some in the office that deals with this at your institution and make sure you document what you were told and when. It is always helpful to have a careful record of all these kinds of conversations in case issues develop down the road.

Animal versus clinical research. Harvard and many other institutions actually make distinctions between animal (or other basic research) and clinical research. In fact, at Harvard, research with a technology that you own can be performed on animals. The only key here is that you need to disclose to the compliance officers in your hospital that you are doing this. They will generally allow you to do what you want here and they will not get excessively involved. But there are some stipulations that still need to be generally put in place, in what they describe as a "management plan." As part of these management plans, they want you to disclose to your research staff that you do have a conflict, ensuring that you are not getting special deals from the company (i.e., discounted equipment or drugs) and that you publically disclose the conflict in all publications and presentations that you give.

The animal-human dichotomy when it comes to what is considered an irreconcilable conflict (humans) and one that can be managed (animals) may at first seem odd. After all biases can end up leading to a great deal of inaccuracy and meaningless data. But I suppose the line has to be drawn somewhere, and at least this gives the opportunity to continue research in your area of interest and expertise.

Patents and conflicts. Another potential area for conflicts to arise is with patents. If you patent an idea, you may be in a similar bind as if you had stock in a company. You may be barred from doing research on that topic. I recall a number of years ago that one of my colleagues at another institution submitted a use patent on a drug—basically a patent describing a new use for a drug—based on research that had been conducted in his and other laboratories. Shortly thereafter, a large clinical trial was started in the disease that used this drug for this specific use. Even though he was basically the guy who came up with the idea, his university barred him from participating in the research on the grounds that he had now a monetary interest in the outcome of the research. This issue is discussed in detail in Chap. 31.

Speaking and travel. Another issue that many universities frown upon is academicians being cajoled into speaking on topics and getting paid for them or receiving in-kind gifts, such as free vacations, travel, or food. To some extent this has been frowned upon for a long time, probably because the connection between work provided and the gift is so close and tangible. Be very cautious if asked to talk for a pharmaceutical company about a product, ensuring that you have not violated any rules and fully disclosing all the conflicts.

Disclosures. What is expected in terms of disclosures varies dramatically from forum to forum. As a neurologist, I generally have to file disclosure when submitting and presenting research at a meeting or when publishing. The American Academy of Neurology, which runs the journal *Neurology*, has one of the most comprehensive disclosures I have seen anywhere, asking for every conceivable conflict that you may have of a biomedical nature, whether or not it is even remotely related to the research, asking you to list every single organization (both for profit and not for profit) that has funded your research or that you have had anything to do with. While one cannot argue with the completeness of this approach, in my view it seems a little over the top. A much better and more widely adopted way is by using the standard form from the International Committee of Medical Journal Editors (ICMJE) that asks a more appropriate set of questions focused on the relevance of the monetary issues to the research. To me, this kind of form makes good sense because as a reviewer or reader of the article, you are not overwhelmed by a litany of unimportant and irrelevant conflicts. There is such a thing as disclosure burnout where if the list is so long, you just stop paying attention. Keeping the disclosures relevant is key.

The point in a disclosure, regardless of the form, is that it be meaningful. It is a simple matter to exclude or understate a potential financial interest, and as a journal associate editor, I have seen more than my fair share of people attempting to understate their relationship to a product or drug. For a meaningful disclosure, you have to simply be honest about your relationship to the technology being studied and what you have to gain or lose by the publication of the work. Many journals, in addition to the ICMJE form, ask that the authors of a publication spell out any potential conflicts of any of the authors on the cover letter in plain English.

University and hospital disclosure requirements. Nearly all institutions now have a yearly mandatory disclosure report where you need to list all of your outside activities for which you are paid. Strictly speaking, any time you have a new activity, you should go to the website and update it as well. Then, when you are applying for funding or doing other activities, you need to confirm that none of the work conflicts with any of these outside activities.

This is also a good time to point out that your institution's job is to ensure that you are reporting all conflicts. So when you apply for a grant from NIH or any other institution or foundation for that matter, your hospital will keep track of your conflicts and make sure there are no potential problems. NIH does not get into this act, fortunately, and leaves the headache of sorting out and disclosing conflicts to the institution in which the investigator works. For publications and other presentations, it is usually the governing body of that organization that takes responsibility, but you still may need to report back to your primary institution that you have made these disclosures during your yearly report.

The Sunshine Act. In 2014, a law went into effect called the Sunshine Act, the goal of which was to make all potential conflicts in medical research easily accessible to all rather than simply dependent on the disclosure by individual investigators. The good news about the Sunshine Act is that it requires little to no effort on the part of the investigators—it is the companies' job to list everything you have been paid for. Thus, there is nothing hidden and all is exposed (hence the term Sunshine). However, there is the possibility of mistakes being made here (and I have already heard of some), so one needs to keep tabs on what is being listed here and there is a government website that physicians and researchers can access to ensure that anything they are getting paid for is correct. I am personally happy to have this disclosure list available. Frankly, it is one less thing I have to worry about.

Conflicts of commitment. One type of conflict that is not strictly financial is a conflict of commitment. This refers to the fact that you should not be spending an excess amount of time on projects/businesses outside of your primary job of being a researcher at the institution at which you work. Harvard Medical School creates an arbitrary 20 % time limit. In other words if you are spending 40 hours per week on your day job, you should not be spending more than additional 8 hours a week on some other effort. Of course, most of us work longer than 40 hours each week, so that number can go somewhat higher. Just remember that as you take on outside activities, be careful not to overdo it.

Summary. Conflict of interest rules are complex and vary from institution, so what I have described may not hold specifically for your situation. Moreover, they seem to be constantly shifting, at one moment becoming more stringent and later becoming more lenient and then flipping back again. Most hospitals and research institutions have official training (usually online) in conflict of interest so that you must come up to speed with it to some extent. But there is usually also a compliance office that can help you navigate anything sticky or complex that develops. Remember, things are generally better when you deal with a potential conflict *before* the conflict develops than after you have created a potentially irreconcilable situation that has the possibility for landing you in hot water.

It is important to remember that these rules exist for a reason and although they may seem arbitrary and some of the specific dollar limits may be especially hard to understand, people have generally put thought into creating them. It is also important to remember that there is nothing shameful or embarrassing about having conflicts—so you should reveal all relevant conflicts whenever you are presenting in public or submitting a paper. Remember that you will care more about this than anyone else. In fact, most people watching a presentation or reading a paper will take them in stride, with the understanding that we are all human and also recognizing that it will come out in the wash, eventually.

I am going to finish this chapter where I began it. While our society focuses on financial conflicts, we all have a deep desire to try to see our work succeed. It is for this reason that many scientific outcomes are overly optimistic, drug effects are found where none actually exist, and mechanistic pathways delineated that are not even remotely associated with disease pathogenesis. By focusing so much on financial conflicts of interest, we are distracted from paying attention to this other ubiquitous issue. We must all keep our eyes vigilant to our own behavior and always question our interpretation of the data if we are to really advance biomedical science.

Chapter 29
Scientific Conduct and Misconduct: What Is Right and Proper, What Is Not, and What Is Somewhere in the Middle

As young children, our parents generally tried to instill in us a sense of what is right and what is wrong. Stealing a toy from a store is wrong, but buying it with money is right; driving through a red light is wrong, but driving through a green is fine; and spreading slanderous lies about some in your class is wrong, but keeping your mouth closed, even though you don't like them, is right. In most things in life, we understand these limitations and most of us try to abide by them. We don't always get it right—we are only human after all—but we can usually stay out of trouble without too much difficulty.

In the practice and performance of scientific research, true and outright scientific misconduct is, thankfully, quite rare. Most of us would never even think of manufacturing data or stealing results from a colleague to create a compelling article or to beat someone else to publication. And yet there are some people, remarkably, who actually do feel comfortable in literally synthesizing impressive data or compelling images in order to win a grant or to be awarded a major prize. What hopefully motivates all of us is not a drive for success or fame, but rather a deep desire to understand the universe better and what I like to view as our "quest for enlightenment": the goal of bringing clarity and brightness to all things opaque and obscure.

But in actuality, the practice of scientific research is far more complex then we would like to imagine. The rules our parents taught us are actually not that easy to apply most of the time, and rather than everything being black and white, most are shrouded in endless shades of gray. So in this chapter, I hope to explore some of the ambiguities of doing science and scientific research correctly and incorrectly, honestly and dishonestly, and where to draw the line.

Fact versus fiction: different types of work require different levels of stringency: working our way down the ladder. Put simply, there is often nothing that is no absolute truth when it comes to science. There are usually varying degrees of truth. Depending on where and how you are saying it greatly determines the amount of stringency that you must apply to your verbiage and to your conclusions. Let's work our way down from the top: from those situations that require the highest level of stringency to those that require the least.

© Springer Science+Business Media New York 2016
S.B. Rutkove, *Biomedical Research: An Insider's Guide*,
DOI 10.1007/978-1-4939-3655-7_29

Research articles. A research article probably demands the absolute highest level of authenticity and integrity. After all, what you are publishing not only has the possibility of changing the way medicine is practiced or research is performed; it actually helps science and scientific understanding advance. So I strongly believe that published research articles must take few liberties, and be exceedingly clean representations of the work that was done, including the results and their interpretation. But even within published research articles, there are different degrees of rigor, as I describe below.

Phase 3 drug studies demand the highest scientific rigor. Now when performing high-level studies, such as multicenter drug efficacy studies aimed at garnering FDA approval (called a phase 3 clinical trial), there are usually endless safeguards put into place to ensure that the work is not altered in any way. Every patient's data set must be accounted for, even those who quit the study early. In fact, after the final data is collected and all the data is rechecked and accounted for, a data "lock" is put into place to ensure that none of the data can be tampered with or otherwise distorted going forward. What has been collected is what it is and nothing can be excluded or removed. The written article on the study then must similarly follow along relatively well-regulated lines. A primary end point was chosen—i.e., a predetermined measure of drug efficacy—and the success of the study must live or die on that predetermined measure, although a variety of secondary outcome measures are always included.

But even in such a strict study, there may be efforts to reinterpret the data to the benefit of the pharmaceutical company or its partners that underwrote the study often to the tune of tens or hundreds of millions of dollars. For example, one of the secondary measures can suddenly be highlighted as actually having been the more appropriate measure (hindsight being 20/20). And it is then possible to try to put a positive spin on the study even though outcome was strictly negative based on the previously well-considered primary outcome measure.

Now this is usually not an issue for a large phase 3 clinical trial; these are fairly well regulated by the Food and Drug Administration. In point of fact, the pharmaceutical company needs to go to the FDA ahead of time to discuss the parameters and get specific language from them supporting the use of the primary outcome measure chosen and the study design needed to prove its value. So if the study failed based on the primary outcome measure chosen a priori, that usually means the drug is not going to move forward to FDA approval, no matter how much reinterpretation the company pursues. But there is still nothing stopping the company from going back and reanalyzing the data—with different statistical tests, subsets of patients, or outcome parameters to see if something turns out positive and then writing this up as a research article and publishing it and then potentially following with a second study aimed at that measure.

Let me be clear: there is absolutely nothing wrong or inappropriate with this. This is not scientific misconduct, but rather honest attempts at reevaluating the data to better understand not only why the drug didn't work, despite promising earlier data, but also because of perhaps study design issues or differences in patient baseline characteristics. Regardless, usually huge amounts of money are spent on these studies, and the potential financial gain of a positive phase 3 study can be great, so it behooves the company to pursue these kinds of analyses and potentially publish them, in part, perhaps to support future research endeavors in the field. It also can help reassure investors.

So in short, these phase 3 studies are huge undertakings and require a degree of scientific rigor and scrutiny that are rarely seen in any other area of science. Everything must be transparent, since not only is the data going to change clinical medical practice, but it can and will be audited by government authorities to ensure that there are no inaccuracies or inconsistencies. Everyone knows that they must be on their best behavior, clean and simple.

Research more generally. Now let's take a step down from the extremely regulated rigor of a multicenter drug trial, the goal of which is to get FDA approval, and focus on perhaps a more typical research scenario. Perhaps you are about to pursue a study evaluating the relationship between a potential mechanism of disease and the development of a new engineering concept as an adjunct to an established imaging system. This is only a study being done under your supervision without other sites. What is to be expected? Certainly not the aggressive controls and predeterminedness of a multicenter drug trial? One can come back and do multiple analyses and try to figure out what is the most compelling data to show and just stick with that, right? Always put your best foot forward, right?

Well, not really. Strictly speaking, any study that you undertake should be performed with the scientific rigor and care with which the most high-level study is performed. The reason the multicenter study design and rules were developed was to help ensure super high quality, so there is very little reason not to undertake such high-quality effort in your own work.

Now this attitude, I believe, is, remarkably, somewhat recent and has been fully maturing in the past couple of decades. There are several reasons for these increasing expectations as to how good lab work should be completed. First, there is increasing recognition of that much of what gets published was either false or partly untrue and that is not repeatable. An excellent article is published in the *Economist* entitled, "Unreliable research, Trouble out at the lab," with a subtitle "Scientists like to think of science as self-correcting. To an alarming degree, it is not." They go on to give examples of the remarkably poor reproducibility of research:

> A few years ago scientists at Amgen, an American drug company, tried to replicate 53 studies that they considered landmarks in the basic science of cancer, often co-operating closely with the original researchers to ensure that their experimental technique matched the one used first time round. According to a piece they wrote last year in *Nature*, a leading scientific journal, they were able to reproduce the original results in just six. Months earlier Florian Prinz and his colleagues at Bayer HealthCare, a German pharmaceutical giant, reported in *Nature Reviews Drug Discovery*, a sister journal, that they had successfully reproduced the published results in just a quarter of 67 seminal studies.

While much of this article actually deals with other issues in scientific research, and not actual strict controls of how experimentation is done, it does point out the fact that much of what goes on in the lab behind closed doors contributes to inconsistency in results. Part of this may be due to inherent variation in any experiment, but anything we can do to help ensure that our work is always of the highest quality is important to pursue at all times. Indeed, there is the long-standing concept of good laboratory practice or GLP. This concept has actually been around since the 1970s and still serves as the basic backbone if a pharmaceutical company wants their drug ultimately to obtain FDA approval. GLP is basically a set of detailed guidelines describing what constitutes appropriate scientific rigor to ensure the accuracy and authenticity of data. The details of GLP go far beyond the scope of this book, but it is worth reading into if you want to understand better what constitutes truly high-quality laboratory work. But GLP is not necessary to get publications accepted into top-notch journals and GLP itself is no guarantee of the value of a study or its interpretation.

Journals actually are starting to focus more on this. For example, *PLoS One* has recently insisted that all data collected be made available on the web so that anyone can go back and do the statistical analyses and confirm or refute the information in an article or perhaps to make it possible to go back and perform additional analyses. Regardless, the idea of putting all the data out there on the Internet not only for transparency's sake but also for the use by other researchers is growing and is likely to keep expanding over the next decade.

There has also been a greater recognition of the failure of animal research to provide data relevant to human studies. Part of the reason for this is that animal studies are often done unblinded and with small numbers of animals. And they are often so easy and fast to do that you can do a dozen experiments and identify the only one with a p value of less than 0.05 and argue that this drug in this dose is clearly effective in disease X. The National Institutes of Health and other funding organizations, however, are becoming increasingly concerned about this kind of work because it ends up wasting huge amounts of money. While funding the initial animal experiments may have been well warranted, the subsequently funded human work based on that initial misleading animal work may dwarf in amount the initial funding. Thus, NIH has issued recommendations as to the way animal research should be performed, including blinding of all investigators, not performing pseudo-replicate studies (i.e., repeating a study ad nauseam until you have a positive result), and not removing outliers arbitrarily, among other suggestions.

Now I fully endorse this approach, but I also worry that if we start mandating how everything is done, we may start suffocating the generation of new ideas. In fact, much of the work that many of us may do is not "hypothesis testing" in the strict sense. It is actually "hypothesis generating," in that we are really not exactly sure what we are looking for, and we first need to make some general observations before generating a hypothesis which we can then test in a second set of experiments — our hypothesis testing. This is the way the scientific method works after all. If we mandate that all studies must live up to the scientific rigor of a multicenter clinical trial and GLP, much less would get completed or accomplished and there simply would be fewer discoveries. There has to be an opportunity for free experimentation in order to generate new ideas and possibilities, in an unblinded fashion without huge numbers of animals or patients, to make that first all-important observation. That then should be followed up with carefully performed studies utilizing the most carefully considered designs and GLP.

My personal take is that you should always keep in mind what is ideal in terms of data gathering and management. If you are doing a study and it is hypothesis testing, not generating, try to do everything you can to do it in the form of a clinical trial. Regardless of the study, plan on making the raw data publically available after the study is completed. Not only may this help spur on new research, but it will also force you to consider that what you are doing is not hidden in the scrawl of some lab notebook, but rather will be available for all to see. This simple step of full disclosure will force you, either consciously or unconsciously, to strive to achieve higher quality. Given the ease with which this has been made possible via the Internet, there is no reason not to do it.

As a final but also important point, when it comes to publishing your work and thinking through study design, things do happen unexpectedly. Perhaps your initial design had a flaw in it, not a killer flaw, but something that limited its value. Or other issues came up in the analysis that you were simply not prepared for. Those flaws or problems should not necessarily make the work unworthy of publication or force you to repeat the whole study. Rather, you can simply point them out honestly in the discussion section of the paper. I almost always add a section on limitations of the study, sometimes to the point of self-degradation, simply to make it clear that I may not have the correct answer.

One further step down the ladder: preliminary data for grant applications. Thus far I have been focusing on publication in a scientific or medical journal. This work demands the highest levels of scientific rigor, and while there are various degrees of quality assurance that should go into a research article for publication, they all should be at or above a certain high level, with the idea that if someone else came in and followed the methods you completed to the letter, they would end up with the similar results.

However, recognize that not all work or analyses you will be doing will be geared for publication. In point of fact, if you are applying for a grant, the level of quality does not necessarily need to be the same as that needed for publication. The point is that in these situations, you are demonstrating *preliminary data*, or data not intended for publication, or at least not yet. In point of fact, when applying for a grant, we really should be putting our best face forward. That does not mean doing an experiment with ten subjects and only using those that had the results that you want—that is essentially fraudulent. But it does mean that you may have only single-case examples or Ns of two or three, and the best you can do is show that you can see a difference between groups or that there is a trend in a certain direction. The reason that you are applying for the grant in the first place is to do the work in a stronger and more consistent and considered way in order to fully to further develop and test a hypothesis.

In short, you can and should take greater liberties when submitting a grant application than when writing a scientific paper. After all, you are asking for money to do the research, and theoretically speaking, you have had to gather the preliminary data that you have by the skin of your teeth, stretching your already thin resources and team (possibly just yourself) to go the extra step to collect some data without virtually no financial support. And don't forget, if you submit too much impressive data in a grant application, you will be accused of already having done the research, so there will be little interest in funding you to do it a second time.

Presentations: somewhere in the middle… depends on what you are trying to achieve. I have discussed conduct of research when aiming to publish a paper and conduct of research when submitting a grant. What about presentations? Well, in my mind, a presentation is somewhere in the middle. In fact, if you are asked to give a talk about your work, you are probably going to show a mix of things. You are not simply going to run through the talk as if you are reading a paper, but you are going to try to tell a story to your audience that has, hopefully, at least a modicum of entertainment value, as discussed in that earlier chapter. Thus, if you have published a few papers on a topic, you will likely include some of the methods, results, and analyses from them. But you may also take some liberties and show some of your more recent "anecdotal" data to emphasize a point or demonstrate a new direction in which you are planning to go. Naturally, it is always good to be sure that if you are called to task during or after the presentation that you will be able to defend what you are doing and that there is strong science and rationale behind it, but you are not locked in the same way as when you are writing a paper.

Scientific misconduct. For much of this chapter, I have been explaining the general attitude one should have when it comes to doing research—how to conduct yourself in a fashion that is reasonable such that the quality of your data is strong, the results real, and that you are contributing to greater scientific and medical knowledge in your own small and hopefully gratifying way. We all may trip up for some reason at some time—perhaps, because we slightly overstep the bounds of reasonableness by claiming too much or doing something a little too sloppily in the end due to time or financial constraints. But in all these efforts, we are trying to be honest with ourselves and won't feel bad when we look at ourselves in the mirror in the morning.

But there is another darker side to biomedical and scientific research that is very different: true scientific misconduct. It means knowingly falsifying data, deleting data, stealing data and ideas, not giving credit where credit is due, or perhaps taking credit where none is due. This can be done unintentionally in some situations, but in others it could imply a certain psychopathology that would allow someone to put career or financial gains above doing good science to help prove a point or to get ahead. There are a number of types of scientific misconduct some more horrible than others, but all fairly bad by any reckoning and are absolute no-no's.

In December 2000, the Office of Science and Technology Policy, a part of the executive branch created by Congress in 1976 to oversee scientific policy broadly in the United States, put out a set of guidelines clarifying what is considered true . scientific misconduct and included the concept of fabrication, falsification, or plagiarism as the cornerstones of misconduct, specifically as follows:

> Research, as used herein, includes all basic, applied, and demonstration research in all fields of science, engineering, and mathematics. This includes, but is not limited to, research in economics, education, linguistics, medicine, psychology, social sciences, statistics, and research involving human subjects or animals. Fabrication is making up data or results and recording or reporting them. Falsification is manipulating research materials, equipment, or

processes, or changing or omitting data or results such that the research is not accurately represented in the research record. The research record is the record of data or results that embody the facts resulting from scientific inquiry, and includes, but is not limited to, research proposals, laboratory records, both physical and electronic, progress reports, abstracts, theses, oral presentations, internal reports, and journal articles. Plagiarism is the appropriation of another person's ideas, processes, results, or words without giving appropriate credit. Research misconduct does not include honest error or differences of opinion.

The report also described whose responsibility this was to evaluate: "Agencies and research institutions are partners who share responsibility for the research process. Federal agencies have ultimate oversight authority for Federally funded research, but research institutions bear primary responsibility for prevention and detection of research misconduct and for the inquiry, investigation, and adjudication of research misconduct alleged to have occurred in association with their own institution."

So to put the basic ideas of scientific misconduct in simpler language, you shouldn't make anything up, steal data or language from other people, or manipulate data to an advantage. Now I think most of us know better than to do this, but I still think it important to spell it out here because the ethics of doing research in any field is often not a topic of great discussion at any time in one's education, in grade school, high school, college, or graduate/professional school. There tends to be an assumption that people understand right from wrong and will always do what is right, unless they are criminals or psychopaths. And if it the latter is the case, there is simply no point in even discussing the matter since those people probably will not be able to change their ways. But the truth is that when one is desperate for research funding or needing to get out an article quickly or simply at a loss for words, it becomes all too easy to manipulate things to one's own advantage.

So while data falsification and fabrication are truly bad, others have pointed out the fact that many people do less unsavory things in their research but that are still problematical. In a study published in *Nature*, entitled "Scientists Behaving Badly," the authors point out that, in fact, many scientists that have practices while not necessarily true at the level of scientific misconduct as described above are actually still highly questionable or problematic. They actually completed a survey of over 3000 individual scientists that showed a considerable number performed activities that were not entirely acceptable or legitimate. And although the survey was anonymous, this still likely represented an underestimation of the true rates. See table below taken from that article (Table 29.1).

Reporting scientific misconduct. Whereas avoiding fraudulent acts or even laboratory misdemeanors may seem straightforward as long as one tries to have high integrity, being a whistle-blower on someone committing fraudulent work is even more daunting. It is all too easy to turn a blind eye to questionable practices that are occurring right in your own backyard. In fact, most of us being social creatures find the idea of tattle tailing on a colleague or another member of your department or laboratory a virtual misbehavior in itself. And such people are often picked out and criticized and ignored. In fact, in most cases of scientific misconduct that have reached high levels of attention, it is not just one person making the accusations of fraud, but rather a group of individuals pointing it out. If only a single

Table 29.1 Percentage of scientists who say that engaged in the behavior listed within the previous 3 years ($n=3247$)

Top ten behaviors	All	Mid-career	Early career
1. Falsifying or "cooking" research date	0.3	0.2	0.5
2. Ignoring major aspects of human subject requirements	0.3	0.3	0.4
3. Not properly disclosing involvement in firms whose products are based on one's own research	0.3	0.4	0.3
4. Relationships with students, research subjects, or clients that may be interpreted as questionable	1.4	1.3	1.4
5. Using another's ideas without obtaining permission or giving due credit	1.4	1.7	1.0
6. Unauthorized use of confidential information in connection with one's own research	1.7	2.4	0.8***
7. Failing to present data that contradict one's own previous research	6.0	6.5	5.3
8. Circumventing certain minor aspects of human subject requirements	7.6	9.0	6.0**
9. Overlooking others' use of flawed data or questionable interpretation of data	12.5	12.2	12.8
10. Changing the design, methodology, or results of a study in response to pressure from a funding source	15.5	20.6	9.5***
Other behaviors			
11. Publishing the same data or results in two or more publications	4.7	5.9	3.4**
12. Inappropriately assigning authorship credit	10.0	12.3	7.4***
13. Withholding details of methodology or results in papers or proposals	10.8	12.4	8.9**
14. Using inadequate or inappropriate research designs	13.5	14.6	12.2
15. Dropping observations or data points from analyses based on a gut feeling that they were inaccurate	15.3	14.3	16.5
16. Inadequate record keeping related to research projects	27.5	27.7	27.3

Note: Significance of χ^2 tests of differences between mid- and early-career scientists are noted by **($P<0.001$) and ***($P<0.001$)
From "Scientists behaving badly" Brian C. Martinson, Melissa S. Anderson, and Raymond de Vries *Nature* **435**, 737-738 (9 June 2005)

person brings up an issue about another researcher's misbehavior, that person may be the one who ends up getting judged harshly and not the person being accused. And while it is usually the institution's responsibility to pursue questions of scientific misconduct, the institution is not sitting in this game as an unbiased observer. In fact, the last thing an institution wants is for one of its faculty members to be making bad headline news. So unless the claims are truly egregious or of an urgent nature, many institutions may respond slowly and with a certain amount of reluctance to the concerns of a potential whistle-blower. But institutions do have ombudspeople whose job it is to deal exactly with these kinds of very complex issues. They are definitely worth speaking to if such issues arise.

Summary. Performing outstanding, high-quality, and honest research is a huge challenge, and for the most part the work that we do every day in the lab, in clinic, and in front of the computer demands our own internal policing on a constant basis. We do not have someone checking over our work daily or confirming that we are constantly working at the highest ethical level from moment to moment. But the level of scientific rigor does depend to some extent on what you are planning to do with that data. I doubt most would consider putting some "examples" of exciting data in a grant application or in a presentation as an example of fraud, but on the other hand, including only that data in a published paper, with the exclusion of the more problematic data, would be considered unethical. The bottom line is that we need to be thinking constantly about what we are doing and why we are doing it and always questioning ourselves. Ultimately, the only way to ensure that there is true scientific progress is to pursue fact and not fiction.

Chapter 30
Article Review and Reading: Being Efficient and Thorough as You Need to Be

The quantity of biomedical literature is astounding. Thousands of articles are published daily and with the advent of online publishing, many new open access journals have sprung up virtually over night. How to read a research article is something you have probably learned about in high school, college, and graduate school. But actually reading an article and digesting its meaning without perusing every word is a critical skill if you are going to succeed in the field of research. This goes not only for reading articles relevant to your field of interest, but also those that you are asked to review for various journals. Like all aspects of biomedical research, article reading and interpretation becomes easier with time and practice, but I hope to put forward a few concepts in this chapter that I believe will help speed you along your way.

Different strokes for different folks. The first major concept I would like to introduce is that *how* you read an article is entirely dependent on *why* you are reading an article. There is no rule that says you should read every article from start to finish. And while articles are constructed hopefully in fairly intelligent ways such that there is a narrative aspect to them, there is no need to feel guilty about skipping parts if you are not interested in all the details. I would break down the *why* of reading into several five different categories, including: exploring topics/ideas with which you are unfamiliar, as background into a new effort that you are undertaking, identifying a specific method or technique that you plan to use in our work, serving as a reference in an article or grant application that you are currently writing, and finally because you have been asked to review the paper for a journal.

1. *Exploring new ideas*. There is no better way of developing new ideas than in reading the scientific literature widely. Learning about an area of research far removed from your own area of study can be a great way of generating new research ideas. But to do so, may also require your delving deeply into an area of study that is unfamiliar to you. For such situations, getting comfortable on your couch with a nice cup of coffee and being prepared to spend an hour or two poring over the article, perhaps reading it and re-reading it in its entirely is a sensible and thing to do.

© Springer Science+Business Media New York 2016
S.B. Rutkove, *Biomedical Research: An Insider's Guide*,
DOI 10.1007/978-1-4939-3655-7_30

The more time and effort you put into this, the more educated and comfortable you will be with the material. This is something that is just so critical to do not only when you are just starting out in your career, but consistently throughout it to help spark new ideas that can be applied to your area of interest. Such articles could include general review articles or perhaps "newsworthy" areas in major journals such as *Science* or *Nature*. Or they could be very detailed specific articles that you came across on a literature search that might inform your thinking in a deeper way. Regardless, it is worth not rushing through these treasures since they could serve as the beginning of a new, exciting direction to your research endeavors.

2. *Background to a new research effort.* A similar category would be those articles you read because you already know what you are trying to do, you are just trying to understand the broader picture or related areas and need to delve into the concepts deeply. For example, you may be in the process of organizing a new study in the lab and you are trying to learn from others. The more deeply and broadly you read in an area, the more versed you will become and the more educated you will be in identifying all the potential problems and all the potential opportunities. Thus in this situation, you will not be reading just one article, but read a number of articles so that you start to become an expert in the area. In truth, one of the most effective ways of becoming an expert is by reading, reading, and reading. Before you know it, you will be the one that everyone will be turning to since you have the most expertise. But the only way to do this is to not give the process short shrift. In our rushed world, it is all too easy to skip this educational adventure as you are rushing to write a grant application or to create a protocol. Your understanding of a topic needs to penetrate far beneath the surface until the concepts become deeply enmeshed in your psyche if you hope to become fluid with a new idea or topic. One excellent way of forcing yourself to do this most effectively is by giving a talk on the topic. There is no better way of synthesizing your understanding of a topic than by having to actually speak on it and teach it. It doesn't have to be a formal talk — perhaps just a talk to your colleagues during a group meeting or, if you are mainly clinically focused, to other members in your department.

3. *Identifying a specific method or procedure or type of analysis.* From this category going forward, you are now no longer focusing on really digesting the innards of an article. You are taking a more pragmatic and focused approach: gleaning only what you need from the article and moving on.

In this category, you may have a specific procedure that you want to copy in the lab or perhaps you want to simply repeat an experiment done by another group either to confirm its results or to get your feet wet in the area. Or perhaps you are writing a grant application and plan to pursue an analogous experiment. There is no need to spend a great deal of time reading the introduction or discussion: your focus may be squarely on the methods section and the results that it generates. And if the methods section seems somewhat superficial, in that you simply cannot make sense of all the steps, make sure to look at related papers by the authors or other papers to which it refers in order to see if you can get all the information you are seeking. The methods section may specifically mention a related paper with the entire procedure delineated. Finally, if you are still stuck, and the paper is not too old, contact the authors by email and see if you can get a more specific, detailed explanation of the procedure or analysis being performed.

4. *As a reference to an article or grant you are writing.* Next, there is what I would call the most superficial review of an article, when you are only trying to identify it to help buoy up a statement you have made in a paper that you are writing or in a grant application. In this situation, there is really no real reason to get too deep into the paper, but rather to simply ensure that it is supporting a statement that you are making. For example, this could be because you need support a method without wanting to give all the details and therefore save space (especially critical in a grant application) or because you need to add a factual basis to a statement you are making, such as the prevalence of a disease or the a mechanistic underpinning of a drug. For these purposes, quickly ensuring the reference works—and this could mean doing nothing more than reading the abstract thoroughly and the single relevant section of the paper and moving on—is fine. There is no value wasting a lot of time with this. You are using the paper only to serve a perfunctory role as a character witness and nothing else.

5. *Reviewing a paper for a journal.* It may seem a little odd to include a section on reviewing a paper for a journal in a book on setting out a career path in biomedical research. But unlike grant reviews, which usually come only after you have already achieved a relative high level of experience, you may be asked to review a paper that has been submitted to a journal for review relatively early in your career. This could be because your mentor has thought it good practice for you and has provided one that he has received for you to review, presumably on a topic related to your research, or because you have received a request to review a paper from a journal directly. Recall that there are so many papers being submitted all the time, it is not unusual to be asked to review a paper in an area even after you have had just a couple of papers in that realm. Journal editors are usually desperate to find reviewers who will agree to review a paper (having been on the other side of this for even one of the more prestigious neurology journals has shown me how truly remarkable it can be to find a person who will say yes), so it is not surprising if they reach out to you after you have only published minimally in one area.

Reviewing a paper for a journal, especially as a junior investigator, is actually valuable for several reasons. The first is that it forces you to be critical about a piece of science writing in a deep and thoughtful way—something that you are probably not going to ordinarily do if you are just passively reading a paper. It is your opportunity to judge the work, from the clarity of the language to the fullness of ideas, to the underlying logic and science, to the intelligibility of the results, and finally, to its general value to the field. By reviewing other people's papers critically, it will teach you how to write better papers yourself.

A second value to reviewing papers is that it may introduce you to information you may not have learned about otherwise. Perhaps you will learn of a new technique or a new approach to data analysis or presentation. Papers you are asked to review are often in the same or related areas of research in which you have published. Thus, usually the work is sufficiently aligned with your interests such that it may also open new directions of research for research for you, forcing you to think "out of the box." This is part of that cross-fertilization of ideas that I had discussed in an earlier chapter. No, I'm not talking about stealing ideas from another researcher, but rather recognizing that some of the tools and ideas that they are utilizing could potentially complement work that you are pursuing.

Third, it gives you a chance to show off your analytical skillset to a group of editors. I glean a great deal of insight from the reviews I receive at the journal, not only about the articles that we are reviewing, but even more so about the reviewers themselves. In general, it is true that the older/more experienced you become, the more superficial or succinct the review, but good scientists and researchers will always try to dig deep in a review, unless they think the paper is just horrible and don't want to waste their time on it. I have learned a considerable amount about my colleagues through this process. Those who give sloppy, thoughtless reviews definitely drop in my estimation; those with detailed well-considered reviews rise. And this could be important, comes the time for future collaborations, being an invited speaker, or when I am in a position of judging their own work. This does not, of course, mean you need to be over the top in all your reviews in terms of the length or detail, but just sufficiently thoughtful to show that you have really spent some time on it. Impressing editors is not a bad thing.

Efficiently reading and critiquing an article. There are no rules about how to do this, but I can give you a general sense as to what I do when I am presented an article for review by another journal. First, I will read the article through quickly from end to end, including all the detailed methods and results section, look through the figures and tables. I will not take notes at this point, because my main interest is simply in seeing the big picture without getting muddled in the details. Sometimes, if it is really outside my area of expertise, I will just skip over areas that are impenetrable. This is OK, because presumably the editors recognize that all reviewers are not experts in the same area. So your goal should be to focus on the areas in which you are expert in and not the areas that are entirely alien.

Once I have completed my initial review, I will then open up a Word document in my computer and quickly jot down any major or obvious concerns generated by my first read of the article. I will then start making my way through the article again, this time jotting down all concerns as I proceed through it.

One of the most challenging issues I find in reviewing articles is not in identifying mistakes or inconsistencies in the text, tables, or figures (which can also be challenging if the article is long, not well written, or far from your area of expertise), but identifying those aspects of the work that are not included but should be. In other words, identifying the *absence* of a concept, data analysis, or result is often challenging since the authors may be guiding you along one specific tack, and recognizing that there is some obvious piece of information is not always easy. At some point during your reading of the article or writing up your review, you may suddenly think to yourself, "Wait … why didn't they do that?" and then look through the article to find out that analysis was never performed or that there is a glaring omission regarding the type or number of animals used. It suddenly seems obvious to you but was perhaps not obvious to the authors.

Once I have worked through the article a second time and have generated a list of concerns, I will usually itemize them in a numbered fashion to make it easier for the editorial staff and the authors to address each concern individually (rather than lumping everything into one huge paragraph that is difficult to follow). I then generally give the entire paper and my comments one quick review, paying especial attention to their figures and tables to make sure all is consistent and comprehensible. It is amazing how these often get short shrift, everyone, authors and reviewers alike, focusing on the narrative text only.

As you finalize your review and make your recommendations, it is useful to remember a few specific issues. If the article is just awful, don't spend a tremendous amount of time creating a litany of concerns, unless you believe there is something salvageable in it and it deserves seeing the light of day once it is fixed. It is better not to waste your own time and simply leave a short, but reasonably thorough review/ commentary and move on. If the article is decent, but in your estimation needs to be considerably reworked, think about not only what is wrong with the article in terms of details or experiments, but also in the actual writing and clarity. If you have struggled to understand what they are writing about, chances are that most other readers will also find it equally inscrutable. Don't be afraid or embarrassed to say so. There is nothing wrong in saying, "I'm sorry... I just don't have a clue what you are talking about." Finally, an article review is not a place to express anger or frustration. Try to always present a poised response, even if you feel your ire rising at some comment or the fact that an important reference of your own has been omitted.

In making your recommendations about acceptance or rejection, be honest and not afraid to suggest rejection of an article if it really is of poor quality in your mind. The editors would rather have a truthful opinion from you rather than a polite response that doesn't provide real guidance. If there are issues that you would rather the reviewers not see, there is usually an area in the online score sheet to complete that includes confidential comments to the editors. You should feel free to utilize this. As a journal editor, I have found that most reviewers are generous and tend to suggest giving the authors an opportunity to revise rather than advocating outright rejection. But if you feel that even if all your suggestions are made the article will still be at best mediocre, it is probably just better to come out and say reject. It will save everyone a lot of work.

Summary. How you read or review an article is really a skill that takes time to develop. While we have all had exposure to reading scientific articles as early as high school (and for many of us nerds, in grade school), it takes time to fully identify the approaches that work best for you. But all articles are not the same and your specific needs should dictate how much time you actually spend working through it. There are some articles that have stood as my "go to" studies or review articles that I find myself referring back to over the years. Few, however, achieve that status. Most play a useful role for a short time—educating me on an area related to my research that will serve as a guide as I take my next few tentative steps. And when it comes to reviewing other people's work, try to always make a good and thorough effort, even if time is short. Such an effort often bears unexpected fruit—from learning new procedures and analyses, to becoming a better writer yourself.

Chapter 31
Patents

Patents are something that many researchers, in fact, I would say most researchers, will never deal with. And yet others may find themselves mired in patent applications and revisions. So a short discussion of patents, just to clear the air on the matter if for no other reason, is useful.

A world unto itself. Not being interested in patent law, I was shocked to learn the complexity of the world of patent and patent litigation. It is not for the faint of heart, since many of the nuances and processes are very complex and yet simultaneously important. Also, there are many players involved in the patenting process, from your institution's technology office to the patent attorneys and their partners, to the international patent examiners to the patent examiners at the United States Patent and Trademark Office. There are also many pieces to a patent, from the specifications, to the figures, to the claims themselves. In short, if you find yourself in the process of applying for a patent, you may be in over your head before you realize it. It is all the more reasonable to have help from people who understand the process well and can help guide you through it—whether it be the patent attorney, friends who have been through the process before, or the people in your institution's technology office.

Why file a patent application? The first question should always be is why bother? And the answer is pretty simple: because your "invention" could have potential commercial and financial benefit down the road. There is no value in filing a patent to claim an invention simply because you want to be able to call yourself an inventor and have a document hanging on your wall. The reason to do it is to protect or claim a concept as your own such that other groups, people, or companies cannot utilize it freely. Thus, your identification of some new minor pathway in the development of atherosclerotic heart disease may not have any apparent value, but your subsequent identification of a class of compounds that has the potential for blocking that pathway could have huge financial impacts. Not patenting that potential class of compounds would seem like a major oversight.

So to reiterate: the only reason to file a patent is because you believe the work will have important financial implications down the road. And as you'll see, filing a

© Springer Science+Business Media New York 2016
S.B. Rutkove, *Biomedical Research: An Insider's Guide*,
DOI 10.1007/978-1-4939-3655-7_31

patent is not always a good thing. It can have major negative consequences, so the decision to do so should be made with great care.

When to file a patent application. For those new to the world of research, one of the greatest problems is that you may not realize the value of filing a patent application until it is too late. The moment you make a public presentation of your work or publish an article, you have already given up certain rights. In the United States, you have 1 year from the date of publication until filing the application. For the rest of the world, you are out of luck the moment you present anything publically. This is the reason that many companies filter all news about potential work and carefully guard all public information. Everything must be kept very close to the chest until all patents are filed. Thus, one mantra in the patent world is that as an academic investigator, by the time you recognize that something is actually worth patenting, you are usually already too late. But that is why I am including this chapter in this book—to make you aware of them just in case there is potential commercial value to something you develop. To some extent every time you are going to give an academic presentation or publish a paper, you should ask yourself very briefly am I giving out some idea that is novel and may have long-term financial value as a potential new product or technology? If both are true, it is probably worth at least a quick discussion with your technology office.

As you can also see, patents and business are at odds with the academic pursuits. If you sit around worrying that everything you are doing is patentable and never present your work publically, you are going to destroy your academic career. Thus, all decisions need to be balanced thoughtfully.

Who files the patent application and who benefits from it? Most institutions own the invention themselves, since you created them under their egis, even though you and whoever else conceived of it are considered the actual inventors. So typically, if you think you have something that is patentable and of commercial interest, it is important that you file first a disclosure with your institution's technology office (these go under various names at different institutions). The individuals in the office may review your official disclosure and try to understand the potential financial value down the road. This will likely also entail some conversations with you to clarify the finer points since these people in those offices are not health care professionals and may not really understand why this invention is important. If the people in the office become convinced of its potential merit and long-term financial value, then they will likely contact a patent attorney to start working on submitting a formal patent application. On the other hand, if they think it not worth their while, they may formally give you the option to proceed with attempting to patent it on your own (this needs to be clearly written out such that if you end up being issued a patent down the road and it ends up being successful, the institution doesn't come back to you demanding their share). If that ends up being the case, it means you would have to take responsibility for filing the application and all costs associated with hiring attorneys, etc.

Now if your institution does want to go forward with submitting a patent, and it eventually gets issued, there is usually some formal set of rules regarding who gets any money resulting from it. That money will come directly from the company that licenses it (see below). At my institution I would personally get 30 %, my lab gets 20 % (i.e., it goes into an account that I can use for research purposes), my department gets 30 %, and the hospital receives the rest. So it is not like all the money goes to the institution. You can end up seeing quite a bit of it personally, but you should also be aware that there is often more than one inventor and so those monies may be split further. Plus, there are often other contingencies and all of these will depend on your institution.

How do those monies get generated? Well if the patent is issued, the holder of the patent is the institution and the institution then licenses it out to a company that wants to use it. The license usually is costly and entails some fixed percentage of the earnings of the company or of a specific product relating to the patent. There may also be additional one-time payments. A variety of different sets of terms can be generated, including having an exclusive license (this means that no other company can have access to his invention) or a non-exclusive license (the license can be given to multiple companies). Obviously, an exclusive license is better for the company, but will also be more costly.

Just to be clear, you usually don't get rich off a patent directly. Patents are valuable in many respects—mainly because you can stave off competitors—but not because of their sales price or the licensing fees they generates. So one take-home-rule from this chapter is this: don't get too excited about coming up with something patentable. It may be valuable, but the value is in its potential to the company not in what it generates directly in income. And many, many years can pass between the patent being issued and it generating any real income for you or your institution.

Types of patents. There are basically two types of patents with which biomedical researchers will become familiar: utility patents and design patents. Utility patents are probably the most common and reflect capturing a process or method to achieve some goal; design patents are just: they protect the design of a specific device or object such that others can't copy that exact design.

The patent submission process. Submitting patents is not free and it is most definitely not easy. Although you don't have to have an attorney submit a patent, they usually get involved fairly early on and their prices are steep (often in $600–$800/hour range). The good news is that the initial patent you submit is what is called a "provisional patent." It is basically a description of what you are going to claim and its potential commercial value. The materials for these provisional applications are pretty simple—anything that you can throw into them is useful, from presentations to preliminary papers. You then have 1 year from the date of filing the provisional application until filing a full application. The provisional does not require much attorney time to put together (perhaps just an hour or two) and the filing fee at the US patent office is cheap—only a few hundred dollars at the time of this writing.

Then you have 1 year to decide whether to pursue a full application. These get considerably more costly, and when you add in attorney costs, can easily reach $20,000–$30,000. Thus, these really have to be worth the time and effort. And if you want to expedite the processing, it costs even more. Since the academic institution is the holder of the patent (with you named as the inventor) these costs fall to them and this is why they negotiate tough bargains with potential companies who may want to license it. If there is a start-up company in the mix that needs those patents, your institution may pass the costs directly onto them.

The full patent application. The original provisional application is filed only in one country and serves to place a flag in the sand. Most of other international countries respect the submission of the provisional as the actual filing date—which becomes critical in determining who was the first to invent an idea or concept. But regardless, when it is time to file the full application rather than applying to the United States Patent office alone, a PCT application (standing for Patent Cooperation Treaty) is created that is considered international. Unfortunately, there is no such thing as an international patent. However, the governing organization, created in 1970 through the PCT, is based in Geneva, Switzerland and they will give a first pass to a patent to determine its likelihood of patentability. Once this initial stage is done, a report is generated and then it is up to the inventors to file for official patents in the countries of their choice. In addition to getting a patent in the United States, there is also a single patent authority for the entire European Union, which makes good sense to obtain. From that point onward, obtaining patent protection in countries is pretty much an individual effort. Since there are filing fees in each country, this can get quite costly. Of course, in practice, most medical inventions won't be stolen in third world countries where there are few resources to produce the invention anyway. However, obtaining patent protection in the United States, Europe, Canada, Japan, Australia, and possibly China, is pretty standard.

The waiting game. Once filed, it may be 18 months or longer before you get your first response regarding your PCT application. You then move forward and submit your patent for specific protection in the United States and other countries where you seek protection. The US patent office is backlogged and at the time of this writing, and it may take 2–3 years (yes, YEARS!) before you get an initial response from the office regarding the status of a patent. Fortunately, patent protection begins from the time of filing, not from the time of actual issuance (that is assuming the actual patent gets issued). Thus if you file on January 2, 2018, but the patent is not issued until November 2021, your patent protection began from 1/2/2018. Note this date applies only to the date of the full patent application, not the provisional. The only downside of this is that it means the life of a patent starts ticking from the moment of filing, not the moment of issuance. In the United States, patents have a total of life of 20 years, and thus it is not always in a company's best interest to file a patent too early. Sometimes, it is better to wait until a product or use is closer to reality in order to ensure that you are getting the most value from the patent.

Who is an inventor? One question that often arises is who actually qualifies for inventorship? Generally, it is people have contributed meaningfully to the actual conceptualization of the idea. To some extent this at the discretion of the principal investigator, but it probably will include any collaborators or advanced graduate students or post-docs, but not every member of the laboratory or research assistants. Generally the patent attorney can help sort this out fairly easily. The more inventors, the more complicated all the paperwork gets, so keeping it as simple as possible is important. Unlike a research article, patents shouldn't include everyone involved in the project including everyone who even contributed nominally.

Patent rejections. Rejections are par for the course with patents. In fact, the examiner may reject the patent because several of the claims are not supported or are stated in prior patents or publications (so-called prior art) or are just obvious. It may simply be a matter of reconfiguring the application to remove or alter the claims that were considered problematical and resubmit the patent. Repeated rejections could lead to a situation where you are continuing to revise the claims until you and the patent examiner are on the same page. This process can also be costly and time-consuming, so if you are finding yourself being unsuccessful, an occasional call to the examiner can help clarify what is needed to see your patent safely through to issuance.

The truth about patents. I started this chapter out saying that there is no point in pursuing a patent unless you think there is going to be financial value to having it. Patenting an idea or concept is not worthwhile if you are not looking to make money off of it. But that is only part of the story. First, it is important to realize that patents can be considered valuable for their perceived benefit. For example, if a company is looking to raise capital through a funding/equity round, having several patents protecting a methodology could be critical to finding investors. If there are no patents, the investors will wonder what is stopping anyone else from walking in and starting a competing business. So patents just *seem* valuable, even if people don't fully understand what they are protecting.

Another major point about patents is that they don't really ensure that your idea is protected. Even if you are issued a patent covering a specific idea and it is licensed to a company, some other company could theoretically start doing the exact same thing, even though they have no patent. The only way would be for the company with the patent to sue the encroaching company. And then it becomes a matter of who has the most money and can hire the most attorneys. Admittedly, this is an unlikely scenario, but I only point it out say that patents are really not the end—they are a means to an end and that even if issued they can still be outmaneuvered.

What is patentable? This is a challenging area and I only will briefly comment on it here. Basically, for something to be patentable, it needs to be new and non-obvious. The concept of "prior art" is important. This refers to any patents, literature (scientific or otherwise), or any other general information that shows that your work may not be sufficiently original or novel to be patentable. This could also mean that if you combine two sources, that together their combination is also "obvious." As you can see, there is a major arbitrary judgment that is being made here, but that is why there are trained patent examiners who evaluate these various claims.

Another important, often misunderstood point is that you cannot patent a biological pathway or other natural phenomena, even if you discovered them. For example, it was decided more than a decade ago that you couldn't patent certain regions of DNA if you discovered their clinical importance. What you can patent, however, are drugs (real or only imagined) or other methods for modulating those new genes or pathways.

What makes a good patent? A good patent is both broad and deep. It is able to protect a variety of possible incarnations of an idea while still being specific and explicit enough such that people cannot tunnel right through it. The wording of patents is usually quite obscure legalistic jargon that attempts to ensure a good breadth. For example, language from a recent patent application that we filed is mind-numbingly complex and obscure. I provide it here in full for humor's sake if nothing else:

"Another embodiment according to the present invention includes a method of determining at least one characteristic of a region of tissue, the method comprising acts of applying a plurality of first electrical signals to the region of tissue, each of the plurality of the first electrical signals being applied at a respective one of a plurality of frequencies, obtaining a plurality of measurements from the region of tissue, each of the plurality of measurements indicative of a respective one of a plurality of frequencies, obtaining a plurality of measurements from the region of tissue, each of the plurality of measurements indicative of a respective one of a plurality of second electrical signals, each of the plurality of second electrical signals resulting from applying a respective one of the plurality of first electrical signals, and determining the at least one characteristic based, at least in part, on the plurality of measurements."

Go figure…

Why not to follow a patent. And if patents are not sufficiently complex, there are even other issue patent law issues that I am choosing to ignore entirely, such as disagreements about inventorship status, what kind of presentation is considered a true disclosure, the length of a patent and ways to extend it, and various additional costs associated with patent applications. And remember, not all good ideas benefit from being patented. The term patent comes from "to make obvious." Thus, when you choose to patent something, you are making the method obvious to the world, such that other people can come in and do the same thing, eventually, but not immediately. Some methods are just left better as trade secrets—the formula for Coca Cola, being the most famous of these.

Another reason for not patenting something is realizing that you might inadvertently tie your own hands to do research in the area. Depending on your institution's policy, the simple act of filing a patent application may prevent you from performing research on humans in which the technology you patent is being utilized. This could be a huge problem if your grant funding is dependent upon it. So before getting overly excited and about filing disclosures and patents, make sure that you know the ramifications of what you are doing and how it is going to impact your own research. Even if you do decide to move forward with the patent, it is better to understand the consequences of what you are doing first, rather than later learning that you have essentially blocked your own ability to do research in the field. This is especially important since some patents they may never end up having any financial value. Once it is done, it cannot be undone.

Summary. If someday you have a great idea that you think could lead to considerable commercial value, talk to your technology office and think through the positives and negative of filing a patent application. As noted above, there are definite downsides to a patent. But if you do decide to move forward with a patent application, you are in for a long, complicated journey with many twists and turns. But in the end it may be very well worth your while, not just because you will have a fancy piece of paper to hang on your wall, but because you will have generated something unique that may ultimately lead to a product or technique that will, hopefully, make the world a better place.

Chapter 32
Working with Industry

The academic medical–industrial complex (to restate President Dwight Eisenhower's concept of the military–industrial complex) is forever growing larger and more complex. Pharmaceutical companies and medical device companies need help from academic physicians and researchers for a variety of reasons. These include: the companies need to learn the conditions that actually need treatment or are being insufficiently treated, new potential mechanistic pathways of pharmacologic relevance, the identification of new therapies or technologies themselves, and then finally the actual application of those in clinical trials to eventually garner approval from federal agencies such as the Food and Drug Administration. And that is not even taking into account that these academic colleagues, after a drug or device is approved, become their main market, as they begin to prescribe these drugs or encourage these institutions to buy new devices. Stated another way, the pharmaceutical and device industries ultimately feed off the medical system. That system helps those companies identify a mission in the first place, understand approaches for undertaking that mission, seeing that mission to completion (i.e., the approval of a new drug or device), and then serving as the major consumer of the product of that mission.

Many people consider industry the "dark side," "opportunistic," or even worse, "parasitic." But I think it is healthier and considerably more accurate to use the concept of commensalism rather than parasitism, since industry benefits academia just as much as academia benefits the pharmaceutical and device industries. It is very much a two-way street. The medical world also receives innumerable benefits from working with industry, including opportunities for young researchers to get their feet wet in research, additional sources of income, the ability to be involved in the evaluation of cutting edge technologies, and to see ideas birthed in their own academic incubators come to full fruition.

However, working with industry requires a special understanding of its goals and culture. In this chapter, I provide a broad overview of industry and some simple suggestions to working with it successfully.

© Springer Science+Business Media New York 2016
S.B. Rutkove, *Biomedical Research: An Insider's Guide*,
DOI 10.1007/978-1-4939-3655-7_32

Thinking like a captain of the industry. The first and most basic thing to understand is that the ultimate goal of any company is to increase shareholder value. In other words, the main goal of any company is to make money for the people who own it, and in the United States, Europe, and Asia, that usually implies a corporation of some sort with a variety of stockholders, whether the company is public or private. The goal is not specifically to do good for the world or to promote individuals or to discover some basic scientific concepts. A successful company is one that grows richer and more dominant in its sector over time.

Now this is perhaps quite obvious, but it does create a tone that is quite distinct from that of the world of academia. Every action by a corporation is guided by that concept. They are not going to do things just for the good of society or because the question being asked is of general scientific interest. It is rather to help a new product or service get to market. And the people in charge of the company, from the chief executive officer to various vice-presidents to other company officers (e.g., chief scientific officer, chief operation officer, chief scientific officer) all have that same goal. Some may be physicians- or scientists-turned-entrepreneurs, but most are actually not from the medical field and may simply be business people whose main ambition in life is to start or run a successful corporation, and in the process, hopefully grow wealthy.

So almost all decisions come down to the financial bottom line. Do we pursue the development of this drug because it will make the company a success? Do we interact with this group of scientists and acquire this patent because it is an important new lead? Do we start working with this consortium of individuals because we may be able to do a clinical trial more effectively? If you want to understand the actions of any corporation, it comes down to understanding the motivation by its very nature has a wholly financial basis.

Now having suggested that all corporations are completely focused on money, I believe that characterization is intrinsically unfair. Companies recognize that they have to be good colleagues to the world of academic medicine, that they have to play by the rules, and that they need to create some really great products that will benefit humanity broadly if they are to be truly successful. They know they need to work with physicians and researchers to help bring in fresh ideas, understand complex biomedical pathways, and to perform successful clinical trials. If they are casting the wrong image, no one is going to want to work with them or help them succeed in their mission. They also have to be good neighbors to the physicians who use their devices or prescribe their treatments and, perhaps most importantly, with the final recipients, the patients themselves.

So most corporations make a strenuous effort to achieve a good working relationship with the entire biomedical community. They may do this through a variety of pathways, including asking physicians and other researchers to consult for them, such that the company managers gain insight and context into their own work, while also making researchers feel more positively about the company and its goals. These consultants become an important point of contact and help serve as liaisons to the general medical community. The companies will also try to work with other investigators who may be interested in studying the company's devices or compounds. For example, the company may offer them a new medication to test in some off-label (non-FDA approved) use of an already approved medication that a researcher is interested in pursuing. Free drug for researchers may not seem like a huge benefit, but it can save lots of money. Or perhaps they will supply drug or a congener to a researcher to do more basic studies on cells in culture or on mice. And then, of course, they are happy to sponsor or help underwrite biomedical conferences and lectures. With the company's plastered up in multiple places, the goal is to help secure the good faith from the biomedical community and to demonstrate that their intentions really are benign.

Companies will also make sincere efforts to provide their drugs to patients who cannot afford them and provide ongoing testing of levels or side-effects as well. They will provide informational pamphlets and web-based information to help ensure everyone taking the drug is getting the care they need. And they will also continue to have post-marketing surveillance to ensure that any new drug doesn't produce unexpected side-effects not caught in its earlier testing.

So while it is true that improving shareholder value is the ultimate goal, most companies are in for the long haul and want to do things right so that everyone benefits.

Companies are not just single, monolithic entities. Whereas a corporation often hopes to act as a single entity, it is not just a single individual or even a group of individuals (i.e., the Board of directors). Depending on the size of the company, there may be hundreds or thousands of people and each of these people has an influence to some extent on the greater whole. And some of these people may be friends or colleagues to many people in the academic world, since nearly all were once graduate or medical students themselves. So when you see these people at meetings or in other contexts, they are very much individual human beings and continue to still see things from multiple perspectives, of both the company and the outside world. Like everything in life, a corporation is more complex than it might first appear. While the goal of making money is the clear, guiding light, it is accompanied by the need to achieve good will and friendly relations with the biomedical community as a whole and also by the fact that much of the workforce is derived from that community itself. Biomedical companies are chimeras: organisms that are intent on enriching themselves through the intake of available resources while still trying to preserve and enrich the environment in which they live.

Corporation structure. With that understanding of the motivation of a corporation, it is worth discussing the structure of a corporation and how it differs so dramatically from an academic institution or department.

First, corporations can come in all sorts of shapes and sizes, from small start-up companies with only a handful of people to huge corporations with subsidiaries in widely varying fields, such as Johnson & Johnson, Pfizer, and GlaxoSmithKline, the three largest pharmaceutical companies in the world in terms of revenue, or Medtronic one of the largest dedicated medical device manufacturers. And with these differences come dramatically distinct cultures and personalities.

Small start-ups are entirely focused on the goal of seeing one medication or device, or perhaps a group of closely related items, through the fire of basic animal and/or clinical testing to ultimate FDA approval. (As an aside, smaller companies have a variety of goals. Some may be just interested in getting a drug through animal testing to the point of clinical application; others may be interested in only initial development and in vitro and in vivo testing of a small set of molecules.) Their investors are looking forward to success on a relatively narrow front of seeing a financial return on just that one small area. They don't want the company to get distracted with unnecessary efforts. And they would like to see a return on an investment as soon as possible, though in the pharmaceutical realm, that could take many years or even decades. So not surprisingly, if you find yourself dealing with a smaller company, for whatever reason, you will usually be dealing with people who are very focused. Usually the structure of the company is small enough such that you'll find yourself talking directly to the chief scientific officer or perhaps the CEO herself.

At the other extreme from these small start-ups with great focus are the mega-corporations. These companies are really huge, often with thousands of employees, frequently spread out across the globe. There are many divisions and vice-presidents and directors and chiefs with a myriad of titles that may seem identical and yet have entirely different meanings. So just because you find yourself talking to one person does not mean that person has any authority to do anything. And more likely than not, any decisions will need to be passed up to higher authority figures who will need to sign off on it. And even if sign-offs happen, say to get a molecule to test in your lab in mice for some different application, a program may be abruptly closed down and you'll find yourself empty-handed. In these large companies, everything seems to move forward very slowly and you are really never sure who is calling the actual shots.

The legal stuff. If you decide to enter into any kind of discussions with a corporation, for example because you are perhaps being asked to serve as a consultant or perhaps because you will be helping participate in a clinical trial that the company is initiating, be prepared to start signing a series of indecipherable documents. Usually even before speaking in any serious way you'll need to sign a confidentiality agreement or a non-disclosure agreement, written up by the company's lawyers. These are usually pretty straightforward documents that say you will not go telling others about the secret information the company is telling you about. These can be either one-way or two-way agreements, the one-way agreement protecting only the corporation, the two-way protecting both sides. It is important to point out that sometimes your own institution may want you to have the company people sign one of these to protect your own work. Who should sign this—you or your institution—depends pretty much on what you are trying to do. If a company asks you to consult on a project and is paying you outside your regular work, that is pretty much a personal decision and you should probably not be involving your institution. On the other hand, if you are planning on becoming part of a multicenter trial or other work that will involve your institution, the institution should be the one signing off on the document.

If you do end up consulting for a company, hence working directly with it yourself rather than through your institution, you will have to deal with these various agreements, from non-disclosure agreements to the actual consulting contracts.

These mostly contain "boilerplate" language and after some careful reading and perhaps a small edit or two, you can probably just go ahead and sign them. On the other hand, if you are unsure, there is no harm in hiring a lawyer to look them over. These will usually result in some modest edits that will require some back-and-forth with the company's lawyers. You will be charged for a couple of hours of time (e.g., $1500 or so), but it may give you peace of mind.

Visiting a company. I think the best way to understand the culture of a corporation is to visit the actual company itself. Larger, successful corporations are usually housed in vast buildings with their own security force. The sign-in procedure can be prolonged, and then you will not be allowed to simply roam free, but will be escorted from entrance to room, and then room to room to ensure that you do not gain access to any sensitive areas. When you leave, you will be escorted out and you will be duly asked to return your temporary ID. You will have a new sense of freedom when you return to the real world. Smaller businesses may not have a strong a "security" feel about them, and are often more comfortable, with less lengthy sign-in procedures and a homey atmosphere. While you still may be escorted around, the whole tenor of the situation usually feels more familiar.

Not the dark side. Let me be completely clear: as I intimated earlier, I do not consider industry the "dark side." There is nothing evil or malignant about corporations seeking financial success. And without for-profit corporations, therapies for hundreds if not thousands of diseases would simply not exist. And the people who work for these businesses are not "sell-outs" or "traitors" but rather decent human beings who are perhaps seeking a change from the grind of grant- and paper-writing and the continual search for new ideas and directions. They are likely to include some of your friends and peers or perhaps old mentors or past students. And perhaps it may even include some future version of you some day.

Summary. My goal here is to simply introduce industry and its culture, at least seen from my perspective, and the strange differences between it and the biomedical academic world this book is mostly focused on helping you navigate. As a biomedical researcher, you will time and time again be interacting with industry and thus having some sense of its mindset and behavior may help you better manage those relationships. Remember that if you have questions about signing any documents, it is always good to confirm whether you are doing it as a private consultant to the company or through your work at your institution. If you have uncertainties, contact the hospital contracting office or consider hiring a lawyer of your own for input. Or talk to a friend or two who have already been through the process. The bottom line is that working with industry is generally a good thing. Don't avoid it because of some idea that it is bad. It isn't. Industry is another partner helping to advance biomedical science.

Part V
Career Choices and Life Lessons

Chapter 33
Jobs in Biomedical Science: Seeking, Landing, and Changing

There are entire books on how to apply for jobs, from writing resumes to interviewing successfully to effective negotiation. I cannot possibly hope to cover all that in a single chapter; indeed, that is not my goal here. Rather, I would like to give an overview of some broad rules governing the road to finding faculty positions in the biomedical sciences, with a focus mainly on the United States, though I suspect certain aspects of this review may hold value abroad as well. Of note, I am also only focusing on academic positions, not industry positions, as I do not believe I am sufficiently versed in that area to provide useful advice (beyond what I described in the previous chapter).

The PhD versus MD dichotomy. The most obvious dichotomy in academic positions, which is especially true in the United States, is between those people with PhDs versus those with MDs. To a great extent, and what I consider quite unfairly, MD degrees offer more freedom and job security than PhD positions, and not to mention, often considerably higher salaries. The main reason for this difference in the United States is that MDs, as long as they have finished residency and fellowship training, can ultimately become licensed to practice medicine and thus demand higher salaries than can PhDs, even if the MD is hired into a position in which he is spending 90 % of his time doing basic science research, which should theoretically pay both types people similarly. On the positive side, it is likely that the higher salary of MDs has actually buoyed up PhD salaries to at least some extent, though the disparity is definitely problematic. I only bring this up here to acknowledge the unfairness and relatively artificial nature of the dichotomy. There is nothing to do but acknowledge it and move on. And recall that if you are a PhD, you are at least not having to take call on weekends, having to deal with difficult patients, worry about being sued for malpractice, or paying back huge loans incurred during medical school.

The job by itself. No two jobs/positions are the same. This is because every institution has its own culture and bylaws, and what is expected from you will mirror the needs of the department and the institution as a whole. Even differences in

© Springer Science+Business Media New York 2016
S.B. Rutkove, *Biomedical Research: An Insider's Guide*,
DOI 10.1007/978-1-4939-3655-7_33

state laws can alter the details of your prospective position. And you will be amazed how much things can vary—from where your salary comes from to the salary itself, to the size of your potential laboratory, to the start-up space available. Whether the institution is in a more rural environment or deep in the heart of a major metropolitan center can also impact important issues that may not seem important when you first start out—like the cost of parking (often inconceivably high in major cities and gratis in many more rural settings). So as you evaluate prospective jobs, make sure that you understand *all* the details and take copious notes as you learn about them. Is the culture at the institution supportive of research or is it a hospital mainly interested in ensuring it is taking adequate care of its patients? Is there a religious affiliation with the institution that could impact your work in some way either now or down the road? It is difficult to give specific suggestions about a job, but thinking really broadly about it, digging up as much information as you can from other people at the institution, and preferentially from someone you know personally, is critical. Only until you are sick of learning about a job should actually feel that you know enough.

Evaluating your prospective boss. Of the myriad of issues that need to be considered, the person under whom you will be directly working—usually a department chair for most faculty positions—is one of the most critical factors in choosing your job and one that is easily undervalued. You should consider the kind of person you would enjoy working under and then as you interview for positions, determine whether that person, as far as you can tell, meets those expectations. This can be achieved, of course, during the interview with the person but also while you are meeting with and talking to other members of your department. Do the faculty honestly like her or do they just barely tolerate her? What are her strong points? What are her weaknesses? Try to dig into things as much as you can. You may also be able to garner additional information by speaking to people outside the department. What is this person's national/international reputation? Were there ever any controversies surrounding the person?

Another important point is to determine the chairperson's tenure in the position. Is he upwardly mobile and looking for a position as a dean or hospital president, or has he been recently appointed to the department, or is he a long-term player with little apparent interest in finding another position? Stability in a chairperson's position may be absolutely critical to your own happiness since an abrupt changing of the guard could mean everything you had anticipated being true is no longer the case. In more than one instance I have had colleagues who had a chairman retire and the new chairman who was brought in was highly problematic. The entire department can get turned upside down and people start leaving because of the new leader's ineptitude or hardline attitude. I, in contrast, have been lucky to have a single, strong chairperson in my department for more than 20 years, providing stability and support, not just to me, but to all of my colleagues as well.

Situations in which a new chairperson comes and completely reorganizes and reprioritizes departmental activities, much to the horror of the established faculty, occur frequently. The way our current academic medical system works is that the department chairperson has relatively unlimited powers, except as relates to breaking of contractual obligations and standard institutional policies. But that gives a chairperson tremendous leverage to make your life wonderful or miserable depending on his whims. Just because you have a contract that ensures a certain salary or office doesn't mean that you can't be made miserable.

Fortunately, most chairman are not crazed, monarchical bigots, but rather generous and caring human beings, who are driven to make their department great while helping you along in your career. So even if there is an unexpected change in chairperson, if you are a hard worker with grant support, you will be one of the valued departmental members.

Where does your salary come from? Institutions have widely varying approaches to paying their employees, and to a great extent, this depends on your specific role at that institution. An entirely salaried position means that you are being paid a fixed sum based on several factors, such as your academic rank and service that you provide. Positions in which your salary is fixed are typical in institutions with larger endowments and other constant sources of income, such as medical schools or large universities. But just because you are salaried does not mean that you have a free ride. That salary may be dependent on your continuing to achieve a certain level of funding for your research, patient care, teaching or other administrative activities within the department. Usually such situations are accompanied by some method of accounting for your time to ensure that you are really earning your keep. One way of doing this is through the concept of an RVU or relative value unit. This is an attempt at housekeeping by assigning an RVU to any activity that you undertake, whether it is research or patient care. You are assigned a minimum number of RVUs to be completed monthly or yearly and you need to stay above that to show that you are truly deserving of your salary. If you are fully salaried, the only situation that may make you entirely free is if you are in a fully tenured position. Even if you can't get grant funding, the institution is forced to pay your salary, as long as you do whatever other contractual obligations you may have, including teaching and administration. Of course, that doesn't stop the university from taking away your lab space or support staff should your funding dry up.

Many positions in the biomedical sciences and medicine in general are not salaried and are made up mostly of what is called "soft money" (as compared to the hard money of a salaried position). What this means is that you will negotiate a salary with your chairman and then "earn" the money to help pay for that. If you are an MD, inevitably that means seeing patients and doing clinical work, from attending on the wards or consult services, to doing surgical or other procedures, and seeing patients in outpatient clinics. It may also mean receiving regular support from the institution for teaching (the amount of support based on how much teaching you do) and administration (e.g., running a division within a department or overseeing a clinical laboratory). This would be considered the "hard money" part of your salary. But you can then add to this grant support. This does not mean that if you land a large grant your salary will abruptly jump up; rather, it means that you can "buy back" some of your time from some of these other activities and devote it to laboratory research instead.

Now the idea of buying back time by getting grant funding is great. It is certainly the way that I have moved my research career forward. But grant support, as ridiculous as it sounds, is a little like having a drug addiction. At first it feels really good, since it frees you up and lets you pursue a line of investigation that you are very excited about. But then the problem becomes that you need to sustain the habit. And it is not a cheap habit. To maintain your lab and your personnel, you need to keep seeking and obtaining funding. Some dry spells or lean years are almost inevitable and can become a source of great and constant anxiety, and you may find yourself seeking other areas of funding (e.g., philanthropy or industry support). Most departments won't throw you to the wolves or kick you out because you have lost your funding, but rather give you an opportunity to eventually find funding or redirect you into another area, if possible (i.e., return to full-time patient care or take on additional administrative responsibilities). But if your true passion is research, this is obviously not ideal; thus, the importance of maintaining a constant and robust line of funding is great.

Of course if you are a PhD and you are mostly living on soft money, you have no choice but to apply for grants and seek other means of supporting your research either through industry partnerships or philanthropy, both of which can also be tricky. Plus, many PhDs don't have the sources of philanthropy open to many MDs who may have a grateful wealthy patient with a disease in that person's area of research who is interested in contributing to push that area of research forward.

Tenure. Tenure in many institutions is becoming increasingly unusual. The concept was gradually introduced into the United States in the late nineteenth and early twentieth centuries as a means of helping to ensure academic freedom by providing job security. Gradually the system evolved such that junior professors, just beginning their academic career, were given non-tenured positions and had to earn the status of tenure through successful academic achievement and after a vetting process that assesses that person's accomplishments. Usually that was accompanied by a promotion from assistant to associate professor. Today, that system still exists for many university departments, but at many institutions, people in medicine (and also in law and business—in other words, other professional programs) live by a somewhat different model. In these situations, while tenure and a title may be granted, there is no guaranteed salary with it, except perhaps a modest contribution from the school for teaching. Most MDs will not find themselves in a classical tenured position and even if it is available, the term "tenure" will describe something other than the classic, guaranteed salary for life concept.

For PhDs, it is quite different. If you are doing lab-based research and teaching, it is most definitely possible to obtain a tenure-track position at the university proper (e.g., within an undergraduate college or medical school), where your salary is essentially guaranteed and supported mostly by hard money—in part because you will be heavily involved in teaching, committee and other university activities. But you could also end up in a position say at a hospital affiliated with a university where your money is mostly soft, since you are dependent on grant funding to keep your research going and are not teaching much or taking part in higher level committee activities. Such positions could still be quite good, but make sure that you are fully cognizant of the stability of your income sources and your overall job security before your sign the contract.

Negotiating. Negotiating your first employment package is probably one of the most challenging things you'll face starting out. Think about it for a moment. Here you are, a total newbie, excited to be finally moving from the rank of trainee to trainer, from mentee to mentor. You are finally going to be independent and not having to have notes co-signed by your attending physician or your work judged by your boss prior to submission for publication. Plus, you are going to earn a real salary for the first time. So *anything* being offered is going to seem like a huge improvement over your current situation. The numbers and specifics in the offer letter may seem unbelievably generous and the whole situation too good to be true. Why would you even consider negotiating or arguing any of the details?

Put on top of that the fact the person that you are negotiating with, namely your future chairperson, has been at this for decades and is tremendously experienced, having negotiated her own position several times as well as negotiating the positions of other faculty members she has hired during her tenure as chairperson. Without having any evil intent or wishing you ill or trying to squeeze you for everything you are worth, this person is going to put forth a position that works for them and that is, hopefully, consistent with what others are doing in the department. And they *know* that you are coming in with relatively low expectations; you are simply excited to be offered a position at all and to start your true adult life, at long last.

Don't be fooled by this situation and try to see the big picture. When you are negotiating for a job, you are definitely in your greatest position of strength. The moment you sign the contract, you have given up a great deal of power and it may be difficult to fix something that you only belatedly recognize as being less-than-ideal. The right way to think about this is a straight line of finite length. The center point of the line is the point of compromise, where you both agree on a set of terms that is mutually advantageous. As someone applying for a job, you may envision that the chairperson's offer letter is fair and generous and therefore is at that center point and that you should simply jump to that point and agree to the terms offered. After all you don't want to be perceived as "difficult" or "demanding" even before starting your job. But that is not the case. In fact, the offer package is usually toward one extreme—say 40% further left than it should be. The chairperson is *expecting* some degree of negotiation and thus is setting out at a position more extreme than the one she is willing to settle on. So you must do the same—you need to take a more extreme position than you think is realistic and plant yourself at the other end of the line (say the right side). By doing so, you have opened up the largest space for negotiation and can manage to move your chairperson more towards the center point corresponding to what is really fair.

What can you negotiate? Well, believe it or not, virtually anything is on the table. That is not to say it will all be possible, but it is worth trying and if perhaps something is not, you will be able to eke out additional concessions in another area. But things to include in a negotiation (depending on the type of position you are seeking) include: salary, vacation time, the size of a start-up package (e.g., money the department or institution puts toward your setting up a lab or applying for grants), the size of your office, an office with a window, the amount of clinical work you will do weekly, the amount of teaching you will do, administrative support, the size and location of your lab space, paid leave, and a host of other things. Obviously, what you negotiate would be highly dependent on the specifics of your position, but realize everything can be on the table, even the type of desk you have or the computer and screen. Of course, you can go a little nutty, and getting into minutia is probably not a great idea. My point here, however, is that you need to think about what you want. You won't get everything, but you should get a lot more than by simply agreeing to what is initially offered. But also remember that many organizations have contracts that are essentially "boilerplate" with many aspects that are non-negotiable and that you shouldn't waste your time debating, such as how much is put in to your retirement account yearly, personal leave policies, and who pays your malpractice insurance. As you negotiate, make sure you know what is potentially negotiable and what is not.

As an aside, you will also often have the chairman come back to you with a line like "That is set by the university and I can't change that." It may be true, but it may not be as immutable as they would like to lead you to believe. Exceptions can always be made and if you feel sufficiently strongly about something you should push on it. But only do it with care.

Also, you shouldn't be aggressive or angry about negotiating. It is something best done very matter-of-factly and coolly. Things can be presented as simple truths not as fiery points of disagreement. The remarkable thing about this is that you might think it will start out your relationship with your chairperson on the wrong foot, and that you have burned your bridges before even walking in the door. But that is really very far from the truth. In fact, it may have the opposite effect. Your ability to negotiate a strong position actually will more likely garner your respect from your chairman from the outset. Of course, if you continue to ask for things and prove a general nuisance, that will change. But if you arrive and hold up your end of the bargain—i.e., work hard, publish, and get funding—all that negotiation will have paid off in spades, with greater respect and good will from your boss than would have been the case had you just submitted unwittingly to the initial package with making a peep.

Get it in writing. You've heard this before, but nothing can be truer than when negotiating a job contract. If you don't have it in writing, it might as well not be in the contract. Any points that you have negotiated on or any other relevant aspects of your position should all be in writing, from the amount of any start-up package to your office with a window, should be in there. Written contracts are the basis of our government, laws, and business practice. Just because you have not dealt with written contracts or respect their power doesn't mean the rest of the world hasn't.

As one example, several years ago, I had an experience in which a line in my contract, that I had signed 15 years earlier, ended up saving the day. Specifically, I had a won a monetary award for some of my research work in amyotrophic lateral sclerosis—not a grant but rather a personal award. When I was told I had won it, I was, of course, delighted. But shortly afterward, I started to get worried about the fact that since I had completed all the work at my institution over a period of many years, that the hospital would be able to fly in and claim all the money or at least demand some split of the funds. After thinking about how to handle this for a couple of weeks, it dawned on me that I should look back at my contract, which I still had tucked away in a drawer in my study. And there, in black and white, was a clause that specifically stated that any personal prizes or other awards that I won as a result of my research were mine and mine alone. Suddenly, I went from worrying about how to proceed, to feeling calm and secure.

Of course, no contract, no matter how detailed, can protect you from every contingency, so a contract is not a panacea to ensure that your position will be great forever. Rather, it just helps ensure that your position will be stable and secure and that you get what you want to start out on the right foot. Ultimately, it is really the character of the person you are dealing with—i.e., your chairman or dean—that determines how good your job is going to be. If you don't trust your boss, no contract is going to save you from having a miserable time. If you trust that person, even if the contract is not perfect, you have little to fear.

Not changing places—transitioning from trainee to trainer without moving. I think it is worth spending just a short time on since this issue since it comes up frequently. Transitioning from being an underling at your institution (e.g., a post-doc, fellow or resident) to a faculty member can be challenging for a variety of reasons. For one, people are used to thinking of you in one way and are unable to suddenly accept the idea that you are no longer in training. While I did not actually have exactly that situation (I actually left the institution for 1 year after completing my residency before returning as an attending), I still recall people being confused by my position for a time as to exactly what role I was serving in the department.

While sometimes being mistaken for someone still in training even after you have obtained a tenure-track position has its humorous aspects, it does underscore that it can be challenging to reinvent yourself when you make the transition to faculty when you don't change institutions. But this does inevitably come with time, and it is something that you simply must accept as part of the reality. Remember you are saving yourself the pain of moving and the difficulty of proving yourself anew to a group of strangers, so it is actually a pretty small price to pay.

But it also may mean you will have a harder time negotiating seriously with your chairman to get everything you want in your position. But remember, from your boss's perspective, if she really wants you to stay, she should be willing to negotiate to at least some extent. Keeping you on is easier and less costly than having a full-fledged search, so you should certainly try to adopt the attitude that you are applying for the job just like anyone else and have the same right to negotiate and ask for what you want even if you are not coming from afar. One way to do this most effectively is to have another job offer in hand as described in the renegotiating section below. But this is definitely an extreme position and one I would probably not recommend.

Changing jobs. One of my colleagues told me a long time ago that the only time people typically leave a position and move into a new one is when there is both a "pull" and a "push." In other words, most people won't actually leave a job unless there is a problem or other issue in their current situation and that the new position offers something more/better than the current one. Now, that "push" could take many shapes, and does not have to relate to a specific problem with your job. It could be your partner's obtaining a great new job offer in a different city, the fact that you just noticed that the housing costs in your area of the country are extraordinarily high now that you are due to have twins, or it could be a difficult new chairman has just taken over the department. And the pulls can be varied as well, from a great offer for more salary and more responsibility or more time to pursue your research. But whatever the case, there is a great deal of inertia associated with being established in a position, and moving is huge, huge, huge undertaking. The more settled you are in one place, the harder it is to uproot yourself even if you have misgivings about being there. After you have been in an institution for a few years, you will have undoubtedly developed a great deal of good will within and without your department and when you arrive at your new place of employment, you'll have to prove yourself all over again.

This is worth realizing since you may often think things are better elsewhere. But the truth is that every position has its good points and bad points and you have to be truly excited about going somewhere else and really frustrated with your current position to go through the pains of uprooting yourself. This only gets more and more difficult, especially when children enter the picture and pulling your teenage daughter out of high school is beyond contemplation. Academic biomedical positions are not like many other jobs, where people change every couple of years when they are looking for something new. Many of us (including myself) are reluctant to change once we find a secure position with plenty of room to grow.

Renegotiating a position. Getting a strong job offer from outside that you seriously entertain accepting can offer a great opportunity to renegotiate your position at your current job. This may seem manipulative, but it is the way business is carried out. Getting an offer of a promotion, additional lab space, additional salary or other goodies from another institution can provide a powerful mechanism for getting one or more of those items currently denied to you at your current job. Now, one has to enter this kind of negotiation carefully since you can't do this without really potentially intending to move; the chairman will know that you are bluffing and won't agree. But don't take for granted the power of a new, real offer and the potential for your leaving. If you have been successful and are well-liked, your chairman would much rather try to keep you around then deal with the often very painful process of having a search and hiring a replacement. But the prospect of your leaving has to be legitimate.

Summary. Landing your first independent job is a major achievement but also a major turning point in your life. Ensuring that you have a good position that provides fertile soil for years of sustainable academic growth is absolutely critical, so don't settle for something that is less-than-ideal and carefully evaluate all angles of the situation, especially the character of your prospective bosses. Do your best to negotiate for what you want, and remember that a good negotiator is respected, not disliked. After all, once you take the position and get settled in, you may find it very hard to leave.

Chapter 34
Academic Promotion and Titles

I have to be honest with you: I have never quite fully understood the significance of the academic hierarchy. Allow me to clarify. I understand that there may be certain coveted accolades that accompany promotion—such as tenure or increased salary—which cannot and should not be belittled or ignored. And I also understand the prestige factor that also goes along with promotion—there is something satisfying about calling yourself a professor. Our culture has invested the title of professor with a certain amount of glamour: it can most certainly be considered a capstone to a career of dedicated work. But when you come right down to it, what does promotion mean and does it really matter?

How promotion works. I believe the promotional process at many institutions was once enshrouded in considerable mystery and arbitrariness. Promotional rules were generally not explicitly stated, leaving the younger faculty trying to grasp exactly what was required to advance up the ladder. However, in the past couple of decades, there has been a major effort at many universities to improve the transparency and thus the legitimacy of the promotional process by making the actual steps much clearer and by removing the sense of its being a weird, unseen ritual. Many universities now post very clearly on their web pages the requirements for promotion so you understand exactly what the rules are how to get there. Others offer educational sessions on the process so that you can have give-and-take with someone from the dean's office who is well versed in the process.

Let's start by just going over the basics. The concept of academic promotion is of course very old but in the past century or so has become solidified to include three basic positions on what would be considered a tenure-track or at least a standard academic track: Assistant Professor, Associate Professor, and Professor. Some institutions may have additional titles, such as "instructor" or "lecturer." And there are also adorned full professor titles, such as a professorship holding an endowed chair or being a "university professor."

Generally, when someone first joins a faculty, it is at the level of Assistant Professor, although some institutions, such as Harvard Medical School, begin all new clinical and most non-clinical faculty out at the level of Instructor, which means

© Springer Science+Business Media New York 2016
S.B. Rutkove, *Biomedical Research: An Insider's Guide*,
DOI 10.1007/978-1-4939-3655-7_34

that yes, you have one additional step to pass on your path upward. The Assistant Professor (or Instructor) title requires no outside stamp of approval, outside of the academic search that accompanied it. And if the person simply stays on at the institution after completing a fellowship or post-doctoral position, she may not even need to have a search to earn that basic title. So step one, in some sense is easy: land the job and you've landed yourself some kind of title.

But then things get a little more complicated. You need to actually achieve something to get promoted to the next rank. But exactly what those specific achievements are may vary considerably depending on your initial position and training, since most medical schools and universities have different "tracks." For example at Harvard Medical School, there are currently three: "Teaching and Education Leadership," "Clinical Expertise and Innovation," and "Investigation," and each of these has different requirements. This is an effort to recognize that not all people who are successful and contribute meaningfully to their institutions are necessarily doing groundbreaking research. Rather, they may be excellent teachers or clinicians who are not writing a litany papers or applying for grants to support a large laboratory. This system is to some extent relatively recent (adopted in the past 15 years or so). At some institutions if you are on a regular investigator track, you will receive the title Assistant Professor, Associate Professor, and Professor but if you are on a clinical track, and usually that means one in which you are not actively applying for grant support, you are given the same titles, but this time with the word "clinical" before professor (e.g., Associate Clinical Professor). Personally, I find this a little degrading; I believe if you are going to go through the annoyances of the process, you might as well all get the same title.

Now one does not need to choose a path and stick to it. In fact, you can switch paths along the way. For example, perhaps you start out pursuing research but realize that really is not your forte and your true love is teaching. And so you might switch from one path to another if you have sufficient evidence that you are now moving up along that path. But having the path chosen ahead of time can help provide you more clear guidance about what kind of work and achievements will be acknowledged with a promotion.

Now in the more standard investigator track, those achievements typically include publishing peer-reviewed papers as a starter. Achieving successful funding is also a key factor, since it is also a peer-reviewed process and is generally considered a mark of success of some sort. Giving presentations at meetings both nationally and internationally are also considered important. Patents are also considered important at many institutions, and being somewhat more unusual and more challenging to get than papers, may be more highly regarded. Being at Harvard, I can tell you that moving up from the basic position of Instructor to Assistant Professor is fairly straightforward. You write a few peer-reviewed papers and maybe a chapter in a textbook and you have probably achieved a sufficient amount of work to meet the criteria for promotion to what would ordinarily be the starting rank at most institutions.

Generally the promotional process begins when you have achieved enough success that your chairman, who presumably is meeting with you on at least a yearly basis, feels that you have accumulated enough accomplishments that she can put you up for promotion. Of course that means immediately more work for you: spiffing up your curriculum vitae in the standard format, providing a list of outside names of people who would be willing to write a letter in support of your promotion, and also possibly writing a few paragraphs describing your accomplishments.

Once that is done, your CV and goods will be sent out to a few different people both within and without the institution (namely some of those people whose names you provided) and then you wait as those letters are received. At some point they do return, though this can take a frustratingly long time, and the goods are forwarded to a promotion committee that then sits down and reviews them and makes a decision as to whether to bestow you with a new title.

The more junior the rank, the more modest and quick the search and approval process is. So at Harvard, moving from the position of Instructor to Assistant Professor is pretty quick and painless, even though it is not a fait accompli. You provide the names of a few colleagues at your institution and elsewhere and hopefully within a few months you find yourself promoted. But moving from Assistant Professor to Associate becomes considerably more challenging. The goal is to show that you have established yourself in one field to the point that your work is taking on national significance. Now, how that works say if your main interest is clinical care is not straightforward, but the idea is that you are making innovations in some fashion that you are publishing or at least teaching about and presenting at national meetings and such. The chairman again is usually the person who makes the determination as to whether or not you are ready for this advancement. This promotion requires additional names both at the institution and from elsewhere. And again the materials are presented to a promotion committee that makes the final decision. Instead of taking just a few months as with promotion to Assistant Professor, it may take a year or a bit longer to move through the whole process.

And finally there is achieving the rank of Professor. At most institutions the rank of Professor is definitely viewed with a great deal of respect, since it is far more challenging to achieve than moving from Assistant to Associate Professor. In fact, at some institutions, many physicians and other researchers can spend an entire career in academia and never achieve the level of Professor. That is because for that level, one really needs to demonstrate that one has done a great deal more than just write many papers (and at Harvard we are talking about 60 or more first- or last-author publications), but also usually have achieved national or international fame for your work and for the potential applications it may have in the field of medicine. Whether it is in teaching or clinical care/innovation or actual investigation, you have to show that you have made major contributions to the advancement of the field. Once again your chairman will make a decision as to whether you are ready to undergo the process and again names are collected. This time you really try to buff up your CV as much as possible. The promotions committee will then consider your application and whether you are ready to take the next step to advancement.

Professorial appointments are unique in that they are usually permanent (unless you die, retire, commit a felony, are convicted of scientific misconduct, or more simply leave the institution for another job) so that you don't need to undergo any kind of reappointment process once you have achieved the rank of Professor. In addition, the university or medical school may try to add some glamour to the event by having a separate ceremony to celebrate the event. Indeed, at Harvard you are awarded the promotion at a formal ceremony by the dean of the medical school. One of the oddities at a number of institutions is that they will also award you a degree from that institution—at Harvard it is a Master of Medicine degree. Why receive a degree with your promotion? Well it is what is considered an "earned degree" meaning that all your work deserves special recognition and the university doesn't want you to be a professor without your having a degree from that institution. Admittedly, the concept is a bit unusual. At the ceremony I attended when I was conferred this degree several years ago, some of the people there were relatively old (think gray hair and slightly stooped posture) and had brought their families along for the event (spouses, grown children and, yes, grandchildren) as the people received their degrees and formal promotions.

Tenure or no tenure. Tenure in the medical and biomedical fields really varies greatly on the university and the school within the university. As noted in the previous chapter, tenure was really created to provide professors job security so that they could not be summarily dismissed from a job just because they were teaching or advocating ideas with which the administration or other university funders or officials disagreed. It has since taken on addition significance in the sense that once you achieve tenure, you do not have to worry about ever being fired, short of committing a criminal act or dying (at which point the position becomes kind of irrelevant anyway).

In many medical schools, tenure is reserved for those on a non-clinical track, or the more standard university track, in which you are mainly teaching and doing grant-supported research. In some schools, there is a difference between doing non-clinical work at a hospital-based affiliate as compared to the medical school itself; in such situations, the hospital-based affiliates don't have a strict tenure policy whereas the medical school, as an intrinsic part of the university, does, even though people are given the same titles. And for most clinical physicians and educators, there really is no tenure to speak of. And maybe this makes sense, since you do not really need the job security that was the original basis for the idea, on the presumption that the teaching you are doing is supporting the standard canon. Plus you have additional sources of income that are not really dependent on your ideas—namely patient care or administrative tasks within the hospital or university.

For positions with the possibility of tenure, tenure is usually not granted automatically and there may be considerable risk associated with this. Generally, when someone is put up for tenure it is after a prespecified period of time (such as 5 or 7 years), regardless of his progress toward that goal. The promotions/tenure committee meets and decides to proceed, obtains reviews from people outside the institution, and a decision is eventually made again as to whether to promote the individual (usually to the role of Associate Professor) and grant them tenure or to simply not offer them any. Sometimes the tenure process happens entirely independently of the promotion process (i.e., you can be promoted to Associate Professor then be evaluated for tenure). Regardless of the timing, if the review committee and university grant you tenure, you are pretty much set: you have job security and you theoretically don't need to do additional work, such as obtaining grant support for your research, although that certainly remains the expectation. But the basic concept is that you can be assured of having a job there until you retire, if you want it.

And what if you are not offered tenure? This usually means that you are pretty much out of a job after a final remaining year, during which time you can work and be paid, and most importantly, job hunt so you have some place to go after that year is over. So obviously, the tenure process, even in the most humble of universities or medical schools, is not something that can or should be taken lightly. It can create considerable stress for the candidate who has a constant sense of job insecurity until he finally lands a fully tenured position.

Why you should or shouldn't care about being promoted. So while there are obvious advantages to achieving tenure, if your institution has such a concept for your specific type of job, the actual titular aspect of the job (i.e., Assistant or Associate Professor) is of less certain value. Clearly, as I noted earlier, there is clearly some prestige that goes along with a higher rank, but beyond that and a modest increase in salary, are there any other truly tangible benefits that go along with it? Well, one advantage of achieving the title of Professor is that you don't have to be appointed every couple of years to your position, which means that once you reach that point, you don't need to keep polishing your CV. While you still need to keep your CV reasonably up to date, since other people may want it before your giving a talk or in case you are applying for jobs elsewhere, that is one very minor irritation that will go away. Another advantage, if you could consider it an advantage, is that you will be asked to serve on additional committees within the university, medical school, or hospital. Though some would consider this extra work a disadvantage, having the opportunity to interact with peers can be fun. Another advantage is that you don't have to think about it anymore. I realize that is not a tangible advantage, but for many of us, if there is a goal out there, such as being Professor, you may not feel satisfied until you reach that goal, even if the benefit of actually achieving it is for the most part illusory. Indeed, I find it a true pleasure to not worry about having to climb the promotion ladder. It is one thing I have hopefully crossed off the to-do list for good.

So my view (and please recognize I am a bit of non-conformist) is that to focus on being promoted is a mistake. Promotion should only be a secondary effect from the outstanding work that you have achieved over a course of many years. I have heard colleagues who reach full professorship, say, "Now I don't have to write any more papers!" Is that really the only reason that you were writing papers and doing research? If so, I think that is a poor testament to that individual's commitment and interest in his work and career. I'd like to think that most of us write papers, teach, try to improve clinical care, and do research, because we love doing it. Not because we are seeking a new moniker.

Summary. I began this chapter saying that I hold what I believe is a healthy skepticism toward the concept of promotion and academic rank. I do believe having some external acknowledgement of your accomplishments is worthwhile, but ultimately, making promotion itself a goal will not give you any kind of real fulfillment. The title itself, in my view, means very little. It is what it stands for—the important and meaningful body of work that produced it—that is actually valuable.

Chapter 35
On Being a Mentor

It may seem a little odd to have a chapter on being a mentor in book geared toward people just starting out on a career in research. But the truth of the matter is that we all start taking on mentoring roles earlier than we might think and by understanding what it takes to be a good mentor also means understanding how to work better with your own mentor. For example, you may find yourself working with a research assistant or medical student or perhaps a high school student during the summer. So just like the chapter on the grant review process from the inside, understanding what it takes to be a good mentor may help you make the most of working with a mentor. In this chapter, I try to provide a handful of ideas about mentoring for people just starting out. Obviously, depending on whom you are mentoring and in what capacity, your roles may be very different, so it is difficult to cover all possibilities here, but I will give it a go nevertheless. And I am going to take a fairly wide definition for the concept of mentoring in this chapter—not only helping guide someone along in their own work, but also how to best supervise the work that they are doing for you.

Guide but don't serve. As a mentor, you don't want to do your mentee's work. Rather, you want to provide general guidelines for doing what that needs to be done. You provide the framework for the project or study and then let them work out the details. But we all have a tendency to not let that happen. In fact, you will be surprised to see how often you will have a sense "of oh, it will just be easier to do it myself rather than having you do it." And in fact, you are probably right, it is probably easier for you to just do it yourself than having someone still just learning the ropes do it for you. Once he has it completed (which in itself might take ten times longer than if you had done it initially), you will have to review it, sit down and talk to your mentee and then let him revise and try again. So there is no question that mentoring is not necessarily time efficient.

One way to help though is avoid the common mentoring mistake of not providing sufficient guidance at the outset. I think we all tend to believe that the person we are instructing fully understands exactly what you are thinking because he says yes and nods his head. Some people actually do get it and will specifically stop you and

© Springer Science+Business Media New York 2016
S.B. Rutkove, *Biomedical Research: An Insider's Guide*,
DOI 10.1007/978-1-4939-3655-7_35

ask for more information as they proceed through a task or project to ensure that they are following your suggestions. But most will be far too timid to show that they did not fully grasp the idea that you had initially laid out. They will muddle along often going in wrong directions until at some point you check in on them and discover that they are off in left field because, in fact, they never grasped the idea when you first presented it. At that point, there is usually some sense of recrimination and frustration—two emotions that are best omitted from any good mentor–mentee relationship.

One way to avoid this is to make sure that your mentee fully understand what you have asked him to do by first taking the time to explain it to him in detail and perhaps going over it two or three times and then asking him to repeat it back to you. If he tells you what he is going to do fully and clearly, and even perhaps writing it down, you can rest assured that it will probably get done right the first time.

Be generous with help. Regardless of the specific position of someone working for you, make it clear that you are there to help them at any time should questions or problems arise. Don't be timid about rolling up your sleeves and actually doing a little bit of the work to set an example as how it should be done if he doesn't understand, whether it is doing some data analysis or running an experiment. But don't just start doing the whole thing because it is easier and faster. Force yourself to delegate, since it is the only way you will both learn in the process. But be there to come in and do damage control on a regular basis. One important corollary to this is to make sure that you are always involved. If you are an absentee landlord, things can really veer far off course and your staff could waste a great deal of time performing entirely useless tasks. See below for more thoughts on this.

Don't micromanage. Micromanaging or getting into the details and nuance of all the work that is being completed is a horrible waste of time both for you as a mentor and also generally is a bad experience for the mentee. You have to give the person ample space to feel that she is in control and can do some of the work without your direct involvement or oversight. To be looking over her shoulder, constantly asking how it is going, or having them make small course adjustments every day is a bad experience. Try to give mentees a fairly long leash so they can learn on their own.

Don't just assume everything is going just fine if you don't hear anything. I tend to have the opposite problem of micromanagement. I let my mentees and research assistants run with something only to find that although they understand the task and started out just fine, they started running at a slight angle to the intended direction and since so much time had passed since I last touched base with them, they are way, way off the target. If there is anything I have learned over the years, don't assume everything is going OK simply because no one is coming to you with questions or concerns. Regular check-ins are mission-critical. Make sure that they are doing the intended procedures or analyses. Better yet, actually observe them doing it. I once had a post-doc gradually alter a procedure over many months such that one day when I stepped in the lab and observed him performing it, it was pretty much unrecognizable from where it had started out. You need to get in there and see what is afoot on at least an intermittent basis. These don't have to be surprise appearances either—which a mentee may find confusing and intimidating. You can let them know that you are planning to drop by just to check in so that they can be prepared.

Don't be passive-aggressive or sarcastic. Sometimes as mentors we feel we have to always put on our best face and not be outwardly critical of someone still in the learning process. We feel that we shouldn't say anything negative or critical of someone's work or efforts. I think this attitude is mostly correct, but the problem with it is that in lieu of being critical, it is all too easy to make some subtle backhanded comments about work that was not completed to the highest standard or to exactly the way you imagined it. You really shouldn't be making comments like: "Great. Now I'll probably just need to redo it myself to make it sure it is correct," or saying something like, "That's fine. We've wasted money in plenty of other ways. So no worries."

It is much better to come out honestly, but at least realize that if there was a mistake, you must take some of the blame. Perhaps you didn't provide sufficiently clear instructions initially or perhaps you didn't check in with them frequently enough to ensure that no mistakes were being made along the way. So be clear and critical and then at the same time turn around and honestly accept some of the responsibility yourself.

Set an example of good behavior. Probably the most important thing you can do to help your mentees and assistants along as they begin their careers is set yourself as an example of model behavior. Of course, none of us is perfect and it is hard to always behave as perfectly as we might like to think we do, but there are some obvious things that will help your mentees someday become outstanding mentors themselves. These are basic ideas they should have been practicing since grade school, but I will reiterate them her for completeness' sake.

1. *Being honest and forthright:* Be honest in your work at all costs. Cutting corners and making analyses look better even when the results are less-than-promising serves no one and only teaches your mentees that deceit is acceptable. Even if what you are doing would not be considered in appropriate by any stretch, it is better to be honest and show that you can take negative results or other disappointments with equanimity and move forward.

2. *Not backstabbing or talking negatively about someone else, especially a colleague or someone else in the lab:* This is probably self evident, but you will find it all too easy at times to be critical of others and the criticism may be very, very well deserved. But that mentee, hearing your frustration, may worry what you say about them when they are not around. It is a two-way street, and being critical of someone behind her back is tantamount to being dishonest in the first place. So no matter how frustrated or annoyed you get, either tell the person to their face that you think they messed up or bite your tongue and let it go. Don't start complaining to others about it.

3. *Being a diligent and timely worker:* The work habits you demonstrate to your mentees set an example for them all to follow, not only in your lab but also when they go off on their own someday. Now as a more senior person, you may have the luxury of not having to work in the office all day, and perhaps you will find yourself

doing much paper and grant writing in the wee hours of the morning or late at night in your home, but regardless of how or when you work, your dedication to the cause should be clear and obvious. If you work hard, they will work hard.

4. *Being timely and prompt and respectful of your mentee's time:* There is nothing more demeaning than having to repeatedly wait for someone, even if that someone is your boss. If you set up a group meeting at 2 PM, you should be there at 2 PM. Don't stroll in at 2:20 with a Starbucks latte in one hand and a scone in the other unapologetically. If you are going to be late for whatever reason, send them a quick text, email or phone call so they can be prepared. Just because they are junior to you does not give you the right to run late. It makes a statement that you simply don't respect them. I think some of my greatest frustrations were with teachers and mentors who seemed to believe that their time was more valuable than mine.

5. *Accepting failure with equanimity:* As I mentioned earlier, being honest is key and not deceiving yourself or others by rewriting the results is an important part of that. But part of research is failure—whether it is having a grant application not be funded, a paper rejected, or disappointing results in a long and costly experiment. Show that you can bounce back and not get angry. All of these failures are just part of the game and standard fare—it is par for the course. Just show your resiliency and try again. There is nothing more impressive than seeing someone take disappointment in stride and immediately bounce back and pursue her next goal.

6. *Being friendly:* This is also self-explanatory. You don't have to create an unnecessary hierarchy in your laboratory. You can joke and pal around with your team. You can ask them about what they are doing for fun on the weekend or whether they are still going out with that girl or how someone's sick parent is doing. You can also tell them about yourself and your family and relate stories from times past. They will enjoy hearing and learning more about you and will consider it a bit of an honor and privilege that you are willing to reveal this information and are interested in them as people, not just as workers.

7. *Not prying into affairs that are best left private*: While it is good to be friendly, don't pry. It is usually pretty clear when people do not want to talk about something and don't force topics that people don't want to share. In my years of being a mentor, I've seen people have plenty of problems—some they are willing to be open about and others they would rather not tell me about. It is not your job to be their therapist or their physician—though some may inadvertently be looking for that. Realize that there is a clear line between what is appropriately kept private and personal and what is OK to discuss. If you start becoming too deeply involved in the affairs of others it may become awkward not only for them but also for you and frankly, also may be against your institution's policies. So keep a distance—it doesn't have to be huge by any means, but don't get too personal. And, I probably don't need to say it but will anyway: avoid getting into any kind of romantic/physical relationship at any cost.

8. *Accept blame and don't be defensive.* The ability to accept blame is difficult for most of us, but just do it when it is appropriate. It is important to show your team that you can acknowledge your own mistakes and are not superhuman. We are not perfect and we will screw up many things. We even repeat mistakes more than once, despite our best efforts to avoid that. That is just how life works. Show that you can embrace that fallibility and that you have humility.

9. *Be a determined optimist*. Biomedical research is hard. Really hard. And it can be really daunting at times, from all the red tape one has to maneuver around to get any project off the ground to the unexpected challenges along the way to having grants and papers rejected. Yet, through all of this, you have to show your resilience and sense of optimism. Research is not for the chronically depressed, dysthymic, or faint of heart, and you need to get that point across. You cannot make someone who has a tendency toward depression into an optimist, but you should make it clear that you really need to be positive if you plan to stick with this line of work for the long run. Reveal to them your own optimism and your ability to remain undaunted both to increase their enthusiasm for what they are doing but also to educate them on one of the most important characteristics that a successful researcher must have.

10. *Celebrate*. There is nothing that a lab group enjoys more than a trip out to a local restaurant or tavern or perhaps a party at your house or a group outing. Don't be afraid to celebrate accomplishments with food or parties, and having fun group meetings every few months can be an important way of celebrating their everyday work. I personally enjoy these outings and always look forward to an opportunity to bond and just relax with the team outside of the work environment.

Summary. You will be a mentor, at least in some fashion, before you know it and the qualities that you seek in a mentor of your own should be those that you try to instill in yourself. Learning to be a good mentor is a lifelong effort, so there is no better time to start than the present. Anytime you have someone working under you, think about how you are behaving and how that person will someday be modeling their own behavior after you, consciously or unconsciously.

Chapter 36
Yardsticks of Success

Ours is a culture of achievement. Many of us focus on proving our success in concrete terms, so that we can quantify how well we are doing, comparing ourselves with our neighbors or friends and family, our work colleagues and our bosses. And in research, this is no different. In this chapter, I would like to explore some of those yardsticks, but also try to emphasize that for the most part, they can be misleading. Indeed, the ultimate success of your work is not its implications today or tomorrow next year or even in the next decade. It is the very long-term consequences of what you do that actually matter.

Prizes. I will start by addressing what I consider the false idols of research: those big "wins" that may bring media attention and considerable amounts of money. Now I write this chapter in part, having won a big myself, as I alluded to in an earlier chapter. In 2011, I won a financial prize from a non-profit organization named Prize4Life for identifying a better method for evaluating disease progression in ALS. In addition to the financial award, there was a large black-tie gala in New York City and a great deal of press around it, including articles in *Science* and in *The New York Times*. It was a wonderful experience, and I believe that the organization's idea of accelerating research into ALS so as to find effective treatments sooner through a prize model is both compelling and valuable. By doing so, they were able to bring additional attention to my work and the technology that I developed. I personally cannot thank them enough.

However, winning this major prize was not the end goal. It was a terrific acknowledgement along a lengthy road. But it made realize that the real satisfaction from my years of research and hard work was actually seeing the technology function and prove itself out. Prizes are not inherently meaningful unto themselves.

I know it may seem perverse or ridiculous to be discussing prizes in a book about launching a career in medical research, but less face it, for most nerdy kids in high school thinking of going into research, the idea of achieving something so great as to win the Nobel Prize is actually not that weird. It was for me and it is true also for many of my colleagues. After all, who doesn't dream of doing something so great that you would get to share the same stage as Einstein, Crick or Salk.

© Springer Science+Business Media New York 2016
S.B. Rutkove, *Biomedical Research: An Insider's Guide*,
DOI 10.1007/978-1-4939-3655-7_36

But first, let's face it: there is going to be a huge amount of luck that leads to your winning a big prize like the Nobel or a MacArthur "genius" award. It is not just a matter of being really smart and creative, but you also need the correct mentors and support and collaborators to see through to completion any project worthy of such a prize. (I note here that Einstein may be the one major exception—his developing theories of special relativity, the photoelectric effect and Brownian motion virtually de novo working alone while serving as patent examiner in Bern, Switzerland.) And you need to enter the correct field at the right time. More than that, there is also a great deal of arbitrariness about it. There are committees and just because they make a decision does not mean they are "correct." And on top of that, you need to stay healthy and, most importantly, alive, since many prizes are not awarded for years or often decades after the work has been completed and, in the case of the Nobel, the award cannot be given posthumously (not that you would care at that point about your success). For example, while Robert Noyce and Jack Kilby probably deserved equal credit for inventing the printed circuit, only Jack Kilby was awarded the Nobel Prize in 2000, since he was still alive, Robert Noyce having died some 10 years earlier.

So while maybe it is good to have something like the Nobel Prize out there as something to vaguely think about in your moments of mania, it is probably not worth focusing on in any way, shape or form. And if you do end up winning it someday, be assured there was a great deal of luck and good fortune that had made that possible. I think most people who win any major prize, if they have any sense of humility, can't help but wonder how much of their success was truly due to their inherent genius or just to a hefty helping of good fortune.

The Institute of Medicine, The Royal Society, and the Howard Hughes Medical Institute. In the United States, for physicians and biomedical scientists, election to the Institute of Medicine is a big deal. The Institute is a non-profit, non-governmental organization that is actually part of the National Academy of Science (which itself is non-profit and non-governmental in nature but its creation was Congressionally mandated in 1863 during Lincoln's tenure) and serves as an advisory board of sorts on biomedical issues of national importance, producing a yearly report. Again, like the Nobel and MacArthur awards, the selection is entirely internal—you don't apply and simply get told one day that you have been elected to the IOM. Unlike the Nobel Prize and the MacArthur Award, however, you are not getting any money out of this, but rather simply the recognition to take part in serious deliberations by an esteemed and serious body. Generally people who are elected to the IOM are senior scientists (read as >55 years of age or so) and thus presumably have greater wisdom and insight than younger individuals. Given its long history and "big picture" work that it does, no wonder it is considered an important accomplishment to be elected to it.

The British Commonwealth's parallel to the National Academy of Sciences and the Institute of Medicine is the Royal Society. Founded in 1660, it has a considerably longer and without a doubt a far more impressive history, including the ranks of Sir Isaac Newton and Charles Darwin amongst its members. Today it continues to elect a small cadre of outstanding scientists in all fields to join its ranks. Like the IOM, it is part honorific and part advisory in nature.

New members of the Howard Hughes Medical Institutes are also always noteworthy. Unlike all the other major awards listed above, you actually apply to the HHMI during one of its intermittent competitions, and if you are selected you actually become an employee of sorts of the HHMI while pursuing all your work at your home institution. Rather than giving a grant for specific work, the HHMI pays all of your salary and laboratory costs for 5 years, freeing you up from the eternal cycle of grant applications. The awards are meant for people only 5–15 years out from their completion of training/fellowship and thus they are aimed at people still building their career and are not meant to represent a capstone to a successful career, such as the IOM or Royal Society knightings. These are great awards and certainly worth keeping an eye out for whenever the competition arises, if you think you may meet their very competitive criteria. So in some ways this is the best—these are huge prizes but they are meant to help your work along rather than merely being honorific.

Academic titles. We covered this for the most part in Chap. 34. However, I think it is worth discussing briefly here again. Probably the most common measure of success that we use is the academic title. Being promoted to Professor serves as a message to all that you have been successful in your work and its importance is recognized by your peers, not only at your institution, but also throughout the country and perhaps throughout the world. But like the awards described immediately above, doing work with the aim of promotion is not exactly the right way to think about it. The promotion should be a by-product of the work and not the main goal of it.

But there can be no question that moving up in rank is a convenient yardstick of success. Certainly to find yourself being at 70 years of age and still at the assistant professor level would be, well, unusual. So if nothing else, you should try to be promoted to not feel entirely left behind.

Chairmanship. In addition to academic titles, there are also additional roles that you can seek. For many researchers in biomedical departments, becoming the head of division or of a department represents the final career achievement. For one, such roles mean that a good portion of your salary is no longer "soft"—you will be given usually a considerable portion of your income from the institution and not be expected to earn all of it through grants, philanthropy, industry relationships, or patient care. For someone who had been applying for grants for 20 or 30 years, it is nice to know that you do not have to keep doing it you do not want to or, at the very least, that you can tone it down a notch. But unlike the titles and awards, this position comes with considerable additional work. In fact, if you become a department chairman, you are likely taking on many new responsibilities.

Simply put, becoming the head of a department also means becoming the captain of your ship. You are not alone, of course, as there are many other departments, so you are more like the captain of your ship in a fleet of ships still under the command of a couple of admirals (the dean, the hospital president, and the university president). But the way you run your ship is, for the most part, your own affair and that is kind of cool.

But don't be deceived: many successful scientists and researchers never seek to become the head of a department. In fact, if you really want to focus on your research efforts, becoming the head of a department means many, many, many more obligations from endless committee meetings, to meeting one-on-one with faculty to ensure career growth, to dealing with complaining patients and major departmental headaches, such as budgets that seem forever to teeter into the red. And you are still ultimately responsible for the behavior of your department within the institution, and ensuring that all of your flock is behaving itself is not easy. Recall that most researchers and physicians within a department like to consider themselves fairly independent. They have their own research labs and interests, so the analogy of "herding cats" is far more apropos than tending to your flock of docile sheep.

At any rate, this chapter is about measures of success and not why or why not you should want to be chairman someday. My reason for pointing this out is that you should be seeking these kinds of positions because you want to do them, not because you are trying to prove how talented or successful you are.

Deanship. For those reading this book have their eyes ultimately on administration, that is a very different kettle of fish than anything else we have been discussing here. Running a medical school or other college or school within a university is a full time job. Attempting to continue to run a lab concurrently with being dean or president becomes virtually impossible. Even trying to serve as a mentor becomes relatively limited.

A number of years ago, I had research fellow who told me point blank that his goal was to become dean of a major medical school some day. I don't think most of us would think along those lines, but I think if you really want to become dean, you do need to start planning early. But I would not focus on that as a career goal, at least not initially. And anyway, if it does happen, you will be in a very different place physically and psychologically than you are today reading this book. But, I don't think my research fellow was off base. I think that if you really want that, you need to start planning early. It will also likely mean that you need to relocate to a different position in a different city possibly more than once, as you work your way up the administrative ladder.

Real measures of success. I do not have the final word on this, but I think the real measure of success is seeing your work and ideas being pursued by others or your insights directly generating new ideas and new direction of research. Seeing your articles being referenced is something meaningful, but it is important to recall that much important work or concepts may not be recognized for many years or decades to come. So just because you have only a few people referencing your work today does not mean that one or two of your papers will be rediscovered decades from now and be considered "seminal." And of course what is considered important and critical today, also may be considered less important as time passes because, while the initial work in one direction was exciting, it led to dead end after dead end and finally was abandoned. Or it became one of a multitude of similar findings.

There is so much risk in scientific research, that ultimately any success we may have will always be due in part to luck and to sheer dint of effort, with only perhaps just a smidgeon of actual preplanning, thought, or theory. It is important to recall so many of the major inventions and innovations that we enjoy today were not preplanned, expected or even sought out but based on discoveries that were entirely accidental or unintended.

Summary. There are many ways to judge success and while receiving a lofty award or prize is not to be taken for granted, those measures are neither the only nor perhaps the most important. If you are lucky enough to see your work and ideas being pursued by others during your lifetime, you should consider that best yard-stick and truest measure of success. And if 100 years from now, all your work ends up being just a forgotten footnote, well, it won't matter horribly to you anyway.

Chapter 37
Research Life Lesson 1: Everything Takes Longer Than You Think, So Plan Accordingly

Named Hofstadter's Law, after the idea was first suggested in the 1970s by Douglas Hofstadter, a professor of cognitive science at the University of Indiana, the idea that everything takes longer than you think, *even* when you take Hofstadter's law into account, should be a mantra you repeat to yourself regularly. But it is not just a matter of things taking longer in the realm of research, but they are always far more complex and far more challenging than you can possibly imagine when you set out. The more general concept that a planned experiment or study will go smoothly and quickly is perhaps more correctly referred to as the Optimism Bias, which states that you are less likely to have a problem or something will go wrong than someone else doing the same experiment or research; or stated conversely, you are more likely to do things correctly than other people in the same position and just because other people may fail at it, you won't.

History is rife with examples of projects taking longer than expected, costing far more, and hitting endless unexpected hurdles. The Sydney Opera House stands as the great monolith in the history of the world for cost overruns and time delays, being completed more than 10 years late (scheduled to be completed in early 1963, its actual completion being in 1973) and horrifically over budget (initial budgeted cost $7,000,000; final total cost, $102,000,000). In fact, the rare exception of something actually finishing ahead of time and being under budget is truly to be marvelled. My favorite example of this is the San Francisco's Golden Gate Bridge, which was completed several months early and was $1.3 million *under budget*. But even this was perhaps circumstantial since it was built during the Great Depression when labor was relatively abundant and cheap, and deflation was causing prices to fall. As you proceed through your work, it is well worth keeping the example of the Sydney Opera House always in your mind.

And there is also the well-known Murphy's Law, "If something can go wrong, it will." While I am not a subscriber to this simplistic negative view, it is very true that when doing science, there are usually so many unknowns, that expecting any experiment or study to provide you the results you expect the first time you try it is highly unlikely. You need to remember that there are usually so many opportunities for failure

© Springer Science+Business Media New York 2016
S.B. Rutkove, *Biomedical Research: An Insider's Guide*,
DOI 10.1007/978-1-4939-3655-7_37

in any scientific experiment—from reagents not working, equipment failing, research subjects not showing up for a specific appointment, or errors being made in the completion of data collection, it is actually a miracle that anything ever gets achieved.

Regardless of terminology and the psychological underpinnings related to these biases, it useful to keep them in mind as you plan out studies, apply for grants, write papers, or prepare presentations. Unless there is a strict deadline, things will tend to run over their anticipated completion dates, often by weeks if not months or even years. Strict deadlines, such as those we commonly encounter for grant applications or abstract submissions for conference can help ensure that we don't extend those out indefinitely, but it still may cause us to severely underestimate the overall investment involved leading to a panicked last few days before submission. The submission of a large grant application can lead to a researcher virtually ignoring all other competing demands, including social interactions with family or friends, for several weeks until the deadline has passed at which point he can again focus on less time-sensitive issues. And by the time he gets to that point, he is so exhausted and so behind on so many other projects, he feels like he will never be able to dig out.

So what does this mean practically speaking? Here are some general tips:

1. **For projects without a specific deadline, create an artificial one**. So if you are trying to submit a paper or a protocol to your IRB, there are usually no specific deadlines. Or if there are, the cycles are so frequent that it is a simple matter to wait just a couple of more weeks. But this is a recipe for never getting anything done. Set an internal deadline for yourself that you can pretend is "a drop-dead submission date." Make everyone work toward that goal whether you really need to or not. Although the sense of urgency created by these kinds of deadlines may be entirely fiction, it can help move the project along or at least get everyone motivated to move it along more quickly.

2. **If you have a specific deadline, try to create a series of interim deadlines to help reach that one final deadline**. Whether or not you have an external deadline (for example a grant application or a large presentation) or have created an arbitrary deadline to speed progress, you then need to consider what interim deadlines you should meet. These generally should not be too detailed, but may relate to different members of your team providing you data or they may be internal and in your head only. For example, perhaps you need to finish x part of the analysis by such-and-such a date so that you can write it up. Try to parse out things in a reasonable fashion, so that there are a series of deadlines over several weeks leading up to the final event. Those Gantt charts discussed back in the section on grant applications are a useful way to do this. Whether they end up becoming reality or not, they will help things move forward in a more ordered way.

3. **Don't set unrealistic deadlines**. There is nothing more demoralizing than setting a deadline that you know is virtually impossible to meet. Perhaps you think you will apply for a grant solicitation that you just discovered with a deadline that is only a week or two away. You are excited because it is theoretically possible to get it accomplished and you figure if you pull a few all-nighters, you'll be able to manage it. These situations usually do not work out well. Shortly after initiating the effort, you'll find that you are missing all sorts of valuable pieces of data, sign-offs

from various collaborators or administrators, and that you can't possibly hope to fashion a coherent research plan in the time allotted. I can almost guarantee you any deadline you set for yourself for a project, even if it is months away, is going to start to seem unrealistic the closer you get to the deadline. Setting unrealistic deadlines is self-torture. Don't do it. There will always be other opportunities.

4. **Try to not let everything else go to hell during the final crunch**. This is tough and if you are fighting an imagined deadline, this is when you might choose to push it off a little longer to get some other work done. My general trick is to make sure I spend say just a short time on a given day (usually first thing in the morning) on work that is unrelated to the project that cannot afford to be ignored any longer. Once you have that done you can focus on your main project and try to move that forward.

5. **You are not a machine**. While I would like to think that anything is possible with determination and effort, the fact of the matter is that it is very hard to keep pushing yourself day in and day out in the hope of completing a project on time. Sometimes, the best thing you can do is actually take a break from a project for a few days and let yourself get more excited about it. In the end, the small respite may allow you to focus more clearly on the tasks at hand and breeze through them in a way that didn't seem possible just a short while before.

6. **Sometimes you need to accept that you can't achieve a deadline**. Sometimes, despite the best of your intentions, you may have to give up meeting a deadline, whether it is imposed from the outside or from the inside. Don't become despondent in these situations. Simply recognize that there are going to be other opportunities and aiming for the next cycle is fine. We are all under considerable pressure to bring in research dollars and publish or perish, etc., etc., but the truth of the matter is that no single grant application or paper submission is critical to your career or life. Take a step back and see the big picture. Recognize that in a few weeks you may have already forgotten about this. It will be just water under the proverbial bridge.

7. **Learn about new methods for achieving efficiency and productivity**. In the past few decades there have been some very clever new approaches to making teams work more effectively. While much of this has really been applied only to business, I think they could work well in the realm of academic research space as well, especially when the entire lab is focusing on one major outcome. One approach, called the Agile technique or Scrum argues that you need frequent daily meetings to determine how to move the project forward most effectively and that while someone needs to be the leader, they are not dictating orders. Rapid movements forward are called "sprints" and require the frequent and well-orchestrated interaction of all the players involved. Two good books to introduce the techniques are *Scrum: The Art of Doing Twice the Work in Half the Time*, by Jeff Sutherland, and *Agile Project Management* by Jim Highsmith. Employing these in a research team, as compared to a product development team, is not something that I have attempted, but I think it is a provocative idea.

Summary. The Optimism Bias often leads us into thinking unrealistically about what we can achieve in a short amount of time, and with a healthy dose of Murphy's Law thrown in, we find ourselves proving again and again the validity of Hofstadter's

Law. Delay is almost always the rule, so while you can try to come up with mechanisms to avoid overly wishful thinking or carefully planning out work toward specific deadlines, you will almost always be impacted by unexpected factors in negative ways. As you go through a research career, try to keep the bigger goals in mind and do not become overly distressed by the fact that things never seem to go as planned.

Chapter 38
Research Life Lesson 2: A Person's Research Is Endlessly Important to Him

Dale Carnegie, in his book *How to Win Friends and Influence People*, provides a variety of life lessons in dealing with people. On the section entitled, "Six Ways to Make People Like You," Carnegie offers a few simple rules about dealing with other people and these include: (1) Becoming genuinely interested in other people; (2) Smile; (3) Remember that a person's name is, to that person, the sweetest and most important sound in any language; (4) Be a good listener and encourage others to talk about themselves; (5) Talk in terms of the other person's interest; and (6) Make the other person feel important—and do it sincerely.

In my view, except for Way 2, smiling, all of these rules have one thing in common: they are entirely about the other person. You are showing interest, kindness, enthusiasm, care, and concern for the other individual. Why does this make the other person like you? Well basically because at a deep level we are all mainly interested in ourselves and our own well-being. Our first thoughts in the morning upon awakening are not feeling sorry for a work colleague's long commute or about our parents' need to hire a new plumber. We think about our immediate needs—like getting that first cup of coffee into our body.

Similarly, whatever one's profession, whether it is in law or masonry or finance, the work that person is doing is uniquely important to him since they have built a life around it. That is how they obtain their self-respect, earn money, and hopefully, receive some enjoyment. Now two caveats: of course that is not true with all professions. Menial or part-time efforts may be relatively disconnected from our psyches and viewed as just temporary situations that only serve to exist until a better position is landed or the individual's true calling identified. And of course we take pride and importance in many things outside of work—family, hobbies, sports, or art.

But for those of us whose main focus is on creative work—and science and medical research is by its very nature creative—the work itself takes on an even greater level of importance and closeness to our selves. The work is a reflection of your own ideas, efforts, dreams, and ideals. Projects are not simple things that you work on for a day or two and then forget about. They are things that take months, years, and often decades of devotion and sweat and toil. They can even become

© Springer Science+Business Media New York 2016
S.B. Rutkove, *Biomedical Research: An Insider's Guide*,
DOI 10.1007/978-1-4939-3655-7_38

entities that start to define us in a certain way and that virtually merge with our egos. In fact our colleagues and friends may even start to associate us with the actual work that we do. And it can become so essential to us that we can start to lose sight of what else is going on out there that we should be considering equally or even more importantly.

Why am I discussing all this? Well for two reasons. The first is that everyone considers what she is working on to be very important. For example, you may have a research colleague who is very enthusiastic about her current line of research and some results that she has recently obtained has led her believe that it might change the world someday. In fact, this person may suggest that the work is so critical and important that it deserves to be highlighted at a major meeting, published in top-tier journal, and snapped up by the media. But when you learn in detail what she is so excited about, you end up not being sure that is really the case, even though you are understandably reluctant to tell her so directly. Similarly, why do people giving presentations go over the time limit so, so often, droning on and on about their work? Or why do so many authors rebut the final rejection by the journal even when the "information for authors" section clearly states, "Rejections are final and will not be reconsidered." The reason for all of these is that people fall in love with what they are working on to the point that they become unable or unwilling to see its faults or limitations.

So, going along with Dale Carnegie's approach to making people like you, it is important to realize that when you are talking to others about their work, you need to be sensitive to their needs and expectations. Even though we are all dealing hopefully with real science and actual truth, we have to be cautious about criticizing another's ideas. Of course in many situations, there is more than one answer or perhaps the way is less than clear. And I am not discouraging honest scientific discourse or disagreement. Rather, I am saying that one has to understand the other's point of view about their work. We become so tightly bound to what we are doing, that a criticism of our work is taken very personally and as a criticism of ourselves.

The second reason for discussing this is to make you consider your own actions and behavior. After all, you are that person too, and you need to be aware of your own loss of perspective and that your own attachment of your research area of interest may make you lose sight of its global importance and what is reasonable and what is not reasonable. In short, you should try to police your own motivations and behaviors. The truth of the matter is that there are very few things that are going to fundamentally change the world. Even those who win Nobel Prizes are not usually making such fundamental contributions.

Of course, that does not mean you should be bored by what you are working on and think pessimistically about its long-term implications. I am just pointing out that when you are passionate about something and it is in part something that you are creating, it becomes very much a reflection of yourself. Keeping a perspective of its actual importance and that it is part of a bigger fabric of science and discovery will be critical to your own ultimate happiness.

Summary. This one is simple. Keep perspective.

Chapter 39
Research Life Lesson 3: Balance, Timing, Cycles, and Seeing the Big Picture

One of the biggest challenges to a biomedical career with a large component of research is trying to figure out how to balance everything. I hinted at some of these issues in earlier chapters, but I want to bring up this issue again in more detail.

The fractal nature of work. A fractal, as you are probably aware, is geometric structure that is made up of ever-smaller units or of the same structure of a similar or analogous structure. While this is spatial, geometric concept, I think it can be applied temporally to a career as well. I believe that the daily or weekly schedule that you may have over a period of time actually mimics the larger monthly or even yearly schedule within which you work.

For example, on a given day, you may try to complete a paper, work on some administrative tasks, and if you are in clinical medicine, take care of some patient-related tasks. The following day, you may have less unscheduled time available and be in committee meetings and spending many hours in clinic. And on the third day, you may have more time to work on a new grant application and perhaps finally finish the paper that you have been trying to cement down for quite some time.

So those 3 days can be mimicked in the larger structure of the month. You may have a week or two of more extended patient care, or find yourself mostly working on a grant application during the beginning of the month and then a paper or talk later in the month. And that same structure can also end up being mimicked across a year, with some months seemingly be entirely eaten up by a grant application or a series of papers or setting up a new project or collaboration and other months entirely devoted to paper writing. Holidays and vacations also follow a similar pattern—occasional weekends supply a much needed respite from the intensity of work during the week; longer vacations offer the same across the year.

I bring up this concept because it helps remind us that when we are in the throes of one type of work, it will eventually shift and that there is natural ebb and flow to one's focus over time. Personally, I find it actually anxiety provoking to spend a great deal of time on just one thing, since I feel like other aspects of my work are falling to pieces as I ignore them. Then as I finally get back to those pieces, I then

© Springer Science+Business Media New York 2016
S.B. Rutkove, *Biomedical Research: An Insider's Guide*,
DOI 10.1007/978-1-4939-3655-7_39

worry about the thing I had just finished. It is valuable to remember that things do vary, and that the month-to-month variations in your work focus are to some extent mirrored in those same day-to-day variations in your efforts.

Cycles. Just like there is a fractal nature to these work patterns, there is also a cyclical nature. In fact, NIH even calls their various grant solicitation times "cycles," and those grant deadlines can in fact start creating a cyclical sense to everything you do. I know that the three NIH grant cycles for me and my lab mean that January–February, May–June, and September–October are mostly grant-focused (not the entire period of course, but much of it), while March–April, July–August, and November–December are more paper and primary work focused. There are certainly times when we are not submitting a grant every cycle (which I strongly suggest you not make a routine or it will drive you crazy), and there are also other types of grants (usually smaller) that get submitted at other times; thus, this is not a strict structure. However, the NIH grant deadlines definitely have a profound influence on the rhythm of the lab. It is also useful to recall that many other good things come out of grant applications besides the grant itself, including new collaborations, new analyses, crazy new ideas, and sometimes cool new papers as you are forced to cement/establish new ideas that you may have not considered before.

Within a grant preparation period there is often building anxiety and pressure too. But it is not usually what you expect. It is not a mad rush to the deadline with the pressure building. Rather, it is often a crescendo up to about 1–2 weeks before the grant is due and then a gradual decrescendo. One reason for this is that the grant is due at our office of sponsored programs (i.e., our administrators who do the actual electronic submission) about a week before it is actually due at the foundation or NIH. Most other institutions now have similar policies. Another reason is that as you approach the deadline, you don't want to be making major alterations. Much of the last week is simply improving the messaging, cleaning up figures and perhaps improving your cover letter or getting your last letters of support.

Paper writing or experimental periods are usually less fraught with anxiety since there are usually no strict looming deadlines. But that can also be problem since there is a natural tendency to let things drag on interminably and Hofstadter's rule comes into play with the submission time seemingly forever retreating into the distance (see previous chapter).

Taking breaks. Obviously, your work may be extremely exciting and interesting, but it is not everything, and it is critical to not become entirely subsumed by it at the loss of everything that is important to life, including family, children, going out with friends, hobbies, travel, books, music, and sports. When you are in the midst of very intense work, usually the thing farthest from your mind is taking a break, but in truth, these are very critical sometimes to improving your own efficiency and idea generation. My wife insists on my taking a few "screen-free days" during the year. I am, of course, naturally resistant to these. But when I do have one, it is actually remarkable how much better I see the big picture. And during a given day it is similarly important to take breaks and not try to push through exhaustion. A short break can go along way in clearing your mind and helping you get back in a true "flow state."

Understanding your own rhythms and working with them—not against them. Along with these rhythms and cycles, another important aspect of successful work life is to understand your internal rhythms and behaviors. You will not feel the same or be in the same mood at every moment of a day. For example, some people are really effective at working in the morning (so called larks) and others are really effective working at night (so called owls). Others find midday the best. And usually there are certain times of the day that are best for creativity (I like the early morning hours, before 7 to get the most creative work done; it is all downhill from there for me). And there are times of day that are best used for menial, mindless tasks like clearing out your email or working on a grant budget or perhaps the painful task of actually uploading a paper and associated files to a journal's website. Maximizing your efficiency by tailoring your tasks to the time of day can be a very effective way for making work not only more efficient, but frankly more enjoyable as well.

These daily rhythms also have their own fractality, with their being mirrored in longer time patterns. You may find yourself simply not in the mood to work on writing for a period of days or longer. Sometimes you need to fight this, for example, when a deadline is looming; but if you can let it go, then you should. It may be that you'll be able to come back to it just a few days later with a much greater zeal than you would otherwise have.

Similarly seasonal effects are also worth considering here briefly. For example, I really feel that the summer is a bad time to be grant writing, especially if you live in a colder climate. This is the one time of year that you want to be out and enjoying the fresh air and not cloistered away in front of your computer struggling with difficult data and wording. I have submitted some fairly large grants on occasion in the summer, and when I reflect back on it in the fall, I feel like I should be kicking myself for having put a pall over the most beautiful time of year in New England. On the other hand, I certainly don't mind cozying up with my laptop in front of a toasty fire on a January evening with a glass of sherry by my side, my dog at my feet as I put the final touches on a grant application or craft the outline of a new paper.

Summary. This chapter has focused on the cyclical and fractal nature of having a research-focused career. Many of the patterns that we experience over months also occur in a smaller fashion during a single day. And the cycles are actually to some extent predictable. The external cycles, introduced by funding agencies, the school year, holidays, and academic traditions, such as the start of residency training programs in July, need to be carefully reconciled with the internal cycles that we, all have. I believe that understanding and working with these cycles will make you more productive, less stressed, and most importantly, happier.

Chapter 40
Research Life Lesson 4: Your Career Is an Ultramarathon, Not a Sprint

Of all the life lessons I would like to present, the idea of going slowly and thinking about the long haul is critical to keeping your sanity and being successful, and is thus probably the most important. As one looks back on a career, it can seem that time goes by very quickly. You can still recall the days when you were just starting out, working with a mentor, perhaps seeing your first paper accepted and your name in print, or submitting your first grant application. And before your know it, 20 or 30 or 40 years have elapsed and you are about to retire.

I have never run an ultramarathon, but from what I understand, there are times when you are running, times when you are walking, and other times when you just sit and take a real break, with some food and drink. Injuries are also almost inevitable, so you may have to get bandaged up a bit or down a few ibuprofen before gearing up for the next segment of the race. Day may pass into night and night into day; it may be sunny early in the race, rainy later, and perhaps the sun will peek out one more time before it comes to its conclusion. In short, running an ultramarathon is different than any other kind of race because you just don't keep going non-stop. Taking breaks, varying up the routine, and constantly recognizing that you are in it for the long haul is what it is all about.

Unlike careers in dance or tennis, if you remain healthy, you will likely be able to work for many, many years on your research. And while getting more sooner is always a good thing, there is also something very meaningful about having something to work toward over many years. In many respects, I feel a little sorry for people who have a very early major success or discovery because they then feel compelled to somehow manage to keep up that level of performance, lest they start to feel defeated. So here I provide some suggestions about how to proceed without moving too fast and how to sustain yourself for many years to come.

1. **Don't give up on an idea until it is fully fleshed out**. One of the most challenging aspects of sustaining a career is to not fall off the pony, so to speak, and keep riding successfully. In other words, if you have a good idea or research agenda, don't abandon it prematurely. Continue to think about other potential applications or other directions it could go in. Most topics can be explored in depth for an extended period

© Springer Science+Business Media New York 2016
S.B. Rutkove, *Biomedical Research: An Insider's Guide*,
DOI 10.1007/978-1-4939-3655-7_40

of time. For example, you may have convinced yourself that you have finally reached the end of a line of research when you may suddenly recognize an unrelated aspect to the research that you had never considered. And it could be that this secondary aspect of the research ends up being more important than the original idea.

2. **Conversely, be an idea generator**. While you should not give up prematurely on an idea, you should also always be looking to try new things. After all, that is the only way truly new innovation occurs. There are, of course, many ways to do this, from reading journals outside your area of expertise, going to lectures within and without your discipline, and perhaps even reading good general non-fiction or fiction. One guaranteed way of not generating new ideas is to only read and focus solely on work closely related to your own.

Discovering new ideas of course does not mean simply throwing out what you were working on. In fact, the new ideas may enhance your current efforts and simply nudge your research into new directions. On the other hand, perhaps you will come across something far afield from your main research thrust, but still relevant to your general area of expertise, and you should not be afraid to pursue it if you are convinced it is worthwhile and excites you.

3. **Don't follow the crowds**. Human beings, like many other animals, exhibit a great deal of herd behavior. An idea or discovery surfaces and then everyone flocks to it, pursuing research on it in the hope of making the next major breakthrough before anyone else. In my view, when everyone is running in one direction, that is an excellent time to actually saunter quietly away in the opposite direction. Being a contrarian can be valuable. Of course, this is not always easy, since it is often very challenging to see group behavior when you are deeply embedded in the group. But not following the moving mass can not only free you up from endless competition and trying to be seen and heard above the throngs, but can also be liberating, providing you with a wonderful sense of independence. So one way of sustaining a career successfully is to try to avoid herd behavior and move out on your own as much as possible.

4. **Mentor people**. Mentoring young investigators is a sure fired way to bring fun and excitement to career. Teaching and helping new investigators grow and blossom into successful independent researchers is very fulfilling. Not only because you feel like you are giving back (and there can be no question that this form of giving is very gratifying), but because these people may give you new ideas as well that perhaps you will work on with them. Moreover, these young investigators can become important collaborators down the road, as they gradually strike out on their own.

It also worth pointing out that mentoring is very different than teaching. While mentoring may encompass some teaching, the joy of mentoring is that it involves more than just presenting the accepted canon. It is alive and constantly changing depending on an individual person's interests, successes, and failures. Every mentee is different and so how you help them successfully navigate the first years of their career is never the same, providing an interesting and hopefully successful adventure for both of you.

5. **Seek out new collaborators**. I consider myself constantly on the prowl for new collaborators. I have discussed in earlier chapters how to set up successful collaborations and the idea that collaborations may eventually come to an end. But that

does not mean that you should not continue to seek out the opportunity to work with people in different areas or with different types of expertise throughout your career. Seeking new collaborations means bringing fresh ideas to your work and continually reinvigorating it. It is very easy to fall into a rut, where the research starts to seem like a dead end. But a new collaboration can mean new ideas and breath of fresh life into your work.

6. **Embrace change**. Perhaps one of the most difficult aspects of life is embracing change. Some work-related changes are, of course, good and desirable—perhaps a new job or a promotion or the start of a major new grant—but others can be difficult, such as the unexpected departure of a colleague or the ending of a grant. One rule that is helpful to remember is that people in general are highly adaptable. What seems inconceivable at one moment becomes OK and perhaps even enjoyable at some later point, simply because we get used to it. Don't fight change, since it is inevitable, but try to understand it and adjust to it in whatever fashion you can. Pining for the past doesn't solve anything.

7. **Appreciate stability**. The status quo is the most difficult thing to appreciate, until we lose it. Having consistent colleagues, an office that you can call your own, a schedule that doesn't change horribly week-to-week, and the absence of nasty surprises really should not be taken for granted. And if things do seem a bit boring at times, that might be OK too—life need not be endlessly exciting all the times. Occasional big talks or exciting experimental results are great, but you should try to accept those as the exception and not the rule. When things are just chugging along quietly without any hoopla, things are generally not so bad.

8. **Be honest**. I spent some time discussing honesty in the conflict of interest chapter and also in the scientific misconduct chapter, but I would just like to reiterate it here. Any small wins you achieve through dishonesty are certain to be illusory and will ultimately cause you to fail. That is why there is no need to rush. Honest work may not always be recognized early or perhaps even be exciting, but in the end, it is what builds a steady career that you can look forward someday to peering back upon with pride. Even one dishonest or disingenuous act can have a host of ramifications that may spiral out of control.

9. **Be generous**. Being generous of spirit and time is ultimately perhaps the greatest gift we can give. For colleagues, it means being that person that people can turn to for advice; it also means helping to ensure that everyone who works with you gets the credit they deserve. For younger people, it means nurturing and sustaining them as they are just starting out on their careers. And they will hopefully mimic your generous behavior some day when they have reached a senior position. Be generous with your collaborators, share credit whenever possible, and try to put yourself second as much as possible.

Summary. While there is no simple rule as to how to lead a successful and fulfilling career, just remember you are in it for the long haul. Rushing, cutting corners, being selfish, being dishonest, turning inward, and being afraid of change, are all certain to make you feel discouraged and ultimately dissatisfied. Every so often, it is worth imagining yourself as that 80-year-old person, who, upon reflecting back on his career, can't help but smile.

Chapter 41
Conclusion: Nothing Satisfies Like Meaningful Work

Thomas Edison once said, "I've never worked a day in my life. It was all fun." Personally, I think he was lying (either to himself or to the reporter who jotted down the comment or both). No matter how much you love what you do, work is not endless fun. And in any career there are sure to be hours or days or weeks or months or even years of drudgery that can at best be considered merely "acceptable" as you seek out your initial funding, work through difficult experiments with conflicting results, have what you consider a great and important paper being rejected repeatedly, and work in deteriorating conditions because of a change in leadership in your department.

But I do understand Edison's basic idea. To find your passion and to work at what you love doing is perhaps one of the greatest gifts you can ever be given in life probably only secondary to having a wonderful family. If life is to have significance beyond its being a simple preparation for the hereafter, as some religions decree, we need to fill our time with meaningful work that not only provides our endlessly inquisitive and creative minds with some enjoyable task, but that also maybe improves or enriches the world in some small but valuable way. Even if you are hardened nihilist or existentialist believing that life and the world have no true meaning or importance and that anything you achieve in your lifetime will have no ultimate value in the greater universe, it is still difficult not to be captured by an interesting puzzle or cool question. Suddenly, despite any misgivings about the importance of what you are doing, you become enthralled and excited about the ideas with which you are working. And while it is true that we each believe that what we are working on may be especially important, that kind of self-deceit, to at least some extent, is probably just fine. It is what we need to keep going in those more difficult times, when the joy of trying to solve the riddle seems less obvious.

I work a great deal on weekends and on vacations, usually with the grudging endorsement of my family (mostly because they know it makes me happy). And when people ask me how I can enjoy taking work home with me, I reply that I view my life as a "seamless tapestry of work and play." I would feel differently if I had to go in to work on the weekends to take call, dictate notes, perform medical

© Springer Science+Business Media New York 2016
S.B. Rutkove, *Biomedical Research: An Insider's Guide*,
DOI 10.1007/978-1-4939-3655-7_41

procedures; that kind of service work, while valuable and important, and undoubtedly enjoyable for some, is not something that I would consider fun since it is not
creative. It is just that: service. But to be able to work on my own projects, gradually
and strenuously moving them along is exactly what Edison was getting at. It *is* fun.

Here is something else worth considering. The advent of the Internet over the
past 20 years has made it possible to create this seamless tapestry. When I was first
starting out doing research in college or even after I finished my medical training,
multiple trips to the stacks of the library were absolutely critical. Nothing could
really be accomplished without spending hours searching articles, finding new references embedded within them and then looking up those articles seemingly *ad
inifinitum*. And that is not to mention the endless photocopying. What a bother that
was. I remember having to grab a book cart (yes, they had book carts just like shop-
ping carts) that I would fill with a stack of bound journals and roll it to the photo-
copy area in the basement of the Countway Library at Harvard Medical School.
Then there would usually be a queue with several other people like myself waiting
patiently for a machine to open. If it was midday and really busy, the smell of the
copiers and the heat they generated made for truly unpleasant working conditions.
Then once you found an open machine there was the endless need to open the
tightly bound journals, trying desperately to split the spine, to ensure that you were
getting the whole page (and even so, you would inevitably miss some, only realizing
after you returned to your office to collate them). And then you also needed to
have an endless collection of pocket change (nickles, dimes, and quarters). While I
must admit there was something mildly romantic about being buried deep in the
lower basement of the library looking through those old, musty bound journals, in
the whole, the experience was a major time-sink.

There were similar headaches, although perhaps not as memorable, whenever
you wanted to order equipment or find new supplies. My office was full of huge
catalogues with enormous indices that you would have to plow through to hopefully
find the one item you needed and ordering it would require a combination of phone
calls, faxes and snail mail.

But now, I can sit comfortably at my desk in my study at home or in at my office
at work or on a porch in a hotel in the Caribbean or at a café in Europe while sipping
a latte or even, remarkably, on board a plane crossing the Atlantic, and do that exact
same work. I can collaborate across vast distances with ease. I can have face-to-face
conversations via Skype and even troubleshoot experiments across the country
without leaving my chair. I can teach other people how to do a measurement on a
mouse or review data simultaneously while we are thousands of miles apart. Talk
about increased productivity! Never has there been a time like this, where we have
virtually the whole world at the tips of fingers.

It is true that this ready access to all of the world's information and to my colleagues and collaborators can create a sense of virtually non-stop work. But that
does not have to be the case. In fact, alternating between enjoyable work and play
can give us heightened pleasure for both. Dan Ariely, author of *Predictably
Irrational* and the *Upside of Irrationality*, in the field of behavioral economics,
makes a strong point about human adaptability. When we do one activity for a

prolonged period of time, we adapt or adjust to it. If it is annoying task, the annoyance starts diminishing, and we just keep working through it. On the other hand, if it is an enjoyable experience, the joy starts to ebb as you again adapt to it. For example, the first piece of chocolate always seems richer and better than the second or third. The moment you walk outside on a spectacular, sunny and warm day in June seems far more miraculous than when you have been outside for a few hours and are used to it. But by varying, by breaking up, and by flipping back and forth between things, we are able to heighten our awareness and enjoyment, reducing the inevitable sense of blasé that develops when exposed to even a very pleasurable experience for a long time.

And in my view this works for doing work that you love, anytime, anywhere, now made so possible through the Internet, laptop computers and tablets, Skype, and nearly universal access via Wi-Fi or cellular networks. It becomes possible to work for just 45 min on a paper and then go outside to go for run or walk the dog, play with the kids and maybe a few hours later, return again to work for another hour. Going back and forth between work and play makes everything constantly fresh and exciting, and as Edison said, "fun."

As I have tried to make clear, a career in research is not about racking up the biggest grants, or winning the Nobel Prize, or becoming dean or by seeing your work on the cover of *Nature*. It is not even about making some significant contribution for the betterment of society or saving the planet. It is not even necessarily doing something that is ultimately meaningful. All of those goals, while lofty, create unnecessary expectation. It is possible that you will pursue an idea or theory that, in the end, will be proven untrue and fail, possibly during your lifetime or long afterward. But that really is just fine. Rather, it is the journey itself. As Steve Jobs reiterated to his team in his early days at Apple, "The journey is the reward."

May your journeys, wherever they take you, provide all the rewards that you need.

ERRATUM TO

Biomedical Research: An Insider's Guide

Seward B. Rutkove

© Springer Science+Business Media New York 2016
S.B. Rutkove, *Biomedical Research: An Insider's Guide*,
DOI 10.1007/978-1-4939-3655-7

DOI 10.1007/978-1-4939-3655-7_42

The print and online versions of the book now contain a brief biography of the Author on the following pages:

1. On page 17 in the Front Matter the Bio of Dr. Rutkove should read as follows:

Dr. Rutkove is Professor of Neurology, Harvard Medical School and serves as Chief of the Division of Neuromuscular Disease in the Department of Neurology at Beth Israel Deaconess Medical Center. He received his medical degree from Columbia University's College of Physicians and Surgeons, and his bachelor *magna cum laude* from Cornell University, College of Arts and Sciences. Dr. Rutkove's research focuses on the application of innovative techniques for the assessment of neuromuscular disease with an emphasis on electrical impedance and ultrasound methodologies. This work has been supported by numerous grants from the National Institutes of Health and multiple foundations and has resulted in nearly 150 peer-reviewed publications. He is currently serving as an associate editor for *Annals of Neurology*. Dr. Rutkove is also a co-founder of Skulpt, Inc, a company commercializing muscle impedance tools for clinical care and consumer use. In 2011, he was awarded the Biomarker Challenge Prize from the non-profit foundation Prize4Life, Inc for his work demonstrating that electrical impedance measurements of muscle could speed clinical therapeutic studies in amyotrophic lateral sclerosis.

The updated original online version for this book can be found at
http://dx.doi.org/10.1007/978-1-4939-3655-7

© Springer Science+Business Media New York 2016
S.B. Rutkove, *Biomedical Research: An Insider's Guide*,
DOI 10.1007/978-1-4939-3655-7_42

Index

A

Academic titles, 271
Agenda, 198
1993 American Academy of Neurology
    Meeting, 197
Amyotrophic lateral sclerosis (ALS), 83
Animal Care Panel, 56
Animal *vs.* clinical research, 214
Animal protocols, 57
Animal research
    animal numbers, 60, 61
    blinding, 60
    euthanasia, 58
    experiment regulation, 56
    oversight within lab, 61
    protocols, 58
Animal Welfare Act, 56, 57
Animal welfare concerns, 180
Approach section, 177
Article reading
    critiquing, 230, 231
    efficiency, 230, 231
    exploring ideas, 228
    procedure identification, 228
    purpose, 227
    reference, 229
    relevance, 227
    research background, 228
Article review, 229, 230
Association for the Assessment and
        Accreditation of Laboratory Animal
        Care International (AAALAC),
        56, 57
Authorship, 100, 101

B

Biomedical research, 3
Biomedical science
    changing jobs, 255
    contracts, 254, 255
    evaluation, 250
    jobs, 249
    negotiation, 253, 254
    PhD *vs.* MD dichotomy, 249
    renegotiation, 256
    salary, 251, 252
    tenure, 252
    trainee to trainer, 255
Biostatistical input, 138
Blinding, 60
Breaks, 282
Budget, 182

C

Career research grants
    evidence, research plan, 156
    investigator grants, 157
    K award, 157
    letters of recommendation and support,
        155
    mentor, 155
    research project, 154
    training and educational plan, 156
Cell culture
    advantages, 65
    ceftriaxone, 65
    and in vitro work, 65, 66
Central IRB mechanism, 48

Printed in the United States
By Bookmasters